AANN
American Association
of Neuroscience Nurses

COMPREHENSIVE REVIEW FOR STROKE NURSING

Edited by
Sarah Livesay, DNP RN ACNP-BC CNS-BC SCRN

American Association of Neuroscience Nurses
8735 W. Higgins Road, Suite 300
Chicago, IL 60631
www.aann.org

AANN COMPREHENSIVE REVIEW FOR STROKE NURSING

ISBN 978-0-9625729-0-6

Notice

Nursing is an ever changing field. Standard safety precautions must be followed, but as new research and clinical experience broaden our knowledge, changes in treatment and drug therapy may become necessary or appropriate. Readers are advised to check the most current product information provided by the manufacturer of each drug to be administered to verify the recommended dose, the method and duration of administration, and contraindications. It is the responsibility of the licensed prescriber, relying on experience and knowledge of the patient, to determine dosages and the best treatment for each individual patient. Neither the publisher nor the editor and authors assume any liability for any injury and/or damage to persons or property arising from this publication.

American Association of Neuroscience Nurses

Joan Kram, Executive Director
Allison Begezda, Marketing Manager
Leah Zamora, Account Manager
Kelly Podkowa, Administrator

AANN Comprehensive Review for Stroke Nursing
Publishing Staff

Katie Macaluso, Managing Editor
Monica Piotrowski, Associate Editor
Danielle Desjardins, Assistant Editor
Sonya Jones, Senior Graphic Designer
Cover design by Matt Santori-Griffith

Printed in the United States of America

Contents

Tables

Figures

Foreword

The delivery of care to individuals at risk for or who have sustained stroke requires nurses to possess a specialized body of knowledge and acquire competence in the management of these individuals. Nurses use their advanced knowledge in stroke when providing education about primary stroke prevention to the public, with the intent to help individuals modify at-risk behaviors and adopt healthy practices. When stroke occurs, individuals entering the stroke system must be managed by nurses and teams delivering advanced stroke care. Highly competent stroke nurses rapidly identify stroke signs and symptoms, work with a team of providers giving expert care to patients as they move through the hyperacute and acute phases, deliver medications safely, minimize potential complications, optimize rehabilitation, and educate about secondary stroke prevention.

Stroke nurses work in emergency departments, critical care units, interventional radiology suites and operating rooms, stroke and rehabilitation units, clinics, and home settings. Wherever stroke nurses choose to work, they can demonstrate their advanced knowledge, skills, and competence in this specific field by attaining a certification. Developed by the American Board of Neuroscience Nurses, the Stroke Certified Registered Nurse (SCRN) certification provides an opportunity for stroke nurses to demonstrate the acquisition of this specialized body of knowledge in stroke by successfully passing an examination. To help nurses prepare for the SCRN exam, the American Association of Neuroscience Nurses (AANN) assembled a team of nursing and pharmacist experts to create a comprehensive study guide. Led by Sarah Livesay, DNP RN ACNP-BC CNS-BC SCRN, the extraordinary authors of this text have assimilated, translated, and integrated a vast body of specialized knowledge in stroke into eight chapters. The text includes chapters dedicated to anatomy and physiology, preventive care, hyperacute care, stroke diagnostics, acute care, medications, postacute care, and systems and quality of care. These chapters will help prepare nurses for the stroke certification exam by identifying the critical elements of stroke knowledge related to ischemic and hemorrhagic stroke. In addition, nurses in all settings will discover that this text can serve as a reference tool and valuable asset for developing nursing competencies or protocols as well as a resource for developing educational offerings.

Every stroke nurse should own a copy of *AANN Comprehensive Review for Stroke Nursing*! It should not sit on a shelf gathering dust but rather be a daily companion in stroke nurses' work environments.

Mary Kay Bader, MSN RN CCNS CCRN CNRN FAHA SCRN
AANN Immediate Past President

Acknowledgments

AANN Comprehensive Review for Stroke Nursing was written by neuroscience nurses and is dedicated to the many nurses and professionals across the globe who work daily to care for patients suffering from stroke. This book was developed primarily for nurses seeking certification as a Stroke Certified Registered Nurse (SCRN), which is offered by the American Board of Neuroscience Nurses and recognizes nurses who demonstrate knowledge and competence in the subspecialty of stroke nursing. This certification review book would not have occurred without the vision and mission of the American Association of Neuroscience Nurses (AANN). I would like to extend a special thanks to Joan Kram, AANN executive director, for her leadership and support of this project, and to Katie Macaluso and Monica Piotrowski, AANN publication staff, for their guidance and organization.

I would also like to acknowledge the tremendous effort and work of the contributing authors. This book simply would not have been possible without the knowledge and wisdom of these individuals, who are leaders in their fields. Personally, I would like to thank the neuroscience nurses who have greatly influenced my own development as a nurse, including Dr. Joanne Hickey, the staff of the Neuroscience Center at Baylor College of Medicine/St. Luke's Episcopal Hospital and University of Texas/Hermann Memorial Hospital in Houston, and Mary Kay Bader, immediate past president of AANN. Finally, I want to thank my family, including my mother, who is my favorite nurse ever, my dad, and my partner. Thank you for your endless love, support, and belief in me.

Sarah Livesay, DNP RN ACNP-BC CNS-BC SCRN
Editor

Contributors

JJ Baumann, MS RN C-CNS
Stanford Hospital and Clinics
Stanford, CA

Gretchen Brophy, PharmD BCPS FCCP FCCM
Virginia Commonwealth University
Richmond, VA

Amber Castle, PharmD BCPS
Yale–New Haven Hospital
New Haven, CT

Millie Hepburn, MPhil MSN RN ACNS-BC SCRN
New York University Langone Medical Center/Rusk Institute
New York, NY

Patricia Garvin Higgins, MN RN CNS CRRN
Long Beach Memorial
Memorial Care Rehabilitation Institute
Long Beach, CA

Mary Kelly, MBA RN CNRN
The Joint Commission
Lombard, IL

Sarah Livesay, DNP RN ACNP-BC CNS-BC SCRN
University of Texas Health–Houston
Houston, TX

Ron Neyens, PharmD BCPS
Medical University of South Carolina
Charleston, SC

Mary Straw, DHA RN ANP CNS
The Joint Commission
Medford, NY

Christina M. Szabo, PhD RN CCRN CNRN
Virginia Commonwealth University Health System
Richmond, VA

Angela West, MSN RN CCRN CNRN
Long Beach Memorial Hospital
Memorial Stroke Center
Long Beach, CA

Susan E. Wilson, MSN RN C-ANP
University of North Carolina
Chapel Hill, NC

Reviewers

Teresa A. Allison, PharmD BCPS
Memorial Hermann Texas Medical Center
Houston, TX

Janice L. Hinkle, PhD CNRN RN FAHA
Nurse Author and Editor
Washington, DC

Elaine M. Kopp, BSN RN
Nurse Consultant
Lodi, NJ

Judi Kuric, DNP RN ACNP-BC CNRN
University of Southern Indiana
Evansville, IN

Linda Littlejohns, MSN RN CNRN FAAN
Integra Foundation
Irvine, CA

Cissi Wimberly Oloomi, MSN APRN CNRN CNS-BC CRRN SCI CNS/NP
Michael E. Debakey VA Medical Center
Houston, TX

Michelle Van Demark, MSN RN ANP-BC CNRN SCRN
Sanford Health
Sioux Falls, SD

Stephanie Vaughn, PhD RN CRRN
California State University at Fullerton
HealthSouth Tustin Rehabilitation Hospital
Tustin, CA

Chapter

1

Anatomy and Physiology

Sarah Livesay, DNP RN ACNP-BC CNS-BC SCRN

Thorough, individualized, and goal-directed care of the patient with stroke is predicated on an understanding of stroke anatomy and physiology. To evaluate and develop an appropriate treatment plan for a patient with suspected stroke, the Stroke Certified Registered Nurse (SCRN), in coordination with the stroke team, must localize the signs and symptoms of stroke to the suspected vessel territory involved, as well as understand likely signs and symptoms of brain herniation and worsening edema when appropriate. This chapter will provide an overview of cerebrovascular anatomy and stroke pathophysiology to serve as a foundation for the SCRN's understanding of caring for the patient with stroke.

Objectives

1. Describe the basic structures of the brain, including cerebral vasculature.
2. Understand stroke pathophysiology.
3. Describe the association between basic brain anatomy and the clinical signs and symptoms of stroke.
4. Discuss various stroke syndromes.
5. Identify common stroke mimics.
6. Discuss the basic principles of neuroplasticity.

Stroke Pathophysiology

A. Ischemic stroke pathophysiology

1. Ischemic stroke occurs when arterial blood flow to brain tissue fails to meet the metabolic demands of the cells, resulting in cell damage or death. Brain cells experiencing decreased blood flow become ischemic. If left uncorrected, brain cells experiencing ischemia will die or become infarct.
2. During the hyperacute phase of an ischemic stroke, a zone of ischemic penumbra surrounds the core infarct or dead tissue (brain cells that are damaged by ischemia but not yet infarcted). In the early stages of ischemic stroke, the penumbral tissue is functionally silent yet metabolically active. The central goal of therapy during the first few hours of ischemic stroke is to restore blood flow to the penumbral tissue (Broughton, Reutens, & Sobey, 2009).
3. The rate at which brain tissue dies after the loss of perfusion and the extent of tissue lost is influenced by several ischemic modifying factors (Livesay & Hickey, 2014).

a. Factors influencing the rate and extent of penumbral tissue and infarcted tissue include the rate of onset and duration of ischemia, degree of collateral circulation perfusing the infarcted zone, functionality of systemic circulation, hematologic factors, and metabolic factors such as elevated temperature and hyper/hypoglycemic states.

4. Hypoxia or anoxia is the central mechanism of neuronal cell death. Cell death occurs via one of two pathways (Livesay & Hickey, 2014):
   a. Necrotic pathway—cell energy failure and rapid cytoskeletal breakdown. This pathway is activated by the loss of oxygen and glucose and cellular electrolyte exchange from the loss of arterial perfusion.
   b. Apoptotic pathway—programmed cell death in the penumbral zone. Apoptosis is a normal biologic function wherein cells are programmed to die in an organized fashion after nearby cell death to dispose of redundant cells (Broughton et al., 2009).

B. Intracerebral hemorrhage (ICH) stroke pathophysiology
   1. ICH occurs when a cerebral blood vessel opens abnormally and spills blood into brain tissue. The abnormal extravasation of blood into brain tissue results in a cascade of damage to surrounding tissue. Tissue damage and cell death occur via two pathways (Belur, Chang, He, Emanuel, & Mack, 2013).
      a. Primary brain injury results directly from pressure incurred from hematoma formation. Deficits seen in the first several minutes and hour after the hemorrhage occurs generally are related to the primary brain injury. The mechanical pressure of hematoma formation and resulting mass effect causes cell damage or death of the tissue directly impacted by the hematoma (Belur et al., 2013).
      b. Secondary brain injury results in the hours to days after ICH. Mass effect from the hematoma causes mechanical disruption to and deformation of neuronal and glial cell membranes. The damage to cell membranes results in the influx of electrolytes such as calcium and excitatory neurotransmitters, causing necrosis and cytotoxic edema. A positive feedback loop forms whereby secondary injury is perpetuated by cellular death, blood brain barrier disruption, vasogenic edema, and upregulation of inflammatory mediators.
         (1) Additional damage is mediated via the activation of the coagulation cascade from thrombin. Thrombin initially is present to limit hematoma expansion. However, after working to stabilize the hematoma, high thrombin levels activate the coagulation cascade and perpetuate multiple destructive pathways, including a proinflammatory state (Belur et al., 2013).

C. Subarachnoid hemorrhage (SAH) stroke pathophysiology
   1. Aneurysmal SAH (aSAH) occurs when an aneurysm forms in the cerebral vasculature and ruptures, resulting in blood spilling into the subarachnoid space. Much remains unknown about the mechanisms of neuronal damage after SAH. The process of cerebral vasospasm occurring in the days to weeks after injury has been known for decades and researched extensively. However, cerebral vasospasm does not fully explain poor patient outcomes after SAH. Recent research suggests early brain injury (EBI) after rupture also plays a key role in morbidity and mortality in SAH (Plesnila, 2013).
      a. Aneurysm formation: Aneurysms are a weakened, bulging section of a cerebral artery. Aneurysms commonly are divided by morphology into saccular—or

berry—aneurysms and nonsaccular aneurysms, including fusiform aneurysms (Hemphill & Smith, 2008).

(1) Saccular aneurysms generally look like a sac or berry, with a narrow neck and widened dome, and account for a large majority of cerebral aneurysms. Saccular aneurysms commonly form at the junction of vessels, particularly at the junction points in the Circle of Willis (COW; Hemphill & Smith, 2008).

(2) Fusiform aneurysms are an outpouching of the vessel without a distinct neck or stem, resembling a cylindrical, longer-length outpouching of the vessel. Fusiform aneurysms are less common than saccular aneurysms and generally are located in the vertebrobasilar vascular system (Park, Yim, Lee, Kim, & Son, 2008).

b. Aneurysm rupture: At the moment of aneurysm rupture, the mechanical injury from blood rushing into the subarachnoid space and the sudden increase in intracranial pressure (ICP) and resulting mass effect cause clinical signs and symptoms of SAH (Hemphill & Smith, 2008).

(1) EBI after rupture: In the hours and first several days after aneurysm rupture, localized and, on some occasions, generalized cerebral edema forms and excitatory neurotransmitter levels begin to rise. EBI results from the severe reduction in cerebral blood flow in the microcirculation of the brain. Additional pathophysiologic processes contributing to EBI include cortical spreading depression, spreading ischemia, and microvasoconstriction (Plesnila, 2013).

(2) Cerebral vasospasm (also called delayed cerebral injury): Large vessel vasospasm generally begins on day four after the hemorrhage occurs and may continue for as long as 21 days.

(a) The exact pathophysiology of cerebral vasospasm remains elusive.

1) Current theories suggest two major physiologic pathways leading to vasospasm. Endothelial nitric oxide is thought to trigger adjacent smooth muscle intracellular calcium channels, resulting in vasoconstriction (Ciurea, Palade, Voinescu, & Nica, 2013).

2) A second endothelian pathway is proposed to be the cause of large vessel vasospasm. Endothelian is a significant vasoconstrictor and is found in higher-than-normal levels in the cerebral spinal fluid of patients with aSAH. Endothelian binds with endothelian receptors on smooth muscles and causes prolonged vasoconstriction (Ciurea et al., 2013).

Basic Vascular Anatomy

A. Cerebral metabolism (Pare & Kahn, 2012)

1. The brain requires 20% of the body's oxygen supply and 15% of the cardiac output. Brain cells do not store oxygen or glucose; rather, they rely on a constant supply of micronutrients from arterial blood flow. Normal cerebral blood flow to cerebral tissue is 50–55 mL/100 g/min.
2. As perfusion begins to decrease, cells become ischemic and, if left uncorrected, become infarct or die. At 15–20 mL/100 g/min, cells experience electrical failure and weakness or other clinical symptoms become apparent. Although the cells are electrically silent, they still are viable for a short period of time should perfusion be restored.

3. Cell membrane failure occurs between 6–10 mL/100 g/min, and complete paresis is observed clinically. Cell death occurs as perfusion drops below 6 mL/100 g/min (Heiss, 2012).
4. The ischemic cascade generally is classified using the following thresholds: oligemia occurs at 30–40 mL/100 g/min; moderate ischemia, also known as the penumbra, occurs at 20–30 mL/100 g/min; and severe ischemia and cell death at the ischemic core occur as the perfusion drops to 0–10 mL/100 g/min (Livesay & Hickey, 2014).

B. Arterial vascular anatomy (Pare & Kahn, 2012)

1. The brain is supplied by four arteries pumping oxygenated blood from the heart. The bilateral carotid arteries supply blood primarily to the anterior circulation of the brain; the bilateral vertebral arteries supply oxygenated blood to the vertebrobasilar territory, or posterior circulation, of the brain.
2. The common carotid arteries originate at the top of the aortic arch and branch into the internal and external carotid arteries. The internal carotid artery (ICA) travels through the neck—feeding multiple cervical branches, the ophthalmic artery, and the superior hypophyseal artery—and terminates at the COW, providing arterial blood flow to the middle cerebral, anterior cerebral, posterior communicating, and anterior choroidal arteries.
3. The vertebral arteries branch from the subclavian artery and travel in the transverse processes of the C6 to C2 vertebrae. Near where the basilar artery enters the cerebral dura mater, the bilateral vertebral arteries join at the lower border of the pons into a single artery, the basilar artery.
4. The basilar artery continues superiorly along the center of the pons, where it divides into the posterior cerebral arteries and the superior cerebellar artery just before the pituitary, forming the posterior section of the COW. The anterior inferior cerebellar artery also branches from the basilar artery and feeds the cerebellum and the pons (Pare & Kahn, 2012).
5. The COW is a circular collection of vessel anastomoses approximately the size of a nickel sitting at the base of the brain in front of the brain stem. Anatomically, the COW serves as the blood supply connection between the anterior and posterior sections of the brain. The circle of arteries also provides redundancy in primary and collateral circulation for the brain.
6. The cerebral arterial system often is divided according to anatomical location into the anterior and posterior circulation. Generally, the anterior circulation includes arterial vessels above and in front of the tentorium, whereas posterior circulation defines the blood vessels below and behind the tentorium.
   a. Anterior circulation
      (1) The carotid artery and ICA feed the COW, then divide into middle and anterior cerebral arteries.
         (a) Middle cerebral artery (MCA): The MCA rises from the COW and feeds a majority of the frontal, parietal, and temporal lobes. Areas supplied include Broca's area, Wernicke's area, the basal ganglia, and the internal capsule. The MCA artery divides anatomically into four different segments: M1 through M4. The lenticulostriate arteries, also known as anterolateral central arteries, arise from the MCA and supply the caudate nucleus and internal capsule (Pare & Kahn, 2012).
         (b) Anterior cerebral artery (ACA): The ACA arises from the ICA via the front of the COW on opposite sides of the anterior communicating artery. The

ACA supplies the medial portion of the frontal and parietal lobes as well as a small section of the corpus callosum and the olfactory bulb and tract. The ACA is divided anatomically into three segments: A1 through A3 (Pare & Kahn, 2012).

(c) Posterior cerebral artery (PCA): The PCA arises from the basilar artery and connects with the ipsilateral margin of the MCA via the posterior circulating artery in the COW. The PCA branches into four anatomical divisions: P1 through P4. The PCA supplies several groups of arteries, including the thalamoperforating, peduncular perforating, and choroidal branches. The PCA provides arterial blood supply to the occipital lobe, midbrain, thalamus, pineal gland, medial geniculate body, choroid plexus, cerebral peduncle, and corpus callosum (Pare & Kahn, 2012).

b. Posterior circulation (Pare & Kahn, 2012)

(1) The vertebral arteries supply the large majority of the posterior circulation with some help from the anterior spinal artery, which feeds a small portion of the brain stem.

(a) The vertebral arteries provide circulation to the caudal portions of the brain stem. They join to become the basilar artery at the level of the junction of the medulla and pons.

1) Just prior to joining together to become the basilar artery, the posterior inferior cerebellar artery (PICA) branches and provides blood supply to the cerebellum, superior section of the medulla, choroid plexus, and fourth ventricle.

2) The anterior inferior cerebellar artery (AICA) branches off the basilar artery just after the bilateral vertebral arteries join to form the basilar artery. The AICA supplies oxygenated blood to the anterior inferior section of the cerebellum.

3) The basilar artery originates at the level of the junction of the medulla and pons and ascends along the pons until the artery branches into the PCA, forming the posterior section of the COW.

7. A second arterial classification scheme describes vasculature according to vessel size and divides ischemic stroke location by large vessel versus small vessel affected. Large vessel occlusions generally are from embolic sources, whereas small vessel occlusions generally are from atherosclerosis. The large vessels of the brain are described above. As vessels branch away from the large vessels and farther into the brain tissue, they become smaller (Livesay & Hickey, 2014).

C. Venous vascular anatomy—venous blood drains away from brain tissue via small venous structures in the pia matter. The venous channels flow into veins that bridge the subarachnoid space and enter into venous sinuses located in the dura mater (Saposnik et al., 2011).

1. Superior sagittal sinus—travels posteriorly between the cerebral hemispheres in the falx cerebri toward the occiput.
2. Straight sinus—travels along the tentorium, draining blood from the superior cerebellar veins and inferior sagittal sinus to the confluence near the occiput.
3. Transverse sinus—travels along the base of the occiput laterally and forwardly with the curve of the skull along the tentorium.
4. Sigmoid sinus—begins beneath the temporal bone and travels to the jugular foramen, where it becomes the internal jugular vein.

5. Convergence near the occiput: The confluence of the sinuses is the connection of the superior sagittal sinus, straight sinus, and occipital sinus in the occipital protuberance of the skull.

Basic Brain Anatomy

A. Cerebrum (Pare & Kahn, 2012)

1. Cortex: The cerebral cortex is the grey matter on the outermost section of the cerebrum and cerebellum that is composed of neuronal cell bodies. Damage to the cortex from ischemia, hemorrhage, or elevated ICP results in clinical presentation corresponding to the loss of anatomical function.
   a. The cerebral cortex and cerebrum are divided into the four lobes of the brain.
      (1) Frontal: The frontal lobe contains the motor cortex in its posterior aspect as well as neuronal networks for behavior and behavioral expression.
         (a) The motor and sensory cortex maps reside at the frontoparietal junction. The maps work in concert with other sensory and motor tracts to control motor movement and sensation. The movement and sensation of various body parts can be mapped to specific areas of the sensory and motor cortex, linking various parts of the body to certain cortical locations.
      (2) Parietal: The parietal lobe is posterior to the frontal lobe and superior to the temporal lobe, and houses the cortex for sensation, optic radiations carrying sensory input from the eyes for visual interpretation, and language centers including Broca's and Wernicke's areas.
         (a) Wernicke's area lies at the temporoparietal junction and is primarily responsible for language comprehension.
         (b) Broca's area lies in the frontal lobe and is primarily responsible for speech production.
         (c) Speech and language comprehension and production represents a complex interplay of several cortical centers and pathways; traditional definitions of Wernicke's and Broca's aphasia, or expressive and receptive aphasia, may represent an oversimplification of aphasia.
         (d) *Dysarthria* is slurred speech and generally reflects poor motor control of the muscles associated with speech and language. Aphasia as a stroke symptom is diagnosed when naming, word choice, comprehension, spelling, or syntax is disrupted (Mesulam, 2008).
         (e) The language network generally is located on the left side of the brain in a large majority of both right- and left-handed individuals.
         (f) Refer to clinical features of aphasias and related conditions. New onset of aphasia should be considered when localizing a stroke lesion. However, aphasia often is mixed by nature and may only generally localize the stroke deficit to a particular vessel (Pare & Kahn, 2012).
      (3) Occipital: The occipital lobe is in the posterior aspect of the brain on top of the tentorium. The occipital lobe is primarily responsible for vision and interpretation of visual sensory signals and contains the primary visual cortex.
      (4) Temporal: The temporal lobe is responsible for coding visual memory and processing auditory and visual sensory input and language comprehension. Wernicke's area spans between the parietal and temporal lobes and Broca's area in the frontal lobe.

2. Basal ganglia: The *basal ganglia* are a group of nuclei serving as the coordinating center for several nerve tracts including coordinating muscle movement as an essential component of the extrapyramidal motor system. The basal ganglia are composed of the striatum, made of the caudate nucleus and putamen, which receives input from the cerebral cortex into the internal capsule. The globus pallidus also is a key component of the basal ganglia and instrumental in control of voluntary muscle movement (Schuenke, Schulte, & Schumacher, 2010).
3. Limbic system: The *limbic system* is a group of nuclei and cortical structures that encode memory and regulate autonomic nervous system and endocrine function in response to emotional stimuli (Schuenke et al., 2010).
   a. Hypothalamus—coordinates autonomic nervous system with endocrine function and participates in the visual pathway; is the main center for control of body temperature, circadian rhythm, and body water or osmolality
   b. Amygdala—plays a crucial role in the management of stress, rage, and anxiety. The center for memory and emotion, the amygdala is often termed the emotional amplifier.
   c. Cingulate gyrus—medial aspect of cerebral cortex; serves as an integral part of the limbic system, receiving input from the thalamus and neocortex to develop emotions and encode memory (Swenson, 2014)
   d. Hippocampus—contains centers for memory and learning, particularly for establishing short-term memory; regulation of corticosteroid production; and the establishment of spatial relations in the environment (Swenson, 2014)

B. Diencephalon: The diencephalon is located between the brain stem and cerebellum and includes the thalamus, hypothalamus, and pituitary and pineal glands. The structures surround the third ventricle and form its lateral wall and floor.
1. Thalamus: Nearly all sensory pathways pass from the cerebral cortex through the thalamus. The thalamus contains approximately 120 nuclei broadly classified into several groups by anatomical location: the anterior nuclei, medial nuclei, ventrolateral nuclei, and dorsal nuclei.
2. Pituitary gland: The pituitary gland sits at the base of the brain as a small protrusion from the bottom of the hypothalamus inside the sella turcica and is covered by a small dural fold. The pituitary gland is divided into two lobes: the anterior lobe responsible for producing hormones and the posterior lobe responsible for releasing hormones. The posterior pituitary is responsible for the release of oxytocin and antidiuretic hormone, and the anterior pituitary is responsible for the release of somatotropin, prolactin, follitropin, lutropin, thyrotropin, and corticotropin.
3. Pineal gland: The pineal gland is located in the epithalamus, produces serotonin and melatonin, and contributes to circadian rhythms and sleep-wake cycles. In adults, the pineal gland often calcifies and calcium deposits may be noted on computed tomography imaging (Schuenke et al., 2010; Swenson, 2014).

C. Cerebellum: The cerebellum lies on the dorsal aspect of the pons and contributes to movement coordination and maintaining balance and position sense. The cerebellum cannot initiate movement; however, it is responsible for the unconscious coordination of movement. The cerebellum has a network of sulci and gyri with grey and white matter. It also may play a role in emotion management and motor learning. However, the cerebellum's role in these functions is less understood than its role in the coordination of muscle movement (Schuenke et al., 2010; Swenson, 2014).

D. Brain stem: The brain stem is the most primitive portion of the brain, containing nuclei and pathways for the most basal neurologic functions and reflexes. The brain stem generally is divided into three sections: the midbrain, pons, and medulla. In addition, the corticospinal and the somatosensory tracts connecting the cerebral cortex with the rest of the body decussate at various places in the midbrain (Schuenke et al., 2010; Swenson, 2014).

1. Medulla: The medulla is the most caudal section of the brain stem, ending at the foramen magnum, where the spinal cord begins.
   a. Several cranial nerves (CNs) originate in the medulla (Hickey & Kanusky, 2014).
      (1) Hypoglossal (CN XII)—motor function; allows for control of the tongue muscles, resulting in normal speech and swallow
      (2) Glossopharyngeal (CN IX)—motor and sensory function; elevates the palate, controls movement of the pharynx and larynx, and contributes to swallowing through control of the stylopharyngeus muscle; controls sensation from the palate and tongue as well as taste from the posterior tongue and pharynx
      (3) Vagus (CN X)—motor and sensory function; controls the muscles and receives sensory input from the pharynx and larynx; provides parasympathetic input to the neck, thorax, and abdomen; provides sensory input from the viscera and external ear
      (4) Portions of accessory nerve (CN XI)—motor function; innervates the muscles of the larynx, pharynx, and trapezius as well as the sternocleidomastoid muscle
2. Somatosensory tracts—pathways of neuronal communication; consists of two significant pathways (Swenson, 2014)
   a. The first system communicates fine touch, proprioception, and vibration via the dorsal column-medial lemniscal system from the peripheral body to the central nervous system (CNS). Peripheral nerves enter the posterior (dorsal) root ganglia of the spinal cord and travel up the spinal cord to the medulla. Just above the medulla, the nerves decussate and form a dense bundle of axons called the medial lemniscus. The tract travels upward to the ventral posterior lateral thalamic nucleus in the thalamus. The track continues to travel through the internal capsule, largely through the postcentral gyrus in the parietal lobe, to the cerebral cortex.
   b. The second system is the anterolateral system (spinothalamic tract), which carries pain and temperature sensation from the periphery to the CNS (Swenson, 2014). Peripheral nerves carry sensation via the posterior (dorsal) root ganglia of the spinal cord and communicate with cell bodies in the dorsal spinal cord. The nerves decussate in the spinal cord and become the anterolateral system. The axons travel upward through the spinal cord to the ventral posterior lateral thalamic nucleus in the thalamus. The axons then travel to the postcentral gyrus of the cerebral cortex, located in the parietal lobe.
3. Pons—located between the medulla and midbrain; acts as message center between the cerebellum and cerebrum
   a. CNs originating in the pons (Hickey & Kanusky, 2014)
      (1) Abducens (CN VI)—motor function; innervates the lateral rectus muscle of the ipsilateral orbit responsible for lateral gaze
      (2) Facial (CN VII)—motor and sensory function; innervates facial muscles; provides parasympathetic supply of the submandibular and sublingual glands; provides taste sensation for the anterior two thirds of the tongue, hard palate, and soft palate, and sensation of the skin around the ear

(3) Vestibulocochlear (CN VIII)—sensory function; divided into two branches: the cochlear branch in control of hearing and the vestibular branch, which is concerned with balance, body position, and orientation in space

(4) Trigeminal (CN V)—both sensory and motor function; divided into three main segments: the ophthalmic division (V1), the maxillary division (V2), and the mandibular division (V3). The nerve communicates pain, temperature, and light touch from the face and scalp as well as the sinuses and oral cavities. The motor fibers innervate the muscles of mastication.

4. Midbrain—cephalic portion of brain stem; coordinates eye movement and reflexes associated with hearing and vision

a. CNs originating from the midbrain (Hickey & Kanusky, 2014)

(1) Optic (CN II)—sensory function; transmits visual cues from the retina to the vision cortex in the occipital lobe. The nerve travels posteriorly from each eye along the inferior aspect of the frontal lobe to the optic chiasm, where the fibers partially decussate. The optic chiasm is located just in front of the pituitary gland. After partial decussation at the optic chiasm, the nerve continues posteriorly to the vision cortex in the occipital lobe. Injury to the nerve pathway may occur at any point along the pathway as a result of stroke or edema and results in different visual field deficits, depending on the location of injury.

(2) Oculomotor (CN III)—motor function; innervates four of the six muscles that move the eye: the medial recti responsible for moving the eye inward or medially, the superior recti that move the eye upward and outward, the inferior recti that move the eye downward and outward, and the inferior oblique responsible for moving the eye upward and inward. The oculomotor nerve also is responsible for pupillary constriction, dilatation, and accommodation.

(3) Trochlear (CN IV)—motor function; innervates the superior oblique muscle of the eye and moves the eye downward and inward

Stroke Syndromes

A. Ischemic stroke (Pare & Kahn, 2012)

1. Large vessel stroke

a. Generally caused by thrombus or embolus. When embolus is the source, the cause generally is either cardiac or artery-to-artery.

b. Stroke syndromes by vessel territory

(1) Carotid: Clinical signs and symptoms associated with stroke involving the ICA include aphasia if the dominant hemisphere is involved; neglect if the nondominant hemisphere is involved; contralateral homonymous hemianopsia; contralateral motor and sensory loss of the face, arm, and leg; and conjugate ipsilateral eye deviation. Patients with carotid territory stroke also may experience transient monocular blindness, or amaurosis fugax, because the ophthalmic artery branches from the ICA (Pare & Kahn, 2012).

(a) Central retinal artery occlusion (CRAO) occurs when the central retinal artery is occluded, usually as a result of ICA atherosclerosis. Patients exhibit sudden, painless, unilateral loss of vision. Relative afferent pupillary defect, also known as Marcus Gunn pupil, is common with CRAO.

(b) Carotid artery dissection also may result in Horner's syndrome, the clinical combination of ptosis, or a drooping eyelid; miosis, or pupillary constriction; and anhidrosis, or decreased sweating.

(2) MCA: Clinical signs and symptoms associated with stroke involving the MCA include aphasia if the dominant hemisphere is involved; neglect if the nondominant hemisphere is involved; contralateral motor and sensory loss of the face, arm, and leg, with the leg less involved than the arm; homonymous hemianopia; and conjugate eye deviation toward the side of the lesion (Pare & Kahn, 2012).

(a) Patients may exhibit anosognosia, known as neglect or lack of self-awareness, particularly when the stroke includes the right hemisphere parietal lobe.

(3) ACA: Clinical signs and symptoms associated with stroke involving the ACA include contralateral motor and sensory deficits impacting the leg more than the arm, with the face and tongue spared; abulia, or a lack of concern or disinhibition, also may be present. In the case of severe injury, primitive frontal lobe reflexes including grasp and suck may be present (Pare & Kahn, 2012).

(4) PCA: The PCA supplies the thalamus and the midbrain, containing major relay centers for several cortical tracks in the brain. Clinical signs and symptoms associated with stroke involving the PCA include contralateral visual field homonymous hemianopia and visual agnosia. If the stroke occurs in the dominant hemisphere, symptoms may include alexia with or without agraphia and prosopagnosia. If bilateral PCA occlusion is present, the patient may exhibit total blindness and may experience amnesia. In general, pure PCA strokes do not include paralysis or aphasia. Sensory loss may be present (Pare & Kahn, 2012).

(a) Weber's syndrome, wherein patients exhibit third nerve palsy and contralateral hemiplegia, may be present if the stroke includes the central territory of the PCA. Patients often exhibit significant bulbar muscle dysfunction.

(b) Parinaud's syndrome is a constellation of symptoms associated with midbrain stroke. Patients exhibit impaired upgaze, convergence-retraction nystagmus, and primary conjugate downgaze.

(5) PICA: Clinical signs and symptoms associated with stroke involving the PICA include Wallenberg syndrome, also known as lateral medullary syndrome, which results from damage to the spinothalamic tract resulting in loss of pain and temperature sensation in the contralateral trunk and ipsilateral face. Patients also may have dysphagia, dysarthria, and dysphonia. In addition, patients may have an ipsilateral loss of the corneal reflex (Pare & Kahn, 2012).

(6) AICA: Clinical signs and symptoms associated with stroke involving the AICA include

(a) AICA syndrome or lateral pontine syndrome, resulting in vertigo, vomiting, nystagmus, falling towards the side of the lesion, ipsilateral loss of sensation to the face, ipsilateral facial paralysis, ipsilateral hearing loss, and nystagmus (Pare & Kahn, 2012).

(b) Stroke involving the AICA and/or PICA will result in cerebellar findings including dysfunction of speech; tremor; and ocular findings such as nystagmus, abnormal gait, and abnormal finger-to-nose or heal-shin testing.

(7) Basilar: The clinical signs and symptoms associated with stroke involving the basilar artery result in vertebrobasilar artery syndrome, a collection of symptoms resulting from the loss of perfusion to the cerebellum, brain stem, pons, thalamus, and occipital lobe. Depending on the extent of the injury, symptoms may include coma, quadriparesis, ataxia, dysarthria, CN dysfunction, and visual deficits (Pare & Kahn, 2012).

(a) Locked-in syndrome: Occlusion of the vertibrobasilar artery resulting in pontine damage rarely may result in locked-in syndrome, in which a patient is quadriparetic and cannot speak, but cognition remains intact (Pare & Kahn, 2012). Akinetic mutism results when patients' cognition remains preserved, but they cannot move or speak. Gaze paresis or intranuclear opthalmoplegia (INO) may be present. Patients may be able to communicate using blinking or lateral or vertical eye movement, depending on the extent of the injury.

1) INO—impaired gaze resulting from damage to the medial longitudinal fasciculus of the pons or midbrain, resulting in weak adduction of the affected eye and abduction nystagmus of the contralateral eye

2) Millard-Gubler syndrome, or ventral-pontine syndrome, represents a constellation of symptoms resulting from pontine damage, including CN VI and VII damage, resulting in diplopia, the inability to rotate the affected eye outward, and ipsilateral weakness of the facial muscles and loss of corneal reflex. If the corticospinal tracts are affected, the patient will exhibit contralateral weakness.

3) Additional symptoms associated with stroke or intermittent ischemia involving the brain stem include nausea and vomiting, diplopia, dysconjugate gaze, gaze palsy, dysarthria, dysphagia, vertigo, tinnitus, hemiparesis or quadriplegia, sensory loss in hemibody or all four limbs, rapidly decreased consciousness, hiccups, and abnormal respirations.

2. Small vessel stroke

a. Also known as lacunar stroke, small vessel stroke often is characterized by a <15 mm infarct resulting from occlusion of the smaller penetrating arteries branching from the large cerebral vessels discussed above. Approximately 25% of strokes are lacunar or small vessel (Toni, Sacco, Brainin, & Mohr, 2011).

b. May result from thrombus or embolus

(1) Atherosclerosis associated with chronic hypertension and diabetes mellitus

(2) Small emboli debris

(3) Other causes of small vessel stroke

(a) Vasculitis

(b) Cerebral amyloid angiopathy

c. Several classic lacunar syndromes or symptoms include (Toni et al., 2011)

(1) Pure motor hemiparesis caused by lacunar stroke of the internal capsule resulting in the loss of motor function in the contralateral face, arm, or leg, with or without dysarthria or dysphagia

(2) Ataxic hemiparesis caused by lacunar stroke of the internal capsule, ACA, or midbrain resulting in contralateral motor and cerebellar symptoms, often affecting the leg more than the arm

(3) Dysarthria and clumsy hand caused by lacunar stroke of the internal capsule, basal ganglia, thalamus, or cerebral peduncle resulting in hand weakness and dysarthria

(4) Pure sensory stroke caused by lacunar stroke of the thalamus, internal capsule, or midbrain resulting in decreased sensation, numbness, tingling, or burning on one side of the body

(5) Mixed sensorimotor stroke caused by lacunar stroke of the thalamus and internal capsule or the pons resulting in hemiparesis with ipsilateral sensory impairment without cortical signs

3. Other stroke causes: Several conditions may rarely result in stroke and should be considered when caring for a stroke patient.

a. Severe hypotension and hypoxia may result in watershed infarct or border zone infarction. The term *watershed* or *border zone stroke* indicates small infarcts occurring between major arterial territories in the brain. Watershed strokes are classified according to their location, with cortical watershed strokes appearing in the territories between the ACA, MCA, and PCA, and internal watershed strokes occurring between the deep MCA territories. Watershed strokes commonly are caused by hypotension but may be caused by other conditions, including a shower of emboli after cardiac or vascular surgery or scattered embolic debris from ICA occlusion (Pare & Kahn, 2012).

(1) Reversible cerebral vasoconstriction syndrome (Singhai & Ducros, 2011)

(a) Represents several conditions, with reversible narrowing of the cerebral arteries associated with severe headaches. Disease processes falling under this heading have a variety of names including vasospasm, angiitis, postpartum cerebral angiopathy, drug-induced arteritis or angiopathy, and Call-Flemming syndrome. The exact pathophysiology and diagnostic criteria for all of the disorders named is unclear, and they likely overlap.

(b) Symptoms include severe headache and focal neurologic deficits, depending on the vessels involved. Patients may report a trigger event or factor such as sexual activity, sneezing, or other stressful or emotional situations.

(c) The exact incidence, etiology, and pathophysiology remain unclear. External factors such as medication or drugs, and physiologic stressors such as changes in hormone status associated with pregnancy and the peripartum period, appear to play a role. At a cellular level, the pathophysiology likely represents interplay between immunologic, biochemical, and sensory pathways.

B. ICH

1. Intraparenchymal hemorrhage symptom presentation generally is associated with the location of the hemorrhage. The location and pattern of the hemorrhage also is associated with its underlying mechanism (Kase, Greenberg, Mohr, & Caplan, 2011).

a. Deep hemorrhages occurring in the brain stem, midbrain, thalamus, and basal ganglia are associated with a rapid decrease in the patient's level of consciousness and lateral focal neurologic deficits, depending on the location and extent of the hemorrhage. Deep hemorrhages often are associated with hypertension and also may be caused by vascular malformations, coagulopathy, or a combination of factors.

b. Lobar hemorrhages occurring toward the periphery of the brain in the cerebral lobes present with signs and symptoms associated with a lobar location and compressed or damaged brain tissue. For example, a lobar hemorrhage in the frontoparietal lobe likely will be associated with contralateral motor and sensory loss, and possibly speech and language difficulty, depending on the location. Lobar hemorrhages more often are associated with amyloid angiopathy, mass with associated hemorrhage, or vascular malformations.

c. Intraventricular hemorrhage: Bleeding into the lateral, third, or fourth ventricles may represent an extension of an ICH into the ventricular space or a primary site of hemorrhage in rare occasions. Blood in the ventricular space is associated with increased ICP.

C. SAH

1. Causes of SAH

a. SAH most often is caused by head trauma or the rupture of a cerebral aneurysm. Other, less common causes of SAH include vasculitis, infectious vascular abnormalities such as mycotic aneurysm, neoplastic lesion hemorrhage, and stimulant drug use such as cocaine and amphetamines (Bershad & Suarez, 2011).

b. aSAH

(1) Cerebral aneurysms tend to form at the bifurcations of large- to medium-sized arterial vessels. A majority (85%) of aneurysms occur in the anterior circulation; the remainder occur in the posterior circulation.

(2) Cerebral aneurysms are classified according to morphology. Saccular or berry aneurysms are responsible for 85% of aSAH and generally occur in the anterior circulation of the brain. The other major classification of aneurysm morphology is fusiform aneurysm, or a dilation of the vessel without a clear neck or stalk to the aneurysm, and generally occurs in the posterior circulation of the brain.

c. Nonaneurysmal SAH: Approximately 15% of patients with spontaneous, or nontraumatic, SAH have no obvious source of bleeding such as an aneurysm, arteriovenous malformation, or other vascular malformation. Case series have reported the frequency of non-aneurysmal SAH between 5%–34%. Nonaneurysmal SAH generally follows a bleeding pattern in which the SAH is concentrated anterior to the midbrain with or without extension into the ambient cistern or basal Sylvian fissure. When this pattern of blood is noted and diagnostic work-up rules out aneurysmal or other vascular malformation as a cause, patient outcomes generally are good. Patients rarely experience cerebral vasospasm. The presence of intraventricular blood or other bleed locations with no vascular source of bleeding is associated with worse outcomes. The cause and mechanism of nonaneurysmal SAH is unknown. Current pathophysiology theories suggest a venous or other non-aneurysmal source of bleeding (Siebert et al., 2011).

(1) Signs and symptoms of aSAH and aneurysm localization

(a) The classic symptom associated with aSAH is a sudden onset headache, with or without signs of elevated ICP including transient or prolonged loss of consciousness, nausea, vomiting, and syncope. In addition, patients may experience focal neurologic deficits and signs of meningeal irritation such as neck stiffness, phonophobia, photophobia, Kernig's sign, or Brudzinski's sign. Kernig's sign is positive when the thigh is flexed at the hip and knee and extension of the knee is painful. Brudzinski's sign is positive when a supine patient exhibits an involuntary lifting of the leg when the head is lifted (Hemphill & Smith, 2008).

d. A clinical exam alone cannot definitively confirm the diagnosis of aSAH or localize the exact location of aneurysmal hemorrhage. However, certain CN deficits are more likely to be found with certain aneurysm locations (Hemphill & Smith, 2008).
   (1) Third nerve palsy with pupillary dilation, loss of ipsilateral light reflex, and pain located behind the eye are associated with an enlarging, generally unruptured, aneurysm located at the junction of the PCA and the ICA (Hemphill & Smith, 2008).
   (2) Hemiparesis, aphasia, and abulia may occur with ruptured ACA or MCA aneurysms, particularly if the rupture produces an ICH resulting in mass effect in addition to the SAH. Pain behind the eye in the temporal region may be associated with an enlarging, generally unruptured MCA aneurysm.
   (3) Sixth nerve palsy is associated with an aneurysm in the cavernous sinus.
   (4) Occipital or posterior cervical pain is associated with PICA or AICA aneurysm.
   (5) Third nerve palsy, sixth nerve palsy, and ataxia may be associated with giant basilar artery aneurysm.

e. Loss of consciousness at the onset of aSAH generally is related to the initial rise in ICP and reduction of cerebral blood flow at the time of hemorrhage. The loss of consciousness may be transient or persistent. Persistent loss of consciousness is associated with prolonged increased ICP.

f. *Sentinel headache* is a severe headache reported in the days or weeks before aSAH. A sentinel headache or sentinel bleed is reported by several case series to occur in anywhere between 15% and 60% of patients admitted with aSAH (Beck et al., 2006). Several theories related to the pathophysiology and significance of sentinel headaches exist. One theory is that the headache signifies a change in the vessel wall structure of the aneurysm without hemorrhage. Other theories proposed that the sentinel headache is associated with a small rupture of blood into the subarachnoid space, serving as a "warning bleed." Retrospective case series suggest that the presence of a sentinel bleed increases the chance of rebleeding (Beck et al., 2006).

D. Cerebral venous thrombosis (CVT): CVT is the thrombosis of the dural sinus or cerebral veins that causes 0.5%–1% of all strokes, particularly in younger individuals. Risk factors contributing to thrombosis formation include prior medical conditions such as thrombophilias and inflammatory bowel disease; medical conditions such as dehydration, pregnancy, and infection; and trauma, including to the head. Any of these conditions may contribute to venous stasis of blood, changes in vein vessel walls, and changes in the viscosity of the blood, increasing the likelihood of thrombosis formation. Patients with CVT exhibit symptoms related to increased ICP due to impaired venous outflow or focal injury from infarction, hemorrhage, or both (Saposnik et al., 2011).

1. Patients with CVT generally present with headache, and 25% of patients exhibit some other focal neurologic deficit such as papilledema or diplopia from sixth nerve palsy (Saposnik et al., 2011). Additional cortical deficits reflect the presence and extent of infarction, hemorrhage, or both.
   a. Superior sagittal sinus—most often involved in CVT; found to be thrombosed in 62% of patients with CVT (Saposnik et al., 2011). Symptoms associated with thrombosed superior sagittal sinus include headache, papilledema, and increased ICP with or without motor deficits and seizure.

b. Transverse or lateral sinus—involved in 41% of CVT cases; symptoms may be associated with an underlying ear infection and enlargement of the draining scalp veins (Saposnik et al., 2011).
c. The straight sinus, vein of Galen, and internal cerebral vein are involved in 16% of CVT cases and are associated with thalamic or basal ganglial infarction and rapid neurologic deterioration (Saposnik et al., 2011).
d. Cortical vein thrombosis is uncommon.
   (1) Seizure is a defining sign and symptom associated with CVT, occurring in approximately 40% of patients with CVT (Saposnik et al., 2011).

Stroke Mimics

A. *Stroke mimics* are diseases that produce symptoms mimicking an acute stroke. Between 6% and 20% of suspected stroke patients are classified as a stroke mimic, depending on the definition and study. One reason for the wide range of reported mimic rates is the difference in measurement methodology. Stroke mimic rates are higher if the clinician has less information. Therefore, practitioners' suspicion of stroke when they have only an onset story will be greater than after imaging and laboratory data is added to the clinical picture. When a healthcare provider has a history of the present illness, clinical exam, radiologic imaging, and laboratory information to complete the clinical picture, mimic rates are at the lower end of the reported range (Magauran & Nitka, 2012).

B. Common stroke mimics include
   1. Toxic metabolic syndromes, including hypoglycemia, severe hyperglycemia, hypernatremia, hyponatremia, hepatic encephalopathy, and Wernicke's encephalopathy (Jauch et al., 2013)
      a. Hypoglycemia, particularly in patients with an extensive history of alcohol abuse, is a classic stroke mimic associated with confusion, decreased level of consciousness, aphasia, and possibly hemiparesis. The symptoms generally resolve rapidly once the hypoglycemia is corrected.
   2. Seizure disorders, particularly in patients with postictal Todd's paralysis following a partial motor seizure. The pathophysiology of hemiparesis in Todd's paralysis is thought to be related to increased metabolic demand and the depletion of excitatory neurons at the seizure focus. A defining factor of Todd's paralysis, in addition to seizure activity, is weakness that cannot be localized to one specific vascular territory.
   3. Migraine headaches, particularly in patients with hemiplegic migraine, may be mistaken for acute stroke. The pathophysiology of hemiparesis in patients with migraine is related to cortical spreading depression with activation of neurons associated with the migraine and subsequent temporary inhibition of neurons in the same region. Similar to Todd's paralysis, a defining factor of migraine-related hemiparesis, in addition to migraine activity, is weakness that cannot be localized to one specific vascular territory.
   4. Degenerative neurologic conditions, including remitting and relapsing multiple sclerosis (MS) or MS with paroxysmal symptoms, which may be mistaken for an acute stroke. Acute inflammatory demyelinating polyneuritis, optic neuritis, and acute myelopathy also may present with signs and symptoms similar to an acute ischemic stroke.
   5. Additional disorders occasionally mistaken for acute stroke include peripheral neuropathies, idiopathic intracranial hypertension; CNS abscess; CNS tumor, particularly when the tumor has evolving mass effect; and drug toxicity (Jauch et al., 2013).

Physiology of Neuroplasticity and Stroke Recovery

A. Importance of neuroplasticity
   1. Neuroplasticity is the process of remodeling of the CNS.
      a. Neuroplasticity is an ongoing process in both healthy individuals and patients with brain injuries, and plays a crucial role in healthy learning and in regaining lost function after injury (Young & Tolentino, 2011).
      b. Historically, damage to neurons and other brain cells was considered irreversible and permanent. However, decades of research demonstrates that the brain has both regenerative and restorative abilities, a concept known as neuroplasticity (Dihne, Hartung, & Seitz, 2011).
      c. Remodeling occurs via two significant pathways: neuronal regeneration through axonal or dendritic sprouting and reorganization or remapping of functional sites to allow for communication via tissue ipsilateral or contralateral to the involved lesion.
         (1) Axonal sprouting occurs in several stages beginning immediately after damage to the brain. In the first 1–3 days after damage, neuronal discharges synchronize. During days 7–14 after a stroke, sprouting is activated and maintained. New connections between neurons are identifiable within 28 days of damage. Axonal and dendritic sprouting results in a change in the number or strength of synapses.
         (2) At a system level, the cellular changes result in changed neural networks and reorganization of communication pathways and maps (Pearson-Fuhrhop & Cramer, 2010).
   2. This concept of neuroplasticity is the foundation for rapid and intense rehabilitation therapies in the days and weeks following a stroke. Neuroplasticity also is thought to explain the varied responses to therapy in stroke survivors. Finally, the concept of neuroplasticity offers new therapeutic targets for research and treatments aimed at stroke recovery (Pearson-Fuhrhop & Cramer, 2010).
      a. Rehabilitation occurring in the initial months after a stroke aims to capitalize on adaptive neuroplasticity based on experience-dependent plasticity mechanisms (Dancause & Nudo, 2011).
   3. The underlying mechanisms contributing to neuroplasticity in individuals are not well-understood (Pearson-Fuhrhop & Cramer, 2010).

B. Types of plasticity
   1. Several types of neuroplasticity exist, and they often work in a complex interplay to develop new neural networks. Plasticity may be adaptive or maladaptive. Functional plasticity is a category of renetworking that occurs in an effort to regain typical human function. Plasticity is further divided into cellular plasticity, systems plasticity, and cortical map plasticity (Dancause & Nudo, 2011).

C. Factors affecting plasticity
   1. Multiple factors affect plasticity in stroke recovery, including genetic makeup, learning, attention to task, depression, and types of rehabilitation interventions (Pearson-Fuhrhop & Cramer, 2010).

D. Several rehabilitation modalities are thought to affect neuroplasticity in stroke recovery, including exercise therapy, brain stimulation therapy, and robotic therapy (Dancause & Nudo, 2011).

References

Beck, J., Raabe, A., Szelenyi, A., Berkefeld, J., Gerlach, R., Setzer, M., & Seifert, V. (2006). Sentinel headache and the risk of rebleeding after aneurysmal subarachnoid hemorrhage. *Stroke, 37*(11), 2733–2737. doi: 10.1161/01.STR.0000244762.51326.e7

Belur, P. K., Chang, J. J., He, S., Emanuel, B. A., & Mack, W. J. (2013). Emerging experimental therapies for intracerebral hemorrhage: Targeting mechanisms of secondary brain injury. *Neurosurgical Focus, 34*(5), E9. doi: 10.3171/2013.2.FOCUS1317

Bershad, E. M., & Suarez, J. I. (2011). Aneurysmal subarachnoid hemorrhage. In J. P. Mohr, P. A. Wold, J. C. Grotta, M. A. Moskowitz, M. Mayberg, & R. Kummer (Eds.), *Stroke: Pathophysiology, diagnosis, and management* (5th ed.). Philadelphia, PA: Elsevier Saunders.

Broughton, B. R., Reutens, D. C., & Sobey, C. G. (2009). Apoptotic mechanisms after cerebral ischemia. *Stroke, 40*(5), e331–e339. doi: 10.1161/STROKEAHA.108.531632

Ciurea, A., Palade, C., Voinescu, D., & Nica, D. (2013). Subarachnoid hemorrhage and cerebral vasospasm—Literature review. *Journal of Medicine and Life, 6*(2), 120–125.

Dancause, N., & Nudo, R. J. (2011). Shaping plasticity to enhance recovery after injury. *Progress in Brain Research, 192,* 273–295. doi: 10.1016/B978-0-444-53355-5.00015-4

Dihne, M., Hartung, H. P., & Seitz, R. J. (2011). Restoring neuronal function after stroke by cell replacement: Anatomic and functional considerations. *Stroke, 42*(8), 2342–2350. doi: 10.1161/STROKEAHA.111.613422

Heiss, W. D. (2012). The ischemic penumbra: How does tissue injury evolve? *Annals of the New York Academcy of Science, 1268,* 26–34. doi: 10.1111/j.1749-6632.2012.06668.x

Hemphill, J. C., & Smith, W. (2008). Neurologic critical care, including hypoxic-ischemic encephalopathy and subarachnoid hemorrhage. In A. S. Fauci & E. Braunwald (Eds.), *Harrison's principles of internal medicine* (17th ed., pp. 1720–1729). New York, NY: McGraw Hill.

Hickey, J. V. & Kanusky, J. T. (2014). Overview of neuroanatomy and neurophysiology. In J. V. Hickey (Ed.). *The clinical practice of neurological and neurosurgical nursing* (7th ed., pp. 48–93). Philadelphia, PA: Lippincott Williams & Wilkins.

Jauch, E. C., Saver, J. L., Adams, H. P. Jr., Bruno, A., Connors, J. J., Demaerschalk, B. M., ... American Heart Association Stroke Council, Council on Cardiovascular Nursing, Council on Peripheral Vascular Disease, and Council on Clinical Cardiology. (2013). Guidelines for the early management of patients with acute ischemic stroke: A guideline for healthcare professionals from the American Heart Association/American Stroke Association. *Stroke, 44*(3), 840–947.

Kase, C. S., Greenberg, S. M., Mohr, J. P., & Caplan, L. R. (2011). Intracerebral hemorrhage. In J. P. Mohr, P. A. Wold, J. C. Grotta, M. A. Moskowitz, M. Mayberg, & R. Kummer (Eds.), *Stroke: Pathophysiology, diagnosis, and management* (5th ed.). Philadelphia, PA: Elsevier Saunders.

Livesay, S. L., & Hickey, J. V. (2014). Transient ischemic attacks and acute ischemic stroke. In J. V. Hickey (Ed.), *The clinical practice of neurological and neurosurgical nursing* (7th ed., pp. 511–541). Philadelphia, PA: Lippincott Williams & Wilkins.

Magauran, B. G. Jr., & Nitka, M. (2012). Stroke mimics. *Emergency Medicine Clinics of North America, 30*(3), 795–804. doi: 10.1016/j.emc.2012.06.006

Mesulam, M. M. (2008). Aphasia, memory loss, and other focal cerebral disorders. In A. S. Fauci & E. Braunwald (Eds.), *Harrison's principles of internal medicine* (17th ed., pp. 162–171). New York, NY: McGraw Hill.

Pare, J. R., & Kahn, J. H. (2012). Basic neuroanatomy and stroke syndromes. *Emergency Medicine Clinics of North America, 30*(3), 601–615. doi: 10.1016/j.emc.2012.05.004

Park, S. H., Yim, M. B., Lee, C. Y., Kim, E., & Son, E. I. (2008). Intracranial fusiform aneurysms: It's pathogenesis, clinical characteristics and managements. *Journal of Korean Neurosurgical Society, 44*(3), 116–123. doi: 10.3340/jkns.2008.44.3.116

Pearson-Fuhrhop, K. M., & Cramer, S. C. (2010). Genetic influences on neural plasticity. *PM & R, 2*(12 Suppl 2), S227–S240. doi: 10.1016/j.pmrj.2010.09.011

Plesnila, N. (2013). Pathophysiological role of global cerebral ischemia following subarachnoid hemorrhage: The current experimental evidence. *Stroke Research and Treatment, 2013,* 651958. doi: 10.1155/2013/651958

Saposnik, G., Barinagarrementeria, F., Brown, R. D. Jr., Bushnell, C. D., Cucchiara, B., Cushman, M., ... American Heart Association Stroke Council and the Council on Epidemiology and Prevention. (2011). Diagnosis and management of cerebral venous thrombosis: A statement for healthcare professionals from the American Heart Association/American Stroke Association. *Stroke, 42*(4), 1158–1192. doi: 10.1161/STR.0b013e31820a8364

Schuenke, M., Schulte, E., & Schumacher, U. (2010). *Thieme atlas of anatomy: Head and neuroanatomy*. New York, NY: Thieme.

Siebert, B., Tummala, R. P., Chow, R., Faridar, A., Mousavi, S. A., & Divani, A. A. (2011). Intracranial aneurysms: Review of current treatment options and outcomes. *Frontiers in Neurology, 2*, 45.

Singhai, A. B., & Ducros, A. (2011). Reversible cerebral vasoconstriction syndromes. In J. P. Mohr, P. A. Wold, J. C. Grotta, M. A. Moskowitz, M. Mayberg, & R. Kummer (Eds.), *Stroke: Pathophysiology, diagnosis, and management* (5th ed.). Philadelphia, PA: Elsevier Saunders.

Summers, D., Leonard, A., Wentworth, D., Saver, J. L.., Simpson, J., Spilker, J. A., ... Mitchell, P. H. (2009). Comprehensive overview of nursing and interdisciplinary care of the acute ischemic stroke patient: A scientific statement from the American Heart Association. *Stroke, 40*, 2911-2944.

Swenson, R. S. (2014). Atlas of the brain: Structure with functional correlates. Retrieved from www.dartmouth.edu/~rswenson/Atlas

Toni, D., Sacco, R. L., Brainin, M., & Mohr, J. P. (2011). Classification of ischemic stroke. In J. P. Mohr, P. A. Wold, J. C. Grotta, M. A. Moskowitz, M. Mayberg, & R. Kummer (Eds.), *Stroke: Pathophysiology, diagnosis, and management* (5th ed.). Philadelphia, PA: Elsevier Saunders.

Young, J. A., & Tolentino, M. (2011). Neuroplasticity and its applications for rehabilitation. *American Journal of Therapeutics, 18*(1), 70–80. doi: 10.1097/MJT.0b013e3181e0f1a4

Chapter

2

Preventive Care

Susan E. Wilson, MSN RN C-ANP

Research has shown that up to 80% of strokes may be prevented by identifying risk factors and reducing personal risks. The Stroke Certified Registered Nurse (SCRN) must recognize stroke risk factors and implement primary and secondary prevention strategies to minimize stroke risk. This chapter is broken into three sections based on stroke subtype: ischemic, hemorrhagic, and subarachnoid. Nursing interventions are covered in depth under the ischemic section and can be extrapolated to the hemorrhagic and subarachnoid section.

Objectives

1. Identify individuals at risk for stroke.
2. Understand the role and use of stroke assessment tools.
3. Identify learning needs and appropriate teaching materials.
4. Identify modifiable and nonmodifiable risk factors.
5. Identify stroke prevention strategies based on clinical practice guidelines.

Stroke Prevention (National Stroke Association, 2013)

A. The National Stroke Association Stroke Prevention Advisory Board published guidelines in 2011 for healthcare providers on how to recognize and reduce stroke risk factors.

B. Risk assessment (Goldstein et al., 2006, 2011)

   1. Risk assessment tools
      a. Understanding risk factors and their effects will guide the appropriate risk-reduction or modification program. Therefore, it is important for the nurse to assist the patient in assessing his or her risk for stroke.
   2. Risk assessment tools are used to
      a. Identify individuals at risk for stroke
      b. Measure risks that can be modified
      c. Estimate risk to assist in selecting treatment
      d. Determine the need for diagnostic testing
   3. Stroke risk-assessment tools exist but have limitations because of the complex interactions of risk factors.
      a. A commonly used tool is the Framingham Stroke Profile (FSP).
         (1) Uses independent stroke predictors
            (a) Age

(b) Systolic blood pressure
(c) Antihypertensive therapy
(d) Diabetes
(e) Current smoking
(f) Cardiovascular disease
(g) Atrial fibrillation (AF)
(h) Left ventricular hypertrophy

(2) 10-year cumulative stroke risk is calculated.

Ischemic Stroke (Goldstein et al., 2006, 2011; Romero, Morris, & Pikula, 2008; Zhang et al., 2008)

A. Nonmodifiable risk factors: The nurse must identify patients at higher risk and those who may benefit from prevention and treatment of modifiable risk factors.
  1. Age: The risk for ischemic stroke doubles for each decade after the age of 55 years.
  2. Sex: Stroke is more prevalent in males.
    a. Men have a higher stroke incidence per age group than women except in the age groups of 35–44 years and older than 85 years.
    b. Factors such as oral contraceptive (OC) use and pregnancy may contribute to the higher rates of stroke in the 35- to 44-year-old age group.
    c. Deaths related to cardiovascular disease in men may contribute to the higher incidence of stroke in older women (i.e., women living longer).
  3. Low birth weight: A study performed in England and Wales found higher rates of stroke among persons with lower birth weights.
    a. A similar study group reviewing South Carolina Medicaid patients younger than 50 years of age compared with population controls found that the odds of stroke were more than double for low birth weights defined as <2,500 g (5 lbs. 8 oz.) compared to birth weights >4,000 g (8 lbs. 13 oz.). The reason for this relationship remains unclear.
  4. Race and ethnicity: Racial and ethnic impact on stroke risk are difficult to determine separately.
    a. In the United States, blacks and Hispanics have higher stroke incidence and mortality rates as compared with those of European descent.
    b. In the Atherosclerosis Risk in Communities (ARIC) Study, blacks had a 38% higher risk of stroke than whites. Possible reasons are increased prevalence of hypertension, obesity, and diabetes in the black population.
    c. The Strong Heart Study (SHS) included 13 American Indian tribes and communities in the southwest. Zhang and colleagues (2008) found that American Indians have a higher incidence of stroke compared with white and black populations, which may be due to increased blood pressure, poor glucose control, and smoking.
  5. Genetic factors: A family history of stroke increases the risk by approximately 30%.
    a. The most established genetic influences are related to hypertension, diabetes, and hyperlipidemia.
    b. Many of the coagulopathies are autosomal dominant traits. Disorders such as protein C and S deficiencies and Factor V Leiden mutations increase the risk of venous thrombosis; however, there has not been a strong association with arterial events such as stroke.
    c. With the exception of sickle cell disease, no treatment based specifically on genetic factors has been shown to reduce stroke risk.

B. Modifiable risk factors

1. Hypertension (American Heart Association, 2010, 2012; Chobanian et al., 2003; Furie et al., 2011; Goldstein et al., 2006, 2011; McGuire, 2008; Romero et al., 2008; U.S. Department of Health and Human Services, 2004, 2006)
   a. Epidemiology: Hypertension affects approximately 76.4 million people, age 20 years and older, in the United States.
      (1) The prevalence of hypertension is increasing due in some part to increasing obesity in the United States.
      (2) Lack of diagnosis and inadequate treatment are more likely to be found in minorities and the elderly.
      (3) The higher the blood pressure, the greater the stroke risk.
      (4) Systolic blood pressure increases with age.
      (5) The Framingham study showed that more than two-thirds of persons age 65 years are hypertensive.
      (6) Seventy-two percent of Americans with hypertension are aware that they have it, 61% are being treated, and 35% have a blood pressure lower than 140/90.
   b. Treatment options: Lowering blood pressure is the most important modifiable risk factor for preventing both ischemic and hemorrhagic strokes.
      (1) Treatment of hypertension is associated with a 35%–44% reduction in the incidence of stroke.
      (2) There is no definitive evidence that any particular class of antihypertensives offer special protection against stroke; therefore, the guidelines recommend following the Seventh Report of the Joint National Committee on Prevention, Detection, Evaluation, and Treatment of High Blood Pressure (JNC 7) classification for treatment of hypertension across the spectrum of age groups.
      (3) The JNC 7 provides a comprehensive, evidence-based approach to the classification and treatment of hypertension, classifying blood pressure into four groupings (see **Table 2-1**).
      (4) When choosing an antihypertensive, cost and tolerability are important because adherence is the strongest risk-reduction measure for vascular events and mortality.
   c. Nursing interventions: Lifestyle changes are recommended as treatment for individuals with *prehypertension*, defined as systolic blood pressure 120–130 mmHg or diastolic blood pressure 80–89 mmHg (**Table 2-2**).
      (1) Lifestyle changes recommended for hypertension
         (a) Weight loss
         (b) Smoking cessation
         (c) Heart-healthy diet—following the Dietary Approaches to Stop Hypertension (DASH) diet, which includes more fruits, vegetables, and low-fat dairy with less saturated and total fat
         (d) Decrease the amount of sodium in the diet to <2,300 mg/day. Decrease the intake of processed or refined foods, including canned and instant soups, and snack items that are low in nutrients and high in salt.
         (e) Calcium, potassium, and magnesium may help lower blood pressure.
      (2) Getting regular aerobic exercise (e.g., brisk walking at least 30 minutes a day or at least several days a week)
      (3) Limiting alcohol to two drinks a day for men and one drink a day for women

Table 2-1. Classification and Treatment of Blood Pressure (JNC 7) (Chobanian et al., 2003)

Classification	Systolic Blood Pressure mmHg	Diastolic Blood Pressure mmHg	No Compelling Indication*	With Compelling Indication*
Normal	<120	<80	No antihypertensive drug	No antihypertensive drug
Prehypertension	120–139	80–90	No antihypertensive drug	Drugs for the compelling indication
Stage 1 hypertension	140–159	90–99	Thiazide-type diuretics for most May consider ACE-Is, ARB, B-blockers, CCB, or a combination	Drugs for the compelling indication Other drugs (diuretics, ACE-Is, ARBs, B-blockers, CCB) as needed
Stage 2 hypertension	>160	>100	Two-drug combination for most++ (usually thiazide-type diuretic and ACE-I, ARB, B-blocker, or CCB)	Drugs for the compelling indication. Other drugs (diuretics, ACE-I, ARB, B-blockers, CCB) as needed.

**Compelling indications include (1) congestive heart failure, (2) myocardial infarction, (3) diabetes, (4) chronic renal failure, and (5) prior stroke.*

++Initial combined therapy should be used cautiously in those at risk for orthostatic hypotension.

ACE-Is indicates ACE inhibitors; ARB, Angiotensin II Receptor Blockers; B-blockers, beta-blockers; CCB, calcium channel blockers; DBP, diastolic blood pressure; SBP, systolic blood pressure.

Reprinted from "Primary Prevention of Ischemic Stroke: A Guideline from the American Heart Association/American Stroke Association Stroke Council," by L. B. Goldstein, R. Adams, M. J. Alberts, L. J. Appel, L. M. Brass, C. D. Bushnell, ... American Academy of Neurology, 2006, Stroke, *37, pp. 1583–1633. © 2006 by the American Heart Association/American Stroke Association. Reprinted with permission.*

Table 2-2. Lifestyle Modification Effects on Blood Pressure

Lifestyle Modification	Approximate Systolic Blood Pressure Reduction
Weight reduction	5–20 mmHg
DASH diet eating	8–14 mmHg
Dietary sodium reduction	2–8 mmHg
Physical activity	4–9 mmHg
Limit to moderate alcohol consumption	2–4 mmHg

Reprinted from "The Seventh Report of the Joint National Committee on Prevention, Detection, Evaluation, and Treatment of High Blood Pressure," by the U.S. Department of Health and Human Services, 2004. © 2004 by the National Heart, Lung and Blood Institute. Reprinted with permission.

2. Exposure to cigarette smoke (Centers for Disease Control and Prevention [CDC], 2014a; Fagerström, 2002; Furie et al., 2011; Goldstein et al., 2006, 2011; Howard et al., 1998; Mayo Clinic, 2014; University of Iowa Hospitals and Clinic, 2006)
   a. Epidemiology: The CDC estimates 19% of U.S. adults 18 years and older smoke cigarettes.
      (1) Cigarette smoking doubles the risk of ischemic stroke.
      (2) Smoking contributes to 12%–14% of all stroke deaths.

b. Etiology and contributing factors increase stroke risk by
   (1) Acute effects on thrombus generation in narrowed arteries
   (2) Chronic effects related to the development of atherosclerosis
   (3) Increasing heart rate
   (4) Increasing mean blood pressure and cardiac index
   (5) Decreasing arterial distensibility
c. Synergistic effects
   (1) Use of OC and smoking—the risk for ischemic stroke is 7.2 times greater in women who smoked and used OC versus those that did not smoke or use OC.
   (2) Exposure to environmental tobacco smoke or passive cigarette smoke is a risk factor for stroke and heart disease because of the development of atherosclerosis.
d. Treatment options
   (1) Quitting without assistance—may take several attempts to be successful. Factors to consider:
      (a) Can be managed alone
      (b) One-step process
      (c) Cost is minimal
      (d) Must be highly committed to the goal of quitting
      (e) Nicotine withdrawal symptoms, such as irritability, headache, or difficulty sleeping, may be severe for some, especially if the cigarettes smoked contain high levels of nicotine.
   (2) Nicotine fading—reduce the nicotine level by 30%, 60%, and 90% during a 3-week period and stop altogether during the fourth week. This method may help reduce the effects of nicotine withdrawal. Factors to consider:
      (a) Easy to follow
      (b) Inexpensive
      (c) Must have a high level of motivation
   (3) Nicotine replacement—comes in several different modes, providing a source of nicotine, and helps reduce withdrawal symptoms: nicotine gum, nicotine transdermal patch, nicotine lozenge, nicotine inhaler, and nicotine nasal spray. Factors to consider:
      (a) Managed alone with gum, patch, and lozenge
      (b) Must have a high level of motivation
      (c) Must stop smoking completely when using nicotine replacement products
      (d) Minor side effects may include lightheadedness, nausea, sore mouth, hiccups, excessive saliva, restless sleep, cough or throat irritation with the inhaler or spray; nasal congestion, sinus irritation, watery eyes, and sneezing with nicotine spray.
      (e) Not recommended during pregnancy or with history of hypertension, heart disease, or joint disease of the jaw if chewing nicotine gum
      (f) Denture wearers may not be able to chew the gum.
      (g) Long-term smokers are more likely to become dependent on the gum.
      (h) Insurance may not cover the cost of the gum and patch.
      (i) Inhaler can keep the smoker's hands busy, which may help with cigarette cravings.
      (j) Nasal spray works faster than the gum, lozenges, and inhaler. Not recommended if a nasal or sinus condition exists

(4) Prescription medications
   (a) Bupropion (Zyban)—approved by the U.S. Food and Drug Administration (FDA) in 1997 for smoking cessation. Although it is not known exactly how Zyban works, it has been shown to help individuals stop smoking, as well as reduce nicotine withdrawal symptoms and cravings. Factors to consider:
      1) Risk of seizure
      2) Should not be prescribed to patients with a history of seizure disorder who are currently taking monoamine oxidase inhibitors, Wellbutrin, or Wellbutrin SR; or who have an eating disorder
      3) Most common side effects are dry mouth and trouble sleeping
      4) Black box warning comes with bupropion (Zyban) because it has been associated with serious mental health problems—such as suicidal thoughts or behavior, hostility, and depression—while taking or after stopping the drug
      5) Available by prescription only
      6) May be used in combination with the nicotine patch; however, blood pressure should be monitored during treatment
   (b) Varenicline (Chantix)—a prescription medication that blocks nicotine receptors in the brain and decreases the pleasurable effects of smoking. Factors to consider:
      1) Most common side effects are vision trouble, fainting, severe skin reactions, vivid or strange dreams, impairment in the ability to drive or operate heavy machinery. Studies have shown an increase in road accidents and falls among people taking varenicline.
      2) Black box warning comes with varenicline (Chantix) because it has been associated with serious mental health problems—such as suicidal thoughts or behavior, hostility, and depression—while taking or after stopping the drug
      3) Use with caution with severe kidney problems
      4) Available by prescription only

e. Nursing interventions (Fagerström, 2002; Goldstein et al., 2006; Howard et al., 1998; University of Iowa Hospitals and Clinic, 2006; Mayo Clinic, 2014)
   (1) Smoking cessation is associated with a reduced risk of stroke and other cardiovascular events to a level that is close to but does not reach the level of those who never smoked. There are effective smoking-cessation approaches through nicotine replacement and behavioral support and training; however, data supporting that participation in such programs reduces stroke is lacking.
   (2) Patients fall into three groups
      (a) Tobacco users willing to quit receive intervention to help quit
      (b) Tobacco users unwilling to quit receive intervention to increase motivation to quit
      (c) Tobacco users who recently quit receive intervention to prevent relapse
   (3) The 5 A's model for treating tobacco use and dependence
      (a) **Ask** about use.
      (b) **Advise** the patient to quit and do so in a clear, strong, and personalized manner. For example, "I think it is important for you to quit smoking because you have had a stroke, your carotid artery is narrowed, you have hypertension, and quitting will decrease your risk for another stroke."

(c) **Assess**. Is the patient willing to quit? Provide intervention.

(d) **Assist**.

1) Set a quit date.
2) Inform family and friends of plan for support.
3) Remove tobacco products from environment.
4) Recommend use of approved medication and discuss use and side effects.
5) Provide counseling by evaluating past attempts and anticipating challenges. Build on past success. Elements of counseling include
   a) Recognize danger situations: stress, other smokers, alcohol, urges.
   b) Develop coping skills: anticipate and avoid temptation, behavioral activities that help cope with smoking urges.
   c) Provide basic information: smoking may cause a full relapse and withdrawal symptoms typically peak within 1–2 weeks after quitting but may persist for months. Symptoms include negative mood, urges to smoke, and difficulty concentrating.
   d) Provide supportive resources: national quit line (1.800.quit.now), American Lung Association.
6) Discuss alcohol use as potential trigger to relapse.
7) Involve social support and ask other smokers in the household to not smoke in the patient's presence.

(e) **Arrange** follow-up.

3. Diabetes (American Diabetes Association, 2013; Collins et al., 2003; Colhoun et al., 2004; Delude, 2010; Diabetes Control and Complications Trial (DCCT) Research Group, 1995; Furie et al., 2011; Gaede et al., 2003; Goldberg et al., 1998; Goldstein et al., 2006, 2011; Heart Outcomes Prevention Evaluation Study Investigators, 2000; Heart Protection Study Collaborative Group, 2002; Hu et al., 2002; Kernan et al., 2002; Klein et al., 2004; Lindholm et al., 2002; ORIGIN Trial Investigators et al., 2012; Sever et al., 2003; Sowers, 2003; Tuomilehto & Rastenyte, 1999)

a. Epidemiology: Since 1990, the prevalence of diabetes has increased by 61% overall and 33% in people with a history of ischemic stroke.

(1) The increase in diabetes across the United States parallels the increase in obesity.

(2) Diabetes has clearly been shown to be a risk factor for first stroke; however, data determining whether it is a risk for recurrent stroke is meager.

(3) Epidemiologic studies evaluating the effects of diabetes on stroke have shown an increased relative risk of stroke ranging from 1.8- to 6-fold.

(4) The risk is present for all ages, but most notable before age 55 years in blacks and before age 65 years in whites.

b. Classification

(1) Normal fasting glucose: <100 mg/dL

(2) Impaired fasting glucose: 100–125 mg/dL

(3) Fasting glucose: >126 mg/dL or HgA1C >6.5% meet threshold for diagnosis of diabetes

(4) HgA1C >7%: inadequate glucose control

c. Associated risks with diabetes

(1) Heart disease

(2) Stroke

(3) Hypertension

(4) Kidney disease
(5) Dental disease
(6) Ocular disease, blindness

d. Treatment options to reduce cardiovascular and stroke risk by 50%
  (1) Blood glucose control: Tight glucose control is controversial in reducing the risk of stroke.
    (a) Although the Action to Control Cardiovascular Risk in Diabetes trial was stopped early due to increased mortality, a meta-analysis found that intense glucose control of HgbA1C <6.5% reduced the incidence of myocardial infarction (MI) and stroke by about 15%.
    (b) The Action in Diabetes and Vascular Disease trial showed no benefit of tight glucose control on decreasing stroke risk.
    (c) Lowering the HgbA1C below 7% appears to reduce the risk of MI and stroke in people who are younger and newly diagnosed with diabetes but not in those who are older, have had diabetes for more than 20 years, are taking insulin, and already have a diagnosis of cardiovascular disease.
    (d) Behavioral risk factor modification for glucose control: Moderate weight loss improves glycemic control and reduces cardiovascular risk associated with diabetes.
    (e) Use of statins: The British Heart Foundation Heart Protection Study showed a 24% reduction in stroke with the addition of a statin.
    (f) Treatment of hypertension: The UK Prospective Diabetes Study Group found tight blood pressure control in people with diabetes decreases the stroke risk by 44%.
    (g) Use of antiplatelet drug if appropriate.
    (h) The American Diabetes Association has adopted the conservative goal of HgbA1C of 7%, but suggests that more aggressive goals be set for younger people with no heart disease. Individualized treatment is important (**Table 2-3**).

Table 2-3. 2013 ADA Recommendations for Glucose, Blood Pressure, and Lipid Control in Most Adults

Measurement	Goal
HbA1c	<7.0%*
Blood Pressure Control	<140/80 mmHg**
Lipids: low-density lipoprotein (LDL)	<100 mg/dL†

**More or less stringent glycemic goals may be appropriate for individual patients. Goals should be individualized based on duration of diabetes, age/life expectancy, comorbid conditions, known cardiovascular disease (CVD) or advanced microvascular complications, hypoglycemia unawareness, and individual patient considerations.*

***Based on patient characteristics and response to therapy, lower systolic blood pressure targets may be appropriate.*

†In individuals with overt CVD, a lower LDL cholesterol goal of 70 mg/dL (1.8 mmol/L), using a high dose statin, is an option.

Reprinted from "Standards of Medical Care in Diabetes—2013," by the American Diabetes Association, 2013, Diabetes Care, *36(1), pp. S11–S66. © 2013 by the American Diabetes Association. Reprinted with permission.*

e. Nursing interventions—provide education regarding
   (1) Diet: Individualize diet teaching to allow for food preferences with the goal of increasing intake of fruits, vegetables, and grains, limiting foods high in saturated fat, decreasing salt, and limiting alcohol intake.
   (2) Reduce portion sizes and consumption of calorie-containing beverages.
   (3) Weight loss: Moderate weight loss improves insulin action and fasting blood glucose levels and reduces the need for diabetic treatment with medication. Weight loss is recommended for overweight (body mass index [BMI] 25–29) and obese (BMI >30) adults with diabetes or those at risk of developing type 2 diabetes. Decrease calorie intake by 500–1,000 kcal/day.
   (4) Decrease time in sedentary behaviors (e.g., watching TV, spending time on the computer, playing video games).
   (5) Encourage exercise, which will improve insulin sensitivity and glycemic control. Encourage 30–45 minutes of moderate aerobic physical activity, such as walking, 3–5 days per week. For inactive individuals, encourage short (approximately 10 minutes per day) activity and gradually increase duration and intensity to tolerance.

4. Dyslipidemia (Amarenco et al., 2006; Amarenco & Labreuche, 2009; CDC, 2012; Collins et al., 2004; Expert Panel on Detection, Evaluation, and Treatment of High Blood Cholesterol in Adults, 2001; Furie et al., 2011; Goldstein et al., 2006, 2011; Horenstein, Smith, & Mosca, 2002; LaRosa et al., 2005; Ridker et al., 2008; Subhi, 2014; U.S. Department of Health and Human Services, 2001; Zhang et al., 2003)
   a. Epidemiology: Seventy-one million (33.5%) American adults (20 years old and older) have high low-density lipoprotein (LDL) cholesterol, and one out of three Americans has their cholesterol under control.
      (1) Elevated total cholesterol increases the risk of heart disease two-fold.
      (2) Race, ethnicity, and gender play a role in hyperlipidemia development (**Table 2-4**).

Table 2-4. Percent of Persons with LDL >130 mg/dL in the United States: 2012

Race/Ethnicity	Men (%)	Women (%)
Non-Hispanic blacks	34.4	27.7
Mexican Americans	41.9	31.6
Non-Hispanic whites	30.5	32.0
All	32.5	31.0

Reprinted from "Cholesterol: Facts," by the Centers for Disease Control and Prevention, 2012, www.cdc.gov/cholesterol/facts.htm. © 2012 by the Centers for Disease Control and Prevention. Reprinted with permission.

   b. Treatment options—Treatments that reduce LDL have been shown to reduce coronary heart disease risk by 25%–45% over 5 years.
      (1) A meta-analysis of 165,000 patients showed that for every 39-mg/dL decrease in LDL cholesterol levels, there was a 21% reduction in the relative risk of stroke.
      (2) In large randomized trials, statins have demonstrated a consistent benefit in stroke prevention in patients with coronary artery disease. Both the Anglo-Scandinavian Cardiac Outcomes Trial (ASCOT) and the Heart Protection Study, which enrolled high-risk patients with prior coronary events, showed a reduction in stroke rates by 27% to 32% compared with placebo.

(3) The Stroke Prevention by Aggressive Reduction in Cholesterol Levels (SPARCL) showed an absolute reduction in ischemic stroke risk of 2.2%.

(4) Non-statin lipid-lowering therapies may also provide a level of stroke prevention, although the data is less certain.

(a) Niacin treatment was associated with a 24% reduction in known or suspected cerebrovascular events (including transient ischemic attacks [TIA]) in the Coronary Drug Project.

(b) The Veterans Affairs HDL Intervention Trial (VA-HIT), which evaluated the effect of gemfibrozil in men with coronary heart disease and low levels of high-density lipoprotein (HDL) cholesterol (<40 mg/dL) found a trend toward reduction in strokes in the treated group (6% vs. 4.6%).

(5) Adult treatment panel (ATP) III classification of LDL, total, and HDL cholesterol (mg/dL) (**Table 2-5**)

Table 2-5. Adult Treatment Panel (ATP) III Classification of LDL, Total, and HDL Cholesterol (mg/dL)

LDL Cholesterol—Primary Target of Therapy	
<100	Optimal
100–129	Near optimal/above optimal
130–159	Borderline high
160–189	High
>190	Very high
Total Cholesterol	
<200	Desirable
200–239	Borderline high
>240	High
HDL Cholesterol	
<40	Low
>60	High

An update to the National Cholesterol Education Program ATP III guidelines recommends aggressively treating LDL cholesterol levels in high-risk patients; For those with established heart disease who also have multiple risk factors, including diabetes, metabolic syndrome, or severe or poorly controlled risk factors, the guidelines recommend aggressively treating LDL levels to less than 70 mg/dL.

Reprinted from "ATP III Guidelines At-A-Glance Quick Desk Reference (NIH Publication No. 01-3305)" by U.S. Department of Health and Human Services, 2001, Bethesda, MD: National Institutes of Health/National Heart, Lung, and Blood Institute. © 2001 by the National Heart, Lung, and Blood Institute. Reprinted with permission.

c. Nursing intervention

(1) Diet—reduce saturated fats, increase plant stanols/sterols (e.g., naturally occurring substances found in plants and in small amounts in fruits, vegetables, nuts, seeds, cereals, and legumes)

(2) Increase fiber (e.g., oats, barley, lentils, beans)

(3) Increase fish consumption for the omega-3 fatty acids

(4) Weight loss/management

(5) Increase physical activity

(6) Smoking cessation

5. Atrial Fibrillation (AF; The ACTIVE Investigators et al., 2009; Albers & SPORTIF Investigators, 2004; Camm et al., 2012; Connolly et al., 2009; Furie et al., 2011; Fuster et al., 2001; Gage et al., 2004; Go et al., 2001; Goldstein et al., 2006, 2011; Healey et al., 2008; Lane & Lip, 2012; Mason et al., 2012 Olsson & Executive Steering Committee on the SPORTIF III Investigators, 2003; Roldán et al., 2013; van Walraven et al., 2002)
   a. Epidemiology: AF causes more than 75,000 strokes per year in the estimated 2.6 million Americans who have AF.
      (1) The number of people with AF is anticipated to double in the future.
      (2) Prevalence increases with age, affecting approximately 5% of those 70 years and older (mean age, 75 years)
      (3) Associated with a four- to five-fold increased risk of stroke, with the average risk for first-time stroke at 2%–4% per year
      (4) Strokes that are caused by AF are usually large and disabling and associated with an increased mortality.
   b. Risk classification—validated stratification schemes
      (1) $CHADS_2$ (acronym for congestive heart failure, hypertension, age older than 75 years, diabetes mellitus, and prior stroke or TIA)
         (a) Derived from independent predictors of stroke risk in patients with nonvalvular atrial fibrillation
         (b) The score gives 1 point each for congestive heart failure (CHF), hypertension, age older than 75 years, and diabetes mellitus and 2 points for prior stroke or TIA.
         (c) Limitation applies to secondary prevention in patients with prior stroke or TIA and no other risk factors. These patients scored a 2 on the scale defining them as moderate risk, but in the validation study, they were found to have 10.8 strokes per year, which means they are at a high risk for recurrence.
      (2) CHA_2DS_2-VASc Score
         (a) Refinement of $CHADS_2$ scoring
         (b) Tested in 8,000 patients and proven to stratify better than $CHADS_2$
         (c) Accounts for vascular disease, younger age (66–74 years), and female sex
      (3) HAS-BLED (hypertension, abnormal renal/liver function, stroke, bleeding history or predisposition, labile international normalized ratio (INR), elderly, drugs/alcohol) Score
         (a) Used to estimate major bleeding risk prior to starting anticoagulants
         (b) Acronym represents each of the bleeding risk factors and assigns 1 point for each that is present.
         (c) Made up of clinical information that is routinely available before therapy is initiated
         (d) Allows the clinician to identify bleeding risks and correct the modifiable ones such as controlling blood pressure, removing concomitant antiplatelet or NSAIDs, and counseling against excessive alcohol intake.
         (e) Used to fully inform patients of risk to assist with their decision making
         (f) Score ranges from 0 to 9, with a score more than 3 indicating a high risk of bleeding, and recommending caution with anticoagulation use and regular patient evaluation.
         (g) Validated against bleeding risk scores (HEMORR2HAGES and ATRIA) with better predictive values

c. Treatment options

(1) Management of patients with AF generally involves three objectives, which are not mutually exclusive:

(a) Rate control, which does not reduce risk of strokes

(b) Prevention of thromboembolism, a mainstay of stroke prevention

(c) Correction of the rhythm disturbance

(2) Clinical trials have established the benefit of antithrombotic therapies for reducing the risk of stroke in patients with a 64% reduction with adjusted-dose warfarin versus 22% reduction with aspirin.

(3) 2010 European Society of Cardiology Guidelines for the management of AF based on scores

(a) $CHADS_2$ score: >2—oral anticoagulant (warfarin [maintain INR 2–3] or direct thrombin inhibitor or direct Xa inhibitor)

(b) $CHADS_2$ score: 0–1

1) CHA_2DS_2-VASc: >2 = oral anticoagulant

2) CHA_2DS_2-VASc: 1 = oral anticoagulant or aspirin (prefer anticoagulant). Assess risk versus benefit and patient preference.

3) CHA_2DS_2-VASc: 0 = truly low risk, aspirin or no antithrombotic

(4) Increased risk for bleeding while on warfarin

(a) Age 75 years and older

(b) Concomitant antiplatelets (aspirin, clopidogrel, dipyridamole) and nonsteroidal anti-inflammatory drugs (NSAIDs)

(c) Uncontrolled hypertension

(d) Supratherapeutic INR

d. Nursing interventions

(1) Hospitalized patients

(a) Recognize symptoms associated with AF

1) Variations in hemodynamic parameters (e.g., blood pressure, heart rate, oxygen saturation)

2) Palpitations

3) Chest pain

4) Dyspnea

5) Weakness, fatigue

6) Syncope

7) Anxiety, restlessness

(b) Provide continuous cardiac monitoring and recognize irregular rhythm or rapid rate, and report to the doctor

(c) Assess vital signs

(d) Assess response to increased activity

(e) Assess mentation

(f) Administer medication as prescribed and evaluate response and side effects

(g) Provide education regarding medication and interventional procedures

1) Explain purpose and side effects of medications prescribed

2) Explain procedures and recovery

3) Discuss progressive activity schedule

4) Discuss diet related to medications

(2) Nonhospitalized patients

(a) Holter monitor—teaching

(b) Medication teaching—compliance is essential
(c) Compliance with lab follow-up if necessary
(d) Education regarding warfarin, appropriate diet
(e) Decrease or eliminate caffeine
(f) Smoking cessation
(g) Weight loss if indicated
(h) Decrease or eliminate alcohol
(i) Obtain regular exercise
(j) Maintain adequate hydration

6. Asymptomatic carotid artery stenosis (Bhatt, 2010; Bogousslavsky, Despland, & Regli, 1986; Executive Committee for the Asymptomatic Carotid Atherosclerosis Study, 1995; Goldstein, Moore, Robertson, & Chaturvedi, 1997; Goldstein et al., 2006, 2011; Halliday et al., 2004; Hobson et al., 1993; Mayo Asymptomatic Carotid Endarterectomy Study Group, 1992; Nederkoorn et al., 2002; Oran & Oran, 2010; Pritz, 2007; Randour et al., 2001; Wolff, Guirguis-Blake, Miller, Gillespie, & Harris, 2007)
   a. Epidemiology: Estimates of carotid artery stenosis from population-based studies range from 0.5% to 8%.
      (1) Approximately 1% of the general American population has clinically significant carotid artery stenosis, defined as 60%–99% narrowing.
      (2) The North American Symptomatic Carotid Endarterectomy Trial (NASCET) found an average annual risk of ipsilateral stroke to be 3% for 60%–74% stenosis, 3.7% for 75%–94% stenosis, 2.9% for 95%–99% stenosis, and 1.9% with a complete occlusion.
   b. Risk factors for carotid disease
      (1) Elevated blood cholesterol levels
      (2) Diet high in saturated and trans fats
      (3) Smoking
      (4) Overweight and obesity
      (5) Sedentary lifestyle or lack of physical activity
      (6) Hypertension
      (7) Insulin resistance
      (8) Diabetes
      (9) Metabolic syndrome—have at least three of the five metabolic risk factors (abdominal obesity, high triglyceride level, low HDL, hypertension, diabetes)
      (10) Older age—before age 75 years, risk is greater in men; after age 75 years, risk is greater in women
      (11) Genetics—family history of atherosclerosis
   c. Treatment options
      (1) Lifestyle changes
         (a) Diet—low-fat and low-salt diet
         (b) Weight loss or maintain healthy weight
         (c) Increase exercise
         (d) Smoking cessation
         (e) Limit alcohol intake
         (f) Take medications as prescribed
         (g) Optimize hyperlipidemia treatment
         (h) Optimize hypertension treatment
         (i) Optimize diabetes treatment

(2) Interventions

(a) Carotid endarterectomy (CEA)—surgically removes plaque from artery

1) The benefit of CEA in symptomatic patients with stenosis of 70% or greater is well established in three major studies: NASCET, the European Carotid Surgery Trial, and the Veterans Affairs Trial of Carotid Endarterectomy in Symptomatic Carotid Stenosis.

2) Benefits of CEA are slightly better in men than women, which may be due to smaller arteries in women.

3) The Carotid Revascularization Endarterectomy versus Stent Trial (CREST) trial established that advanced age is not a contraindication to surgery.

4) Data from three randomized clinical trials found no benefit of CEA in asymptomatic patients.

5) The benefit of endarterectomy in the setting of asymptomatic carotid artery stenosis (CAS) is highly dependent on surgical risk.

(b) CAS—stent placement to expand and maintain blood flow through the artery

1) CREST found similar stroke endpoints between the two procedures.

2) Younger patients (69 years or younger) responded better to CAS and those 70 years and older to CEA.

7. Postmenopausal hormone therapy (Furie et al., 2011; Goldstein et al., 2006, 2011; Hulley et al., 1998; Lisabeth & Bushnell, 2012 Simon et al., 2001; Rossouw et al., 2002)

a. Epidemiology: Natural menopause usually occurs between the age of 45 and 55 years.

(1) During this time women develop cardiovascular risk factors, and the risk of stroke roughly doubles in women.

(2) Framingham Heart Study (FHS; **Table 2-6**) stroke rate in women

Table 2-6. Framingham Heart Study (Lisabeth & Bushnell, 2012)

Race	Age Range (Years)	Percent Per 1,000 Person-Years
White	45–54	0.82
Mexican American	45–59	1.94
African American	45–54	2.47

b. Treatment options: Studies of women transitioning through the menopausal phase have shown changes associated with increased cardiovascular risk, which include abdominal obesity and increased body mass index, blood pressure, blood sugar, triglycerides, cholesterol, and LDL, along with a decrease in HDL.

(1) Use of estrogen plus progestin or estrogen alone increases stroke risk.

(a) The Women's Health Initiative randomized 16,608 postmenopausal women and reported that the combination of estrogen plus progestin increased ischemic stroke risk by 44% with no effect on hemorrhagic stroke risk.

(b) In addition, 10,739 postmenopausal women with a hysterectomy receiving estrogen alone had a 55% increased risk of ischemic stroke with no hemorrhagic stroke risk.

(2) Use of transdermal estrogen may be safer with regard to stroke risk because it does not increase clotting factors and inflammatory markers or involve first-pass liver metabolism since it is delivered across the skin.
(3) The Nurses' Health Study showed a dose relationship between oral estrogen and stroke risk. Women taking 0.625 mg of estrogen were 35% more likely to develop a stroke while those taking 1.25 mg were 63% at risk. Those taking 0.30 mg were not at increased risk.
(4) The American Heart Association (AHA) guidelines state that hormone therapy should not be used for heart disease or stroke prevention.
(5) If the decision is made to treat, the lowest effective estrogen dose should be used and transdermal therapy should be first choice.

c. Nursing interventions
(1) Lifestyle counseling to decrease cardiovascular risk
(a) Heart-healthy diet
(b) Maintain a healthy weight.
(c) Participate in physical activity.
(d) No smoking
(e) Discuss measures to control blood pressure, cholesterol, and glucose.
(2) Lifestyle counseling to combat menopausal symptoms
(a) Lifestyle changes
1) Dress in cooler clothing.
2) Sleep in a cooler room.
3) Avoid spicy foods and caffeine.
4) Reduce stress through relaxation techniques, meditation, and deep breathing.
5) Get plenty of rest. If the patient suffers from insomnia, try
a) Over-the-counter sleep aids
b) Glass of milk or cup of yogurt prior to bedtime
c) Physical activity in morning or early afternoon, not in the evening
d) Hot shower or bath prior to bedtime
e) Mental exercises to assist with memory
f) Phytoestrogen (found in soy beans and soy-based products)
g) Antidepressants have shown some benefit in clinical trials (venlafaxine, paroxetine, and fluoxetine).

8. Use of OC (Chan et al., 2004; Gillum, Mamidipudi, & Johnston, 2000; Goldstein et al., 2006, 2011; Zuber, Toulon, Marnet, & Mas, 1996)
a. Epidemiology: Population-based studies, which controlled for smoking and hypertension, showed an additional 4.1 ischemic strokes per 100,000 women on low-dose estrogen OCs.
b. Risks: Some groups of women appear to be at higher risk for stroke if they use OCs.
(1) Older than 35 years of age
(2) Smoke cigarettes
(3) Hypertension
(4) Diabetic
(5) Migraines
(6) Hypercholesterolemia
(7) Obese
(8) Prothrombin mutations, such as factor V Leiden

c. Treatment options: The AHA Stroke Prevention Guideline recommends aggressive therapy for stroke risk factors for those women who use OCs.
   (1) Blood pressure measurement is recommended prior to the initiation of hormonal contraception.
d. Nursing interventions
   (1) Discuss stroke risk associated with taking OCs.
   (2) Smoking cessation or counsel never to start
   (3) Discuss measures to control blood pressure, cholesterol, and glucose.
   (4) Weight loss teaching
   (5) Increase physical activity.

9. Diet and nutrition (American Heart Association Nutrition Committee et al., 2006; Appel et al., 1997; Ding & Mozaffarian, 2006; Goldstein et al., 2006, 2011; He et al., 2004; John et al., 2002; Joshipura et al., 1999; Larsson & Orsini, 2011; Sacks et al., 2001; Sauvaget, Nagano, Allen, & Kodama, 2003; Threapleton et al., 2013)
   a. Risks
      (1) Increases blood pressure
         (a) Excess salt intake
         (b) Low potassium intake
         (c) Increased alcohol consumption
         (d) Poor diet
      (2) Blacks are especially sensitive to the effects of increased salt, low potassium, and poor diet on blood pressure.
      (3) Increased intake of fruits and vegetables is associated with a decreased stroke risk.
         (a) The Nurses' Health Study and the Health Professionals' Follow-Up Study found for each single serving per day of fruit and vegetable intake, the risk of stroke was reduced by 6%.
         (b) A prospective study of more than 40,000 Japanese men and women assessed fruit and vegetable intake during an 18-year follow-up period.
            1) Daily intake of vegetables was associated with a 26% reduction in the risk of death from stroke.
            2) This protective effect was observed for both ischemic and hemorrhagic stroke and was slightly stronger for ischemic.
            3) Daily fruit intake was associated with a 35% reduction in stroke risk of stroke in men and a 25% reduction in women.
         (c) A Mediterranean diet, which incorporates legumes and olive oil, may prevent stroke. Evidence is limited regarding optimal levels for stroke prevention.
         (d) A meta-analysis of 15 prospective studies found that three servings of fish a week were associated with a 6% reduction in stroke risk.
         (e) Dietary fiber intake is inversely associated with risk of ischemic and hemorrhagic stroke. This may be due to soluble fibers helping lower LDL and regulate blood sugar levels. Seven grams per day was associated with a relative reduction; however, 4 grams per day was not.
   b. Nursing interventions: Provide culturally sensitive diet teaching.
      (1) DASH diet
         (a) Decreases sodium
         (b) Increases potassium

(c) Increases fruits and vegetables
(d) Decreases fat intake
(2) Promote decreased red meat intake and increased fish intake.
(3) Encourage increased fiber intake.
(4) Teach food labeling.
(5) Assist with referral to dietician.
(6) Provide resources, including free tools to better nutrition.
(a) U.S. Department of Agriculture Food and Nutrition Service's Super Tracker: www.supertracker.usda.gov
(b) Nutritional Analysis Tool 2.0: www.myfoodrecord.com/mainnat.html

10. Physical inactivity (American Heart Association Nutrition Committee et al., 2006; Artinian et al., 2010; Blair et al., 1996; CDC, 2013a, 2014b; Furie et al., 2011; Goldstein et al., 2006, 2011; Kokkinos et al., 1995; Lakka & Salonen, 1993; Pate et al., 1995; Ruppar & Conn, 2010; Sacco et al., 1998; U.S. Department of Health and Human Services, 2008)
a. Epidemiology
(1) Forty-eight percent of adults in the United States do not meet the 2008 physical activity guidelines
(a) Two and a half hours of moderate intensity aerobic exercise per week
(b) Two or more days per week of muscle strengthening activity
(2) Rates of inactivity vary according to region; for example, the southern states are the most sedentary states.
(3) Physical activity differs by groups according to ethnicity, sex, educational level, and poverty status.
b. Sedentary lifestyle increases the risk of
(1) Stroke
(2) Heart disease
(3) Type 2 diabetes
(4) Obesity
(5) Hypertension
(6) Depression
(7) Some cancers
(8) Early death
c. Benefit of physical activity on stroke risk
(1) Moderately active = 20% lower stroke risk
(2) Highly active = 27% lower stroke risk
(3) Improves heart function
(4) Improves lipid profile
(5) Lowers blood pressure and resting heart rate
(6) Increases insulin sensitivity
d. Benefit of physical activity for stroke survivors
(1) Improves strength
(2) Improves balance
(3) Improves endurance
(4) Reduces depression and anxiety
(5) Improves self-confidence
(6) Improves independence

e. Nursing interventions
   (1) Behavioral approaches
      (a) Incorporate rewards for performing more physical activity (e.g., a trip, clothing).
      (b) Set up a patient contract (e.g., perform physical activity at a specified level for a specified duration).
      (c) Set goals (i.e., help the patient set realistic goals with specific outcomes).
      (d) Self-monitor (e.g., keep a record of daily activity, use pedometers to record daily steps).
      (e) Provide stimuli and cues (e.g., calendars, diaries, phone calls from family and friends as reminder to exercise, placing exercise shoes by front door).
   (2) Cognitive approaches
      (a) Educate patients on how to avoid obstacles or deterrents to physical activity.
      (b) Chart the benefits of physical activity.
      (c) Provide motivational counseling; help the patient resolve their lack of readiness.
      (d) Solve individual barriers to exercise.
         1) Identify and define the problem.
         2) Have the patient brainstorm solutions.
         3) Evaluate the pros and cons of solutions.
         4) Implement the plan.
         5) Evaluate the success.
   (3) Self-efficacy—belief in capabilities to obtain goals
      (a) Mastering—achieve a goal, such as walking one mile
      (b) Modeling—observe another patient performing an exercise routine or speak to someone who has been successful
      (c) Verbal persuasion—express belief in the person's capability to exercise and meet goals
      (d) Physiological feedback—educate the patient that he or she will feel better with exercise; for example, exercise will help the patient feel less fatigued
   (4) Supervised exercise—encourage group exercise classes, but financial resources may be a limiting factor
   (5) Address cultural influences.
      (a) Use church, work, or community settings to promote exercise.
      (b) Use cultural beliefs and values when developing strategies.
   (6) Tailor exercise plans to meet individual needs.
   (7) Provide exercise prescription with written-out instructions on intensity, duration, and frequency.
   (8) Encourage fitness testing and provide a fitness baseline and a motivating goal.
   (9) Prevent relapse by teaching patients to recognize situations that place them at risk for preventing exercise and using behavioral or cognitive strategies to deter relapsing.

11. Obesity and body fat distribution (Cavill & Ells, 2010; CDC, 2013a, 2013b; Faith & Kral, 2006; Flegal, Carroll, Ogden, & Johnson, 2002; Furie et al., 2011; Goldstein et al., 2006, 2011; Hamdy, 2013; Isozumi, 2004; Lavizzo-Mourey & Levy, 2013; Lopez, Stefan, Schulman, & Byers, 2008; Mathew, Francis, Kayalr, & Cone, 2008; Neter, Stam, Kok, Grobbee, & Geleijnse, 2003; NHLBI Obesity Education Initiative Expert Panel on the Identification, Evaluation, and Treatment of Obesity in Adults, 1998; Suk et al., 2003)
   a. Epidemiology
      (1) In the United States, 35.7% adults are obese.
      (2) Obesity by race: Blacks have the highest obesity rates, followed by Hispanics and then whites
      (3) Estimated annual U.S. medical cost for obesity is $147 billion
   b. Screening tool
      (1) Use BMI (i.e., weight divided by height) to assess weight status.
         (a) Higher BMI equals higher disease risk
         (b) Limitations include
            1) An overestimate of body fat in athletes who have muscular build
            2) An underestimate of body fat in older people who have lost muscle
      (2) Abdominal obesity waist circumference measurements
         (a) Greater than 102 cm (40 inches) in men
         (b) Greater than 88 cm (35 inches) in women
   c. Comorbidities associated with obesity
      (1) Fat distribution—abdominal adiposity correlates with negative metabolic and clinical effects of obesity
      (2) Waist circumference—increased morbidity with larger waist circumference
      (3) Age of obesity onset—higher BMI during childhood is strongly associated with increased risk of disease
      (4) Intra-abdominal pressure—increased intra-abdominal pressure is associated with comorbidities, including thrombophlebitis, lower-limb circulatory stasis, and hypertension
      (5) Increased risk of stroke
         (a) Obesity associated with ischemic stroke risk but not hemorrhagic stroke
         (b) Abdominal fat is a stronger predictor of stroke risk.
         (c) Direct relationship of stroke mortality to BMI above 25; and no relationship below 25
         (d) Currently, there are no clinical trials evaluating the effect of weight reduction on decreasing stroke risk.
      (6) Increased hypertension
         (a) Increased prevalence of hypertension in BMI above 30
         (b) Increased blood pressure equals 12% increased risk for cardiovascular heart disease and 24% for stroke
         (c) Pathophysiology of obesity-associated hypertension
            1) Increased vascular resistance
            2) Increased cardiac output
            3) Increased blood volume
            4) Sodium retention

(7) Dyslipidemia—associated with BMI above 25
  (a) Increased cholesterol
  (b) Increased triglycerides
  (c) Decreased HDL
(8) Diabetes
  (a) Relative risk increases by 25% for each BMI unit over 22
  (b) Twenty-seven percent of new cases attributed to weight gain of 5 kg or more in adults
  (c) Abdominal obesity is a major risk factor for type 2 diabetes.
(9) Coronary artery disease
  (a) Risk of MI and cardiovascular death increases with increasing BMI
  (b) Weight gain of 5–8 kg increases the risk by 25%
(10) CHF
  (a) A common complication of severe obesity
  (b) Duration of obesity increases the risk of CHF
  (c) Obesity alters the cardiac structure
(11) Electrolyte disturbance—hypokalemia is the most common
  (a) Cardiac arrhythmias
    1) Increased risk of sudden cardiac death
    2) Prolonged QTc interval
    3) Affects myocardial repolarization because of increased fatty acid levels
    4) Changes in autonomic system
      a) Decreases parasympathetic tone
      b) Increases heart rate
(12) Obstructive sleep apnea (OSA)
  (a) Underdiagnosed
  (b) The incidence of OSA increases as BMI increases.

d. Influences on obesity
(1) Environment
  (a) Communities designed for automobiles that do not promote walking or biking
  (b) Few parks
  (c) Safety issues that prevent activity
  (d) Abundance of high-calorie foods
(2) Social
  (a) Large portions served
  (b) Fast food industry influence
(3) Behavioral
  (a) Long hours spent watching TV, on the computer, or using other electronics
  (b) Physical inactivity
  (c) Poor diet
  (d) Food intake behaviors
  (e) Physical inactivity
(4) Genetic
  (a) The number of genes known to be associated with obesity has increased dramatically over the past 10 years.
  (b) Obesity is not associated with a single gene but with a complexity of many genes and environmental factors.

(c) Genetic factors may affect 25%–75% of body mass or body fat.
(d) Obesity-promoting genes become active at different stages of the lifespan.
(e) Genes that are linked to obesity are also part of energy intake and expenditure pathways.

e. Treatment
   (1) Comprehensive lifestyle management
      (a) Diet
      (b) Physical activity
      (c) Behavior modification
   (2) Weight reduction programs
      (a) Clinicians involved
         1) Healthcare provider
         2) Dietician
         3) Psychologist
         4) Physical and exercise therapist
      (b) Weight loss tends to be short term, with goal to lose 10% over 12–24 weeks
      (c) Weight regain common
   (3) Pharmacologic therapy
      (a) Drugs that impair dietary intake
      (b) Drugs that impair dietary absorption
      (c) Drugs that increase energy expenditure
      (d) Antidepressants
      (e) Herbal products or nutraceuticals (not FDA approved)
   (4) Bariatric surgery
      (a) Patient selection
         1) BMI greater than 40 kg/m^2
         2) Weight greater than 45 kg above ideal weight
         3) BMI 35–40 with one major comorbidity
      (b) Outcomes are procedure- and surgeon-specific

f. Nursing interventions
   (1) Dietary component teaching
      (a) Reduced-portion, low-calorie diet
      (b) Low-fat diet (e.g., Ornish diet)
      (c) Low-carbohydrate diet (e.g., Atkins, South Beach)
      (d) Midlevel diets (e.g., Zone diet—fat, carbohydrate, and protein eaten in similar proportions)
   (2) Reduce portion sizes.
   (3) Reduce calorie intake.
   (4) Aim for a 600 calorie/day deficit.
   (5) Ensure that diet is balanced and nutritious.
   (6) Decrease calorie-dense and nutrient-deficient foods.
   (7) Involve family members for support.
   (8) Individualize diet changes by taking into account
      (a) Food preferences
      (b) Cultural beliefs
   (9) Increase water intake.
      (a) Drink water before each meal.

(b) Adults who drank 500 mL of water before each meal had a 44% decrease in weight.

(c) Will add to resting energy expenditure

(10) Increase exercise

(a) Aerobic exercise gives the greatest results in obesity.

(b) Perform a minimum of 30–60 minutes of aerobic exercise 5–7 days per week.

(c) Resistance training is important to prevent muscle mass loss.

(d) Mobility will improve with exercise.

(11) Behavioral component

(a) Set goals.

(b) Keep a diary.

(c) Slow eating rate.

(d) Add physical activity.

(e) Ensure support is available.

(f) Develop strategies for relapse prevention.

(g) Develop strategies for dealing with weight gain.

(h) Encourage 7–8 hours of sleep; less than 6 hours and more than 9 hours of sleep have been associated with increased weight.

(i) Offer referrals to assist with weight loss.

1) Dietician

2) Psychologist

3) Exercise or physical therapist

C. Potentially modifiable risk factors

1. Migraine headache (Bushnell, 2001; Chawla, 2013; Dalkara, Nozari, & Moskowitz, 2010; Dowson et al., 2008; Etminan, Takkouche, Isorna, & Samii, 2005; Gibson, 2000; Goldstein et al., 2006, 2011; Kruit et al., 2004; MacClellan et al., 2007)

a. Epidemiology

(1) Seventeen percent of women and 6% of men have migraine headaches

(2) Of people who suffer migraines, 30%–40% have migraines with auras.

(3) Association with stroke is seen in young women.

(4) Approximately 18 million working days are lost each year due to migraines.

(5) No association between migraine and stroke in those older than 60 years.

b. Stroke risk

(1) A University of Maryland study found that odds for ischemic stroke are 1.5 greater for women with migraine plus visual aura.

(2) If smoking and OC use is present, stroke risk is increased seven-fold.

(3) Migraine frequency and duration is associated with stroke risk, but severity is not.

c. Pathophysiology of migraine with aura related to stroke

(1) Reduced blood flow

(2) Decreased blood volume

(3) Cortical spreading depression—short-lasting depolarization that alters brain activity, involving changes in neural and vascular function

(4) Increased platelet activation and platelet-leukocyte aggregation, which increases the risk of emboli formation

(5) Possible relationship between patent foramen ovale (PFO) and migraine due to paradoxical embolism

d. Treatment
  (1) No data that treatment will reduce the risk of first stroke
  (2) Nonpharmacologic treatment options
    (a) Biofeedback
    (b) Relaxation therapy
    (c) Cognitive behavioral therapy
  (3) Abortive therapy
    (a) Uses a stepped-care approach
    (b) Drugs used depend on severity of headache
    (c) Acute treatment is most effective when taken within 15 minutes of pain starting.
  (4) Treatment for nausea and vomiting
  (5) Preventive therapy
    (a) Antiepileptic drugs
    (b) Antidepressants
    (c) Antihypertensive drugs
  (6) Alternative therapy
    (a) Massage
    (b) Yoga
    (c) Acupuncture
    (d) Chiropractic
    (e) Herbal supplements
    (f) Biofeedback

e. Nursing intervention
  (1) Assist the patient in identifying triggers to avoid
    (a) Foods and drink
      1) Alcohol—wine, beer
      2) Caffeine—high use, withdrawal
      3) Chocolate
      4) Aspartame—NutraSweet, Equal
      5) Monosodium glutamate
      6) Fruits—bananas, dried fruit, citrus fruits, avocados
      7) Nuts—peanuts, soy nuts
      8) Tyramine (found in aged foods)—cheese, bacon, lunch meats, smoked or cured meats, pickled foods, heavily yeasted breads (e.g., sourdough)
    (b) Stress
    (c) Fatigue
    (d) Skipped meals
    (e) Lack of sleep
    (f) Vasodilator use
    (g) Fluctuating hormone levels
  (2) Encourage the patient to keep a headache diary describing patterns and associations.
  (3) Provide education about over-the-counter medications.
  (4) Encourage regular exercise, which reduces pain intensity.
  (5) Teach relaxation techniques.
  (6) Offer support.

2. Sleep-disordered breathing (SDB; Goldstein et al., 2006, 2011; Martinez-Garcia et al., 2009; Peppard, Young, Palta, & Skatrud, 2000; Punjabi, 2008; Yaggi & Mohsenin, 2003; Yanti & Neatherlin, 2005)
   a. Epidemiology
      (1) Prevalence ranges 3%–7%
      (2) Underdiagnosed
   b. Risk factors
      (1) Age—increases with age, especially older than 65 years
      (2) Male
      (3) Obesity
      (4) Family history
      (5) Menopause
      (6) Cigarette smoking
      (7) Alcohol use
   c. Stroke relationship
      (1) Snoring is a marker for SDB, which may increase stroke risk by leading to or worsening the following
         (a) Hypertension
         (b) Heart disease
         (c) Cardiac arrhythmias, such as AF
         (d) Reductions in cerebral blood flow
         (e) Impaired endothelial function
         (f) Accelerated atherogenesis
         (g) Hypercoagulability
         (h) Inflammation
         (i) Paradoxical embolism in patients with PFO
      (2) The Sleep Heart Health Study (2000) found a relationship between SDB and hypertension. For each additional apneic event per hour of sleep, the odds of developing hypertension were increased by 1%, and for each 10% decrease in oxygen saturation the odds were increased by 13%. The association of SDB with drug-resistant hypertension is particularly high (Nieto et al., 2000).
   d. Treatment
      (1) Recommended treatments for SDB
         (a) Continuous positive airway pressure (CPAP) ventilation
         (b) Bilevel positive airway pressure
         (c) Automatic control of airway pressure delivery with CPAP devices
         (d) Surgical interventions
         (e) Prosthetic oral devices
      (2) Those with obstructive sleep apnea who were treated with CPAP did not differ with regard to fatal or nonfatal cardiovascular events as compared with healthy participants. Data on stroke was not reported separately.
      (3) Martinez-Garcia (2009) enrolled 223 patients with ischemic stroke, performing sleep studies on 166 with CPAP treatment offered for moderate to severe cases. The study found that long-term CPAP treatment reduced the risk of mortality.
   e. Nursing interventions
      (1) Identify risk factors
         (a) Excessive daytime sleepiness
         (b) Headaches

        (c) Difficulty with work
        (d) Alcohol intake
        (e) Smoking
        (f) Snoring and apnea occurring during sleep
        (g) Changes in personality or mood
    (2) Encourage patient to maintain a sleep diary
        (a) Hours of sleep
        (b) Bedtime rituals
        (c) Frequency of awakenings
        (d) Number of naps
        (e) Daytime sleepiness
    (3) After diagnosis
        (a) Provide education on CPAP devices.
        (b) Advise to avoid alcohol before bedtime and sedating medications to promote airway patency.
        (c) Encourage the avoidance of nasal sprays.
        (d) Encourage weight loss.
        (e) Monitor vital signs and pulse oximeter.
        (f) Evaluate medication list for sedating medications.
        (g) Administer oxygen as necessary.
        (h) Raise the head of the bed.
        (i) Position patient on side.

Intracranial Hemorrhage (ICH; Ariesen, Claus, Rinkel, & Algra, 2003; Cantu, Arauz, Murillo-Bonilla, López, & Barinagarrementeria, 2003; Elzawahry, 2013; Flaherty et al., 2005; Fric-Shamji, Shamji, Cole, & Benoit, 2008; Gill, Zezulka, Shipley, Gill, & Beevers, 1986; Hart, Boop, & Anderson, 1995; Howard et al., 2013; ICH; Juvela, Hillborn, & Palomaki, 1995; Klatsky et al., 2005; Labovits, Halim, Boden-Albala, Hauser, & Sacco, 2005; Magistris, Bazak, & Martin, 2013; Martini et al., 2012; Morgenstern et al., 2010; Nolte, Brass, & Fletterick, 1996; Pisters et al., 2010; Rannikmäe et al., 2014; Standridge, 2004; Torres Duarte, Dong, Young, Abi-Younes, & Myers, 1995)

Evidence supporting risk factors for ICH is not as clear as with ischemic stroke, however, there are a few risk factors that leave no doubt. Ariesen and colleagues (2003) performed a systematic review of 14 case-control and 11 cohort studies on ICH risk factors from 1966 to 2001. Primary risk factors for ICH were age, male sex, hypertension, and high-alcohol intake.

A. Nonmodifiable risk factors
  1. Age
    a. Risk of ICH increases with every 10-year increase in age
    b. Blacks have higher risk of ICH compared with whites at age 45 years, with a greater than five times increased risk of ICH, but only one-third risk at age 85 years.
  2. Sex: ICH is more common in men than women, with three times higher risk of ICH in men.
  3. Race—increased risk of ICH in blacks, Mexicans, and Asians compared with whites.
  4. Genetics—Apolipoprotein E (APOE) is a specific type of very low-density lipoprotein (VLDL) that removes excess cholesterol from the blood and carries it to the liver for processing.
    a. There are three different alleles (versions) of the APOE gene called ε2, ε3, and ε4.

b. ε3 is the most common, occurring in half the population.

c. ε2 and ε4 have been associated with lobar ICH through the promotion of cerebral amyloid angiopathy (CAA).

d. Inherited disorders of the clotting factors, including factors V, VII, X, XI and XIII, can lead to cerebral hemorrhage.

5. CAA

   a. Important cause of spontaneous ICH

      (1) Associated with amyloid-beta AB protein deposits in the brain, which damage blood vessels, causing microhemorrhages

      (2) Deposited in small- or medium-sized vessels

      (3) Often causes lobar ICH

      (4) Rarely seen in people younger than 55 years

   b. Pathogenesis

      (1) AB deposition causes vasculature to become brittle and fragile

      (2) Impairs regulation of cerebral blood flow

      (3) Disrupts blood brain barrier

      (4) Causes inflammation

   c. Use of antiplatelet or anticoagulant therapy

      (1) Increases risk of hemorrhage with anticoagulation therapy

      (2) Must weigh risk/benefit ratio

   d. Prevention

      (1) The Perindopril Protection Against Recurrent Stroke Study (PROGRESS; 2010) trial showed lowering blood pressure protected against CAA-related ICH, regardless of the presence of hypertension (Arima et al., 2010).

      (2) Statin should be avoided in the setting of recent CAA-related ICH

      (3) A phase 2 study showed tramiprosate might delay or inhibit the progression of CAA. Tramiprosate is an ionic compound that binds soluble AB and interferes with the amyloid cascade.

B. Modifiable risk factors

1. Hypertension—the most important modifiable risk factor for ICH

   a. Contributing factors

      (1) Damages the tunica media of arteries in the brain

      (2) Weakens the walls leading to rupture

      (3) Causes ICH in cerebral hemispheres: thalamus, putamen, and deep white matter. Also common in pons and cerebellum

   b. Treatment options

      (1) Follow JNC 7 guidelines for hypertension treatment

      (2) In the PROGRESS trial, the ICH risk was reduced from 2% to 1% over 3.9 years of follow-up.

      (3) Prevention of recurrent ICH—target blood pressure is lower than 140/90 or 130/80 in diabetic or chronic kidney disease

2. High alcohol intake

   a. Pathophysiology that might contribute to ICH

      (1) Increased blood pressure

      (2) Impaired hemostasis

      (3) Decreased circulating clotting factor produced by the liver

      (4) Excessive fibrinolysis

b. Arieson and colleagues (2003) found an odds ratio of 3.36 of having an ICH with high alcohol intake

c. The AHA guidelines recommend that avoidance of heavy alcohol use can be beneficial (Class IIa, Level of Evidence B).

3. Oral anticoagulation (OAC) treatment

a. Epidemiology

(1) Approximately 10% of ICHs due to anticoagulant use

(2) More common in elderly due to increased OAC use

(3) Mortality doubles for OAC-associated ICH

b. Risk factors associated with OAC

(1) Hypertension

(2) Advanced age

(3) History of prior stroke

(4) No absolute safe INR—Seven- to ten-fold increased risk in the conventional therapeutic range of 2.5–4.5

(5) More likely to require surgical intervention.

(a) In a retrospective chart review by Fric-Shamji, Shamji, Cole, and Benoit (2008) of 315 patients with spontaneous ICH, 65 patients received OAC therapy and 25% of patients required surgical intervention compared to 14% of the non-OAC patients

c. Prevention strategies

(1) Screen patients for increased risk of ICH associated with OAC prior to starting anticoagulation using a validated assessment tool.

(a) HAS-BLED assessment tool, which has a better predictive value than other scores

(2) Consider risk of CAA.

(3) Review imaging for leukoaraiosis, which indicates small vessel disease and is associated with increased risk of bleeding.

(4) Evaluate carefully the risk versus benefits of anticoagulation after ICH.

(a) The effects of antiplatelet therapy on ICH recurrence and severity are smaller than the effects for anticoagulation and may be an alternative

(b) Use of direct factor Xa inhibitors or direct thrombin inhibitors have lower hemorrhage rates compared with warfarin

(5) The AHA guidelines recommend avoiding long-term anticoagulation as treatment for nonvalvular AF after spontaneous lobar ICH because of the relatively high risk or recurrence (Class IIa, Level of Evidence B).

(6) According to the AHA guidelines, anticoagulation following nonlobar ICH and antiplatelet therapy following any type of ICH may be considered, particularly when there are indications for these agents (Class IIb, Level of Evidence B)

4. Use of sympathomimetic drugs

a. Physiological effects

(1) Increased heart rate

(2) Blood vessel contraction

(3) Reduce digestive secretions

b. Nonprescription over-the-counter drugs (contain ingredients such as ephedrine or phenylpropanolamine)

(1) Cold remedies

(2) Weight loss drugs

(3) Illegal substances
    (a) Cocaine
    (b) Amphetamines
    (c) Methamphetamine
    (d) Ecstasy
(4) An autopsy study examined all fatal nontraumatic ICH from 1989–1990
    (a) Cocaine is a significant risk factor for fatal ICH.

5. Hemorrhagic transformation of ischemic stroke
   a. Pathophysiology is not fully understood, but is believed to be associated with the following
      (1) Vascular injury
      (2) Reperfusion
      (3) Disruption of the blood-brain barrier
      (4) Altered permeability
   b. Attributed to thrombolysis if occurs within 24–36 hours post treatment
   c. Risk is approximately 5.9% compared with 1.1% in controls
   d. Risk factors
      (1) Increased age
      (2) Stroke severity
      (3) Hypertension
      (4) Hyperglycemia
      (5) Early computed tomography changes
      (6) Large baseline diffusion lesion volume on magnetic resonance imaging
   e. Prevention strategies
      (1) Carefully screen patients while reviewing all clinical data
      (2) Strictly follow tissue plasminogen activator guidelines
      (3) Blood pressure control
6. Reperfusion syndrome
   a. Rare complication following revascularization
   b. Defined as an increase in ipsilateral cerebral blood flow above brain tissue needs
   c. Can occur with the following
      (1) Thrombolytic therapy
      (2) Complication of CEA
      (3) Complication of intracranial stenting
   d. Risk factors of reperfusion syndrome
      (1) Postoperative hypertension
      (2) High-grade stenosis with poor collateral flow
      (3) Recent contralateral CEA (<3 months)
      (4) Intraoperative distal carotid pressure less than 40 mmHg
   e. Prevention strategies
      (1) Use of transcranial doppler to measure cerebral blood flow
          (a) Used to predict patients at risk
          (b) Early identification of hypertension and treatment
          (c) Used to select patients for aggressive postprocedure observation
      (2) Use agents that do not cause excessive vasodilatation
          (a) Labetalol
          (b) Nicardipine

(c) ACE inhibitors, calcium channel blockers, and vasodilators such as nitroprusside are less favored

(3) No specific parameters or guidelines established for hyperperfusion-related hypertension

(4) Use American Stroke Association and ICH guideline recommendation of mean arterial pressure of less than 110 mmHg

7. Smoking—Unlike ischemic stroke, current smoking behavior is a weak risk factor for ICH. The data is inconsistent.
8. Diabetes—Unlike ischemic stroke, having a diagnosis of diabetes is a weak risk factor
   a. OC use
      (1) OC use combined with smoking increases risk of hemorrhagic stroke by 3.7 times
10. Hypercholesterolemia—possible protective association
   a. Low cholesterol is theorized to contribute to fragile vasculature
   b. The Multiple Risk Factor Intervention Trial (MRFIT) found the risk of death from hemorrhagic stroke showed a three-fold increase in men with total cholesterol of 160 mg/dL compared with higher levels.
   c. The Rotterdam Scan Study—patients with the highest level of triglycerides had the lowest rate of deep and infratentorial bleeds
   d. SPARCL trial found an increased risk of recurrent ICH among patients with prior stroke randomized to high-dose atorvastatin. In the atorvastatin group, 2.3% had hemorrhagic strokes compared with 1.4% of the placebo group.
   e. There is insufficient data to recommend restrictions on use of statin agents (Class IIb, Level of Evidence C)

Aneurysmal Subarachnoid Hemorrhage (aSAH; Bederson et al., 2000, 2009; Broderick et al., 2003; Chang et al., 2013; Connolly et al., 2012; Conway & Tamargo, 2001; Feigin et al., 2005; Gaist et al., 2000; Gill, Zezulka, Shipley, Gill, & Beevers, 1986; International Study of Unruptured Intracranial Aneurysms Investigators, 1998; Isaksen, Egge, Waterloo, Romner, & Ingebrigtsen, 2002; Juvela, 2000; Kissela et al., 2002; Qureshi, et al., 2001; Standridge, 2004; Teunissen, Rinkel, Algra, & van Gijn, 1996; Torres Duarte, Dong, Young, Abi-Younes, & Myers, 1995; University of Minnesota, Boynton Health Service, 2013; van Gijn & Rinkel, 2001; Wiebers et al., 2003; You et al., 2010)

Ruptured aneurysm is the cause of subarachnoid hemorrhage (SAH) in 85% of cases and is a significant cause of morbidity and mortality. Incidence in the United States ranges from 9.7–14.5 per 100,000 but may be higher because approximately 12%–15% die prior to hospital admission.

A. Nonmodifiable risk factors
   1. Sex
      a. Women have a 1.6 times higher risk of aSAH.
      b. Posterior-communicating aneurysms are more likely to rupture in men.
   2. Age
      a. Risk increases with age, with the mean incidence at 50 years old
      b. Anterior-circulation aneurysms are more likely to rupture in people younger than 55 years old.
   3. Race: Blacks have a 2.1 times higher risk than whites.
   4. Genetics

a. History of previous aSAH
    (1) Increased risk of aneurysmal rupture is 11 times that of no prior history of SAH
b. Family history of aneurysm
    (1) Five percent to 20% have a family history of aneurysm
    (2) First-degree relatives have a three- to seven-fold increased risk, but second-degree relatives have risk similar to the general population.
    (3) First SAH occurs at an earlier age.
    (4) More likely to have large or multiple aneurysms
c. History of certain genetic diseases, such as autosomal dominant polycystic kidney disease, Ehlers-Danlos syndrome type IV, and neurofibromatosis type 1

B. Modifiable risk factors
1. Cigarette smoking—most important modifiable risk factor
    a. Qureshi (2001) found an odds ratio of 5.2 risk of developing SAH
    b. Risk is doubled in former smokers compared with those who never smoked
    c. Increased risk of developing multiple aneurysms
    d. Increases blood pressure for approximately 3 hours
    e. Smoking associated with increased size of aneurysm due to degradation of blood vessel walls and increased dilatation from increased blood pressure
2. Hypertension
    a. Chronic blood pressure higher than 160/95 mmHg is a risk factor for development of SAH.
    b. May increase risk of developing multiple aneurysms
    c. Untreated hypertension is an independent risk factor for poor outcome following a SAH
3. Heavy alcohol intake
    a. More than 150 g/week was a significant risk. Fourteen grams of pure alcohol equals 0.6 ounces.
    b. Binge drinking may increase risk.
4. Sympathomimetic drug use
    a. Several studies have found high cocaine use in young SAH patients, however, direct association is lacking.
    b. Increases risk of aneurysmal rupture and mortality
    c. There is increased risk of vasospasm with recent cocaine use.
5. BMI—lower BMI (<23)
    a. Possible association
6. Diet
    a. Increased consumption of vegetables is associated with lower aSAH risk
7. Increased caffeine intake
    a. Possible association with more than five cups a day
8. Unruptured cerebral aneurysm
    a. Natural history depends on
        (1) Previous aSAH
        (2) Family history
        (3) Age
        (4) Coexisting medical history
        (5) Aneurysm characteristics
            (a) Size
            (b) Location

(c) Form and structure

b. Screening as prevention strategy

(1) Not recommended in the general population for asymptomatic intracranial aneurysms

(2) Cost of screening versus risk and consequence of aSAH

(3) Two large observational studies showed there may be a cost benefit and improved quality of life to screen patients with family history of aSAH

(4) The Cerebral Aneurysm Re-rupture after Treatment Study

(a) Incomplete aneurysm obliteration increases risk of recurrent SAH with a median occurrence at 3 days but rarely after 1 year

(b) Complete obliteration has a low risk of recurrence for the first 5 years.

(c) Repeated screening in these patient groups may not be cost effective.

Nursing Responsibility and Role in Stroke Prevention (Hanger & Wilkinson, 2001; Ostwald, Davis, Hersch, Kelley, & Godwin, 2008; Rodgers, Bond, & Curless, 2001; Vecchione, 2011)

A. Studies have shown that stroke patients and their caregivers do not feel adequately educated about the disease process and feel less informed about the consequences and what to expect physically and emotionally.

B. A randomized trial ($n = 36$) evaluated the distribution of personalized stroke education booklets.

1. No differences were found in basic stroke knowledge and only 50% of respondents felt the booklet was useful.

C. A larger study ($n = 93$) evaluated a stroke association information packet given at discharge or 1 month after stroke (whichever came sooner) versus conventional education.

1. The packet contained stroke association educational leaflets, information about local services, and contact information.
2. No differences were found in knowledge or satisfaction.

D. A randomized trial evaluating three options: 1-hour educational classes for caregivers starting 3 weeks post-admission ($n = 64$); counseling sessions with a trained counselor during and post-admission plus the educational program ($n = 63$); and conventional education ($n = 61$).

1. The dual program of education and counseling was found to improve stroke knowledge.
2. Counseling was more effective than education alone.

E. Identify components of a stroke educational program

1. Goal of education
   a. Inform
   b. Empower—develop self-management skills
   c. Prevent illness progression through behavior change
   d. Prevent illness complications
2. Education process
   a. Timing—educational needs change over time
      (1) Acute phase
      (2) Rehab phase
      (3) Discharge phase
      (4) Community phase

b. Key components to an evolving educational process
   (1) Active interaction
      (a) Repeat the material
      (b) Provide opportunities to apply and practice the information
      (c) Problem-solving information, such as lifestyle changes
      (d) Provide feedback on patients learning
   (2) Relevant material—sources of information dependent on the patient's learning needs and style
      (a) Written
      (b) Lecture
      (c) Multimedia
      (d) Group sessions
      (e) Peer support
   (3) Personalized information
   (4) Counseling—discuss new information and coping strategies to adjust to diagnosis.

c. Measuring understanding and retention
   (1) Recall
   (2) Reinforcement
   (3) Functional outcome assessment of information provided
      (a) Did the information improve participation in activities of daily living?
      (b) Did the information improve quality of life?
      (c) Did the information decrease anxiety?

d. Components of an educational program
   (1) Basic stroke education
      (a) Types of stroke
      (b) Signs or symptoms
      (c) Calling 911
      (d) Risk factors and prevention of stroke
      (e) Medical follow-up
      (f) Treatment options—medications, intervention, rehabilitation
   (2) Stroke recovery
      (a) Fatigue
      (b) Intimacy
      (c) Anger management
      (d) Behavioral issues
      (e) Stress
      (f) Depression
      (g) Grief—functional loss, death, and dying
   (3) Promotion of a healthy lifestyle
      (a) Work
      (b) Social activities
      (c) Physical fitness
      (d) Nutrition
      (e) Sleeping patterns
      (f) Sexual activity

(4) Functional limitations
  (a) Aphasia
  (b) Paralysis
  (c) Bladder/bowel function
  (d) Dysphagia
  (e) Emotional changes
  (f) Pain
  (g) Spasticity
(5) Coping
  (a) Problem-solving activities of daily living
  (b) Safety—home and community
  (c) Use of equipment
  (d) Support system
  (e) Coping strategies
  (f) Relaxation exercises
(6) Community networks
  (a) Financial assistance
  (b) Local agencies
  (c) Support groups
  (d) Respite resources for caregivers
(7) Community education
  (a) FAST (Face, Arms, Speech, Time) program
  (b) Give Me Five
  (c) Stroke screenings

Stroke Prevention Resources

A. National Stroke Association: www.stroke.org
B. American Heart Association and American Stroke Association: www.strokeassociation.org
C. CDC Division for Heart Disease and Stroke Prevention: www.cdc.gov/dhdsp/
D. National Institute of Neurological Disorders and Stroke Brain Basics: Preventing Stroke: www.ninds.nih.gov/disorders/stroke/preventing_stroke.htm

References

The ACTIVE Investigators, Connolly, S. J., Pogue, J., Hart, R. G., Hohnloser, S. H., Pfeffer, M., ... Yusuf, S. (2009). Effect of clopidogrel added to aspirin in patients with atrial fibrillation. *New England Journal of Medicine, 360*(20), 2066–2078.

Albers, G. W., & SPORTIF Investigators. (2004). Stroke prevention in atrial fibrillation: Pooled analysis of SPORTIF III and V trials. *American Journal of Managed Care, 10*(14 Suppl), S462–S473.

Amarenco, P., Bogousslavsky, J., Callahan, A., III, Goldstein, L. B., Hennerici, M., Rudolph, A. E., & The Stroke Prevention by Aggressive Reduction in Cholesterol Levels (SPARCL) Investigators. (2006). High-dose atorvastatin after stroke or transient ischemic attack. *New England Journal of Medicine, 355*(6), 549–559.

Amarenco, P., & Labreuche, J. (2009). Lipid management in the prevention of stroke: Review and updated meta-analysis of statins for stroke prevention. *Lancet Neurology, 8*(5), 453–463.

American Diabetes Association. (2013). Standards of medical care in diabetes—2013. *Diabetes Care, 36*(1), S11–S66.

American Heart Association. (2010). High blood pressure statistics. Retrieved from www.americanheart.org/presenter.jhtml?identifier=4621.

American Heart Association. (2012). Statistical Fact Sheet 2012 Update. Retrieved from www.heart.org/idc/groups/heart-public/@wcm/.../ucm_319587.pdf

American Heart Association Nutrition Committee, Lichtenstein, A. H., Appel, L. J., Brands, M., Carnethon, M., Daniels, S., ... Wylie-Rosett, J. (2006). Diet and lifestyle recommendations revision 2006: A scientific statement from the American Heart Association Nutrition Committee. *Circulation*, 114(1): 82–96.

Appel, L. J., Moore, T. J., Obarzanek, E., Vollmer, W. M., Svetkey, L. P., Sacks, F. M., ... Karanja, N. (1997). A clinical trial of the effects of dietary patterns on blood pressure. DASH Collaborative Research Group. *New England Journal of Medicine, 336*, 1117–1124.

Ariesen, M. J., Claus, S. P., Rinkel, G. J. E., & Algra, A. (2003). Risk factors for intracerebral hemorrhage in the general population: A systematic review. *Stroke, 34*, 2060–2065.

Arima, H., Tzourio, C., Anderson, C., Woodward, M., Bousser, M. G., MacMahon, S., ... PROGRESS Collaborative Group. (2010). Effects of perindopril-based lowering of blood pressure on intracerebral hemorrhage related to amyloid angiopathy: The PROGRESS trial. *Stroke, 41*(2): 394–396.

Artinian, N., Fletcher, G. F., Mozaffarian, D., Kris-Etherton, P., Van Horn, L., Lichtenstein, A. H., ... American Heart Association Prevention Committee of the Council on Cardiovascular Nursing. (2010). Interventions to promote physical activity and dieting lifestyle changes for cardiovascular risk factor reduction in adults: A Scientific Statement from the American Heart Association. *Circulation, 122*, 406–441.

Bederson, J. B., Awad, I. A., Wiebers, D. O., Piepgras, D., Haley, E. C., Jr., Brott, T., ... Caroselli, C. (2000). Recommendations for the management of patients with unruptured intracranial aneurysms: A statement for healthcare professionals from the Stroke Council of the American Heart Association. *Circulation, 102*, 2300–2308.

Bederson, J. B., Connolly, E. S., Jr., Batjer, H. H., Dacey, R. G., Dion, J. E., Diringer, M. N., ... American Heart Association. (2009). Guidelines for the management of aneurysmal subarachnoid hemorrhage: A statement for healthcare professionals from a special writing group of the Stroke Council, American Heart Association. *Stroke, 40*, 994–1025.

Bhatt, D. L. (2010). Carotid revascularization endarterectomy vs stenting trial (CREST). Retrieved from www.cardiosource.com/clinicaltrials/trial.asp?trialID=1907

Blair, S. N., Kampert, J. B., Kohl, H. W., III, Barlow, C. E., Macera, C. A., Paffenbarger, R. S., Jr., & Gibbons, L. W. (1996). Influences of cardiorespiratory fitness and other precursors on cardiovascular disease and all-cause mortality in men and women. *JAMA, 276*, 205–210.

Bogousslavsky, J., Despland, P. A., & Regli, F. (1986). Asymptomatic tight stenosis of the internal carotid artery: Long-term prognosis. *Neurology, 36*, 861–863.

Broderick, J. P., Viscoli, C. M., Brott, T., Kernan, W. N., Brass, L. M., Feldmann, E., ... Hemorrhagic Stroke Project Investigators. (2003). Major risk factors for aneurysmal subarachnoid hemorrhage in young are modifiable. *Stroke, 34*, 1375–1381.

Bushnell, C. D. (2001). Migraine and risk of ischemic stroke: An evidence-based medicine review. *Journal of Clinical Outcomes Management, 8*, 33–39.

Camm, A. J., Lip, G. Y., De Caterina, R., Savelieva, I., Atar, D., Hohnloser, S. H., ... ESC Committee for Practice Guidelines (CPG). (2012). 2012 focused update of the ESC Guidelines for the management of atrial fibrillation: An update of the 2010 ESC Guidelines for the management of atrial fibrillation. Developed with the special contribution of the European Heart Rhythm Association. *European Heart Journal, 33*, 2719–2747.

Cantu, C., Arauz, A., Murillo-Bonilla, L. M., López, M., & Barinagarrementeria, F. (2003). Stroke associated with sympathomimetics contained in over-the-counter cough and cold drugs. *Stroke, 34*, 1667–1672.

Cavill, N., & Ells, L. (2010). Treating adult obesity through lifestyle change interventions. A briefing paper for commissioners. Oxford, UK: National Obesity Observatory.

Centers for Disease Control and Prevention. (2012). America's cholesterol burden. Retrieved from www.cdc.gov/cholesterol/facts.htm

Centers for Disease Control and Prevention. (2013a). Adult obesity facts. Retrieved from www.cdc.gov/obesity/data/adult.html

Centers for Disease Control and Prevention. (2013b). U.S. obesity trends. Retrieved from www.cdc.gov/obesity/data/trends.html

Centers for Disease Control and Prevention. (2014a). Smoking prevalence. Retrieved from www.cdc.gov/nchs/fastats/smoking.htm143

Centers for Disease Control and Prevention. (2014b). Facts about physical activity. Retrieved from www.cdc.gov/physicalactivity/data/facts.html

Chan, W. S., Ray, J., Wai, E. K., Ginsburg, S., Hannah, M. E., Corey, P. N., & Ginsberg, J. S. (2004). Risk of stroke in women exposed to low-dose oral contraceptives: A critical evaluation of the evidence. *Archives of Internal Medicine, 164*, 741–747.

Chang, T. R., Kowalski, R. G., Caserta, F., Carhuapoma, J. R., Tamargo, R. J., & Naval, N. S. (2013). Impact of acute cocaine use on aneurysmal subarachnoid hemorrhage. *Stroke, 44*(7), 1825–1829.

Chawla, J. (2013). Migraine headache. *Medscape*. Retrieved from http://emedicine.medscape.com/article/1142556-overview

Chobanian, A. V., Bakris, G. L., Black, H. R., Cushman, W. C., Green, L. A., Izzo, J. L., Jr., … National High Blood Pressure Education Program Coordinating Committee. (2003). The Seventh Report of the Joint National Committee on Prevention, Detection, Evaluation, and Treatment of High Blood Pressure: the JNC 7 Report. *JAMA, 289*, 2560–2572.

Colhoun, H. M., Betteridge, D. J., Durrington, P. N., Hitman, G. A., Neil, H. A., Livingstone, S. J., … CARDS investigators. (2004). Primary prevention of cardiovascular disease with atorvastatin in type-2 diabetes in the Collaborative Atorvastatin Diabetes Study (CARDS): Multicentre randomised placebo-controlled trial. *Lancet, 364*, 685–696.

Collins, R., Armitage, J., Parish, S., Sleigh, P., Peto, R., & Heart Protection Study Collaborative Group. (2003). MRC/BHF Heart Protection Study of cholesterol lowering with simvastatin in 5963 people with diabetes: A randomised placebo-controlled trial. *Lancet, 361*, 2005–2016.

Collins, R., Armitage, J., Parish, S., Sleight, P., Peto, R., & Heart Protection Study Collaborative Group. (2004). Effects of cholesterol-lowering with simvastatin on stroke and other major vascular events in 20,536 people with cerebrovascular disease or other high-risk conditions. *Lancet, 363*, 757–767.

Connolly, S. J., Ezekowitz, M. D., Yusuf, S., Eikelboom, J., Oldgren, J., Parekh, A., … RE-LY Steering Committee and Investigators. (2009). Dabigatran versus warfarin in patients with atrial fibrillation. *New England Journal of Medicine, 361*(12), 1139–1151.

Connolly, E. S., Rabinstein, A. A., Carhuapoma, J. R., Derdeyn, C. P., Dion, J., Higashida, R. T., … Council on Clinical Cardiology. (2012). Guidelines for the management of aneurysmal subarachnoid hemorrhage: A statement for healthcare professionals from a special writing group of the Stroke Council, American Heart Association. *Stroke, 43*, 1711–1737.

Conway, J. E., & Tamargo, R. J. (2001). Cocaine use is an independent risk factor for cerebral vasospasm after aneurysmal subarachnoid hemorrhage. *Stroke, 32*(10), 2338–2343.

Dalkara, T., Nozari, A., & Moskowitz, M. A. (2010). Migraine aura pathophysiology: The role of blood vessels and microembolisation. *Lancet Neurology, 9*(3): 309–317.

Delude, C. (2010). Reducing cardiovascular risk in diabetics. *L.A. Times*. Retrieved February 22, 2010 from http://articles.latimes.com/2010/feb/22/health/la-he-0222-glucose-control-20100222.

Ding, E. L., & Mozaffarian, D. (2006). Optimal dietary habits for the prevention of stroke. *Seminars in Neurology, 26*(1), 11–23.

Dowson, A., Mullen, M. J., Peatfield, R., Muir, K., Khan, A. A., Wells, C., ... Rickards, A. (2008). Migraine Intervention With STARFlex Technology (MIST) Trial: A prospective, multicenter, double-blind, sham-controlled trial to evaluate the effectiveness of patent foramen ovale closure with STARFlex septal repair implant to resolve refractory migraine headache. *Circulation, 117*, 1397–1404.

Elzawahry, H. (2013). Reperfusion injury in stroke. *Medscape*. Retrieved July 18, 2013 from http://emedicine.medscape.com/article/1162437-overview#a1.

Etminan, M., Takkouche, B., Isorna, F. C., & Samii, A. (2005). Risk of ischaemic stroke in people with migraine: Systematic review and meta-analysis of observational studies. *BMJ, 330*, 63–67.

Executive Committee for the Asymptomatic Carotid Atherosclerosis Study. (1995). Endarterectomy for asymptomatic carotid artery stenosis. *JAMA, 273*, 1421–1428.

Expert Panel on Detection, Evaluation, and Treatment of High Blood Cholesterol in Adults. (2001). Executive Summary of the Third Report of the National Cholesterol Education Program (NCEP) Expert Panel on Detection, Evaluation, and Treatment of High Blood Cholesterol in Adults (Adult Treatment Panel III). *JAMA, 285*, 2486–2497.

Fagerström, K. (2002). The epidemiology of smoking: Health consequences and benefits of cessation. *Drugs, 62*(Suppl 2), 1–9.

Faith, M. S., & Kral, T. V. E. (2006). Social environmental and genetic influences on obesity and obesity-promoting behaviors: Fostering research integration. In L. M. Hernandez, D. G. Blazer, & Institute of Medicine (US) Committee on Assessing Interactions Among Social, Behavioral, and Genetic Factors in Health (Eds.), *Genes, behavior, and the social environment: Moving beyond the nature/nurture debate*. Washington, DC: National Academies Press.

Feigin, V. L., Rinkel, G. J., Lawes ,C. M., Algra, A., Bennett, D. A., van Gijn, J., & Anderson, C. S. (2005). Risk factors for subarachnoid hemorrhage: An updated systematic review of epidemiological studies. *Stroke, 36*, 2773–2780.

Flaherty, M. L., Woo, D., Haverbusch, M., Sekar, P., Khoury, J., Sauerbeck, L., ... Broderick, J. P. (2005). Racial variations in location and risk of intracerebral hemorrhage. *Stroke., 36*, 934–937.

Flegal, K. M., Carroll, M. D., Ogden, C. L., & Johnson, C.L. (2002). Prevalence and trends in obesity among US adults, 1999–2000. *JAMA, 288*, 1723–1727.

Fric-Shamji, E. C, Shamji, M. F., Cole, J., & Benoit, B. G. (2008). Modifiable risk factors for intracerebral hemorrhage. *Canadian Family Physician, 54*, 1138–1139.

Furie, K. L., Kasner, S. E., Adams, R. J., Albers, G. W., Bush, R. L., Fagan, S. C., ... Interdisciplinary Council on Quality of Care and Outcomes Research. (2011). Guidelines for the prevention of stroke in patients with stroke or transient ischemic attack: A guideline for healthcare professionals from the American Heart Association/American Stroke Association. *Stroke, 42*, 227–276.

Fuster, V., Rydén, L. E., Asinger, R. W., Cannom, D. S., Crijns, H. J., Frye, R. L., ... North American Society of Pacing and Electrophysiology. (2001). ACC/AHA/ESC Guidelines for the Management of Patients with Atrial Fibrillation: Executive Summary A Report of the American College of Cardiology/American Heart Association Task Force on Practice Guidelines and the European Society of Cardiology Committee for Practice Guidelines and Policy Conferences (Committee to Develop for the Management of Patients With Atrial Fibrillation). *Circulation, 104*, 2118–2150.

Gaede, P., Vedel, P., Larsen, N., Jensen, G. V., Parving, H. H., & Pedersen, O. (2003). Multifactorial intervention and cardiovascular disease in patients with type 2 diabetes. *New England Journal of Medicine, 348*, 383–393.

Gage, B. F., van Walraven, C., Pearce, L., Hart, R. G., Koudstaal, P. J., Boode, B. S., & Petersen, P. (2004). Selecting patients with atrial fibrillation for anticoagulation: stroke risk stratification in patients taking aspirin. *Circulation, 110*(16), 2287–2292.

Gaist, D., Vaeth, M., Tsiropoulos, I., Christensen, K., Corder, E., Olsen, J., & Sørensen, H. T. (2000). Risk of subarachnoid haemorrhage in first degree relatives of patients with subarachnoid haemorrhage: Follow up study based on national registries in Denmark. *BMJ, 320*, 141–145.

Gibson, F. (2000). The nurse's role in the management of migraine. *Nursing Times.Net, 96*(44), 37.

Gill, J. S., Zezulka, A. V., Shipley, M. J., Gill, S. K., & Beevers, D. G. (1986). Stroke and alcohol consumption. *New England Journal of Medicine, 315*, 1041–1046.

Gillum, L. A., Mamidipudi, S. K., & Johnston, S. C. (2000). Ischemic stroke risk with oral contraceptives: A meta-analysis. *JAMA, 284*(1), 72–78.

Go, A. S., Hylek, E. M., Phillips, K. A., Chang, Y., Henault, L. E., Selby, J. V., & Singer, D. E. (2001). Prevalence of diagnosed atrial fibrillation in adults: national implications for rhythm management and stroke prevention: The AnTicoagulation and Risk Factors in Atrial Fibrillation (ATRIA) Study. *JAMA, 285*(18), 2370 –2375.

Goldberg, R.B., Mellies, M. J., Sacks, F. M., Moyé, L. A., Howard, B. V., Howard, W. J., ... Braunwald, E. (1998). Cardiovascular events and their reduction with pravastatin in diabetic and glucose intolerant: Myocardial infarction survivors with average cholesterol levels: Subgroup analyses in the cholesterol and recurrent events (CARE) trial. *Circulation, 98*(23), 2513–2519.

Goldstein, L. B., Adams, R., Alberts, M. J., Appel, L. J., Brass, L. M., Bushnell, C. D., ... American Academy of Neurology. (2006). Primary prevention of ischemic stroke: A guideline from the American Heart Association/American Stroke Association Stroke Council: Cosponsored by the Atherosclerotic Peripheral Vascular Disease Interdisciplinary Working Group; Cardiovascular Nursing Council; Clinical Cardiology Council; Nutrition, Physical Activity, and Metabolism Council; and the Quality of Care and Outcomes Research Interdisciplinary Working Group: The American Academy of Neurology affirms the value of this guideline. *Stroke, 37,* 1583–1633.

Goldstein, L. B., Bushnell, C. D., Adams, R. .J, Appel, L. J., Braun, L. T., Chaturvedi, S., ... Council on Peripheral Vascular Disease, and Interdisciplinary Council on Quality of Care and Outcomes Research. (2011). Guidelines for the primary prevention of stroke: A guideline for healthcare professionals from the American Heart Association. *Stroke, 42,* 517–584.

Goldstein, L. B., Moore, W. S., Robertson, J. T., & Chaturvedi, S. (1997). Complication rates for carotid endarterectomy. A call to action. *Stroke, 28,* 889–890.

Halliday, A., Mansfield, A., Marro, J., Peto, C., Peto, R., Potter, J., ... Asymptomatic Carotid Surgery Trial (ACST) Collaborative Group. (2004). Prevention of disabling and fatal strokes by successful carotid endarterectomy in patients without recent neurological symptoms: Randomised controlled trial. *Lancet, 363,* 1491–1502. [published correction appears in *Lancet.* 2004;364, 16].

Hamdy, O. (2013). Obesity. *Medscape.* Retrieved August 26, 2013 from http://emedicine.medscape.com/article/123702-overview.

Hanger, H. C., & Wilkinson, T. J. (2001). Stroke education: Can we rise to the challenge? *Age and Ageing, 30,* 113–114.

Hart, R., Boop, B., & Anderson, D. (1995). Oral anticoagulants and intracerebral hemorrhage. *Stroke, 26,* 1471–1477.

He, K., Song, Y., Daviglus, M. L., Liu, K., Van Horn, L., Dyer, A. R., ... Greenland, P. (2004). Fish consumption and incidence of stroke: A meta-analysis of cohort studies. *Stroke, 35,* 1538–1542.

Healey, J. S., Hart, R. G., Pogue, J., Pfeffer, M. A., Hohnloser, S. H., De Caterina, R., ... Connolly S. J. (2008). Risks and benefits of oral anticoagulation compared with clopidogrel plus aspirin in patients with atrial fibrillation according to stroke risk: The atrial fibrillation clopidogrel trial with irbesartan for prevention of vascular events (ACTIVE-W). *Stroke,39*(5), 1406–1408.

Heart Outcomes Prevention Evaluation Study Investigators. (2000). Effects of ramipril on cardiovascular and microvascular outcomes in people with diabetes mellitus: Results of the HOPE Study and MICRO-HOPE Substudy. *Lancet, 355,* 253–259.

Heart Protection Study Collaborative Group. (2002). MRC/BHF Heart Protection Study of cholesterol lowering with simvastatin in 20 536 high-risk individuals: A randomised placebo-controlled trial. *Lancet, 360,* 7–22.

Hobson, R. W., II, Weiss, D. G., Fields, W. S., Goldstone, J., Moore, W. S., Towne, J. B., & Wright, C. B. (1993). Efficacy of carotid endarterectomy for asymptomatic carotid stenosis. The Veterans Affairs Cooperative Study Group. *New England Journal of Medicine,* 328, 221–227.

Horenstein, R. B., Smith, D. E., & Mosca, L. (2002). Cholesterol predicts stroke mortality in the Women's Pooling Project. *Stroke, 33*(7), 1863–1868.

Howard, G., Cushman, M., Howard, V. J., Kissela, B. M., Kleindorfer, D. O., Moy, C. S., ... Woo, D. (2013). Risk factors for intracerebral hemorrhage: The REasons for Geographic and Racial Differences in Stroke (REGARDS) study. *Stroke, 44,* 1282–1287.

Howard, G., Wagenknecht, L. E., Burke, G. L., Diez-Roux, A., Evans, G. W., McGovern, P., ... Tell, G. S. (1998). Cigarette smoking and progression of atherosclerosis: The Atherosclerosis Risk in Communities (ARIC) Study. *JAMA, 279,* 119–124.

Hu, F. B., Stampfer, M. J., Haffner, S. M., Solomon, C. G., Willett, W. C., & Manson, J. E. (2002). Elevated risk of cardiovascular disease prior to clinical diagnosis of type 2 diabetes. *Diabetes Care, 25*(7), 1129–1134.

Hulley, S., Grady, D., Bush, T., Furberg, C., Herrington, D., Riggs, B., & Vittinghoff, E. (1998). Randomized trial of estrogen plus progestin for secondary prevention of coronary heart disease in postmenopausal women. Heart and Estrogen/progestin Replacement Study (HERS) Research Group. *JAMA, 280*, 605– 613.

Implementation of treatment protocols in the Diabetes Control and Complications Trial. (1995). *Diabetes Care, 18*, 361–376.

International Study of Unruptured Intracranial Aneurysms Investigators. (1998). Unruptured intracranial aneurysms—Risk of rupture and risks of surgical intervention. *New England Journal of Medicine, 339*(24), 1725–1733.

Isaksen, J., Egge, A., Waterloo, K., Romner, B., & Ingebrigtsen, T. (2002). Risk factors for aneurysmal subarachnoid haemorrhage: The Tromsø study. *Journal of Neurology, Neurosurgery, and Psychiatry, 73*(2), 185–187.

Isozumi, K. (2004). Obesity as a risk factor for cerebrovascular disease. *Keio Journal of Medicine, 53*, 7–11.

John, J. H., Ziebland, S., Yudkin, P., Roe, L. S., Neil, H. A., & Oxford Fruit and Vegetable Study Group. (2002). Effects of fruit and vegetable consumption on plasma antioxidant concentrations and blood pressure: A randomised controlled trial. *Lancet, 359*, 1969–1974.

Joshipura, K. J., Ascherio, A., Manson, J. E., Stampfer, M. J., Rimm, E. B., Speizer, F. E., ... Willett, W. C. (1999). Fruit and vegetable intake in relation to risk of ischemic stroke. *JAMA, 282*, 1233–1239

Juvela, S. (2000). Risk factors for multiple intracranial aneurysms. *Stroke, 31*, 392–397.

Juvela, S., Hillborn, M., & Palomaki, H. (1995). Risk factors for spontaneous intracerebral hemorrhage. *Stroke, 26*, 1558–1564.

Kernan, W. N., Inzucchi, S. E., Viscoli, C. M., Brass, L. M., Bravata, D. M., & Horwitz, R. I. (2002). Insulin resistance and risk for stroke. *Neurology, 59*, 809–815.

Kissela, B. M., Sauerbeck, L., Woo, D., Khoury, J., Carrozzella, J., Pancioli, A., ... Broderick, J. (2002). Subarachnoid hemorrhage: A preventable disease with a heritable component. *Stroke, 33*(5), 1321–1326.

Klatsky, A. L., Friedman, G. D., Sidney, S., Kipp, H., Kubo, A., & Armstrong, M. A. (2005). Risk of hemorrhagic stroke in Asian American ethnic groups. *Neuroepidemiology, 25*(1), 26–31.

Klein, S., Sheard, N. F., Pi-Sunyer, X., Daly, A., Wylie-Rosett, J., Kulkarni, K., ... American Society for Clinical Nutrition. (2004). Weight management through lifestyle modification for the prevention and management of type 2 diabetes: Rationale and strategies: A statement of the American Diabetes Association, the North American Association for the Study of Obesity, and the American Society for Clinical Nutrition. *Diabetes Care, 27*(8), 2067–2073.

Kokkinos, P. F., Holland, J. C., Pittaras, A. E., Narayan, P., Dotson, C. O., & Papademetriou, V. (1995). Cardiorespiratory fitness and coronary heart disease risk factor association in women. *Journal of the American College of Cardiology, 26*, 358–364.

Kruit, M. C., van Buchem, M. A., Hofman, P. A., Bakkers, J. T., Terwindt, G. M., Ferrari, M. D., & Launer, L. J. (2004). Migraine as a risk factor for subclinical brain lesions. *JAMA, 291*(4), 427–434.

Labovits, D. L., Halim, A., Boden-Albala, B., Hauser, W. A., & Sacco, R. L. (2005). The incidence of deep and lobar intracerebral hemorrhage in white, blacks, and Hispanics. *Neurology, 65*(4), 518–522.

Lakka, T. A., & Salonen, J. T. (1993). Moderate to high intensity conditioning leisure time physical activity and high cardiorespiratory fitness are associated with reduced plasma fibrinogen in eastern Finnish men. *Journal of Clinical Epidemiology, 46*, 1119 –1127.

Lane, D. A., & Lip, G. (2012). Use of the CHA_2DS_2-VASc and HAS-BLED scores to aid decision making for thromboprophylaxis in nonvalvular atrial fibrillation. *Circulation, 126*, 860–865.

LaRosa, J. C., Grundy, S. M., Waters, D. D., Shear, C., Barter, P., Fruchart, J. C., ... Treating to New Targets (TNT) Investigators. (2005). Treating to New Targets (TNT) Investigators. Intensive lipid lowering with atorvastatin in patients with stable coronary disease. *New England Journal of Medicine, 352*, 1425–1435.

Larsson, S. C., & Orsini, N. (2011). Fish consumption and the risk of stroke: A dose response meta-analysis. *Stroke, 42*(12), 3621–3623.

Lavizzo-Mourey, R., & Levi, J. (2013). F as in fat: How obesity threatens America's future 2013. *Robert Wood Johnson Foundation*. Retrieved from www.rwjf.org.

Lichtman, J. H., Krumholz, H. M., Wang, Y., Radford, M. J., & Brass, L. M. (2002). Risk and predictors of stroke after myocardial infarction among the elderly: Results from the Cooperative Cardiovascular Project. *Circulation, 105*, 1082–1087.

Lindholm, L. H., Ibsen, H., Dahlöf, B., Devereux, R. B., Beevers, G., de Faire, U., ... LIFE Study Group. (2002). Cardiovascular morbidity and mortality in patients with diabetes in the Losartan Intervention for Endpoint Reduction in hypertension study (LIFE): A randomised trial against atenolol. *Lancet, 359*(9311), 1004–1010.

Lisabeth, L., & Bushnell, C. (2012). Stroke risk in women: The role of menopause and hormone therapy. *Lancet Neurology, 11*(1), 82–91.

Lopez, P., Stefan, B., Schulman, C. I., & Byers, P. M. (2008). Prevalence of sleep apnea in morbidly obese patients who presented for weight loss surgery evaluation: More Evidence For Routine Screening For Obstructive Sleep Apnea Before Weight Loss Surgery. *The American Surgeon, 74*(9), 834–838.

MacClellan, L. R., Giles, W., Cole, J., Wozniak, M., Stern, B., Mitchell, B. D., & Kittner, S. J. (2007). Probable migraine with visual aura and risk of ischemic stroke: The stroke prevention in young women study. *Stroke, 38*, 2438–2445.

Magistris, F., Bazak, S., & Martin, J. (2013). Intracerebral hemorrhage: Pathophysiology, diagnosis, and management. *McMaster University Medical Journal, 10*(1), 15–22.

Martinez-Garcia, M. A., Soler-Cataluña, J. J., Ejarque-Martínez, L., Soriano, Y., Román-Sánchez, P., Illa, F. B., ... Durán-Cantolla, J. (2009). Continuous positive airway pressure treatment reduces mortality in patients with ischemic stroke and obstructive sleep apnea: A 5-year follow-up study. *American Journal of Respiratory and Critical Care Medicine, 180*, 6–41.

Martini, S., Flaherty, M. L., Brown, W. M., Haverbusch, M., Comeau, M. E., Sauerbeck, L. R., ... Woo, D. (2012). Risk factors for intracerebral hemorrhage differ according to hemorrhage location. *Neurology, 79*, 2275–2282.

Mason, P. K., Lake, D. E., DiMarco, J. P., Ferguson, J. D., Mangrum, J. M., Bilchick, K., ... Moorman, J. R. (2012). Impact of the CHA2DS2-VASc score on anticoagulation recommendations for atrial fibrillation. *The American Journal of Medicine, 125*, 603.e1–603.e6.

Mathew, B., Francis, L., Kayalr, A., & Cone, J. (2008). Obesity: Effects on cardiovascular disease and its diagnosis. *Journal of the American Board of Family Medicine, 21(6)*, 562–568.

Mayo Asymptomatic Carotid Endarterectomy Study Group. (1992). Results of a randomized controlled trial of carotid endarterectomy for asymptomatic carotid stenosis. *Mayo Clinic Proceedings, 67*, 513–518.

Mayo Clinic. (2014). Quit-smoking products: Boost your chance of quitting for good. Retrieved from www.mayoclinic.org/healthy-living/quit-smoking/in-depth/quit-smoking-products/art-20045599?footprints=mine

McGuire, R. (2008). Results of the ONTARGET study comparing ramipril with telmisartan, and its combination in high-risk individuals without heart failure. Retrieved from www.cardiosource.com/rapidnewssummaries/summary.asp?SumID=299.

Morgenstern, L. B., Hemphill, J. C., III, Anderson, C., Becker, K., Broderick, J. P., Connolly, E. S., Jr., ... American Heart Association Stroke Council and Council on Cardiovascular Nursing. (2010). Guidelines for the management of spontaneous intracerebral hemorrhage: a guideline for healthcare professionals from the American Heart Association/American Stroke Association. *Stroke, 41*, 2108–2129.

National Stroke Association. (2013). Stroke prevention. Retrieved from www.stroke.org/site/PageServer?pagename=prevent.

Nederkoorn, P. J., Mali, W. P., Eikelboom, B. C., Elgersma, O. E., Buskens, E., Hunink, M. G., ... van der Graaf, Y. (2002). Preoperative diagnosis of carotid artery stenosis: Accuracy of noninvasive testing. *Stroke, 33*, 2003–2008.

Neter, J. E., Stam, B. E., Kok, F. J., Grobbee, D. E., & Geleijnse, J. M. (2003). Influence of weight reduction on blood pressure: A meta-analysis of randomized controlled trials. *Hypertension, 42*, 878–884.

NHLBI Obesity Education Initiative Expert Panel on the Identification, Evaluation, and Treatment of Obesity in Adults (US). (1998). *Clinical guidelines on the identification, evaluation, and treatment of overweight and obesity in adults: The evidence report.* (NIH Publication No. 98-4083). Bethesda, MD: National Heart, Lung and Blood Institute. Retrieved from www.nhlbi.nih.gov/guidelines/obesity/ob_gdlns.pdf.

Nieto, F. J., Young, T. B., Lind, B. K., Shahar, E., Samet, J. M., Redline, S., ... Pickering, T. G. (2000). Association of sleep-disordered breathing, sleep apnea, and hypertension in a large community-based study. Sleep Heart Health Study. *JAMA, 283*(14), 1829–1836.

Nolte, K. B., Brass, L. M., & Fletterick, C. F. (1996). Intracranial hemorrhage associated with cocaine abuse: A prospective autopsy study. *Neurology, 46*(5), 1291–1296.

Olsson, S. B., & Executive Steering Committee on the SPORTIF III Investigators. (2003). Stroke prevention with the oral direct thrombin inhibitor ximelagatran compared with warfarin in patients with non-valvular atrial fibrillation (SPORTIF III): Randomised controlled trial. *Lancet, 362*, 1691–1698.

Oran, N. T., & Oran, I. (2010). Carotid angioplasty and stenting in carotid artery stenosis: neuroscience nursing implications. *Journal of Neuroscience Nursing, 42*(1), 3–11.

ORIGIN Trial Investigators, Gerstein, H. C., Bosch, J., Dagenais, G. R., Díaz, R., Jung, H., ... Yusuf, S. (2012). Basal insulin and cardiovascular and other outcomes in dysglycemia. *New England Journal of Medicine, 367*, 319–328.

Ostwald, S. K., Davis, S., Hersch, G., Kelley, C., & Godwin, K. M. (2008). Evidence-based educational guidelines for stroke survivors after discharge home. *Journal of Neuroscience Nursing, 40*(3), 173–191.

Pate, R. R., Pratt, M., Blair, S. N., Haskell, W. L., Macera, C. A., Bouchard, C., ... King, A. C. (1995). Physical activity and public health. A recommendation from the Centers for Disease Control and Prevention and the American College of Sports Medicine. *JAMA, 273*, 402–407.

Peppard, P. E., Young, T., Palta, M., & Skatrud, J. (2000). Prospective study of the association between sleep-disordered breathing and hypertension. *New England Journal of Medicine, 342*, 1378–1384.

Pisters, R., Lane, D. A., Nieuwlaat, R., de Vos, C. B., Crijns, H. J., & Lip, G. Y. (2010). A novel user-friendly score (HAS-BLED) to assess 1-year risk of major bleeding in atrial fibrillation: The Euro Heart Survey. *Chest, 138*(5), 1093–1100.

Pritz, M. B. (2007). Usefulness of catheter angiography in evaluation of common carotid artery origin occlusion. *Journal of Stroke and Cerebrovascular Disease, 17*(1), 42–46.

Punjabi, N. M. (2008). The epidemiology of adult obstructive sleep apnea. *Proceedings of the American Thoracic Society, 5*(2), 136–143.

Qureshi, A. I., Suri, M. F., Yahia, A. M., Suarez, J. I., Guterman, L. R., Hopkins, L. N., & Tamargo, R. J. (2001). Risk factors for subarachnoid hemorrhage. *Neurosurgery, 49*, 607–613.

Randour, B., Marro, B., Koskas, F., Duyme, M., Sahel, M., Zouaoui, A., & Marsault, C. (2001). Carotid artery stenosis: Prospective comparison of CT, three-dimensional gadolinium-enhanced MR, and conventional angiography. *Radiology, 220*(1), 179–185.

Rannikmäe, K., Kalaria, R. N., Greenberg, S. M., Chui, H. C., Schmitt, F. A., Samarasekera, N., ... Sudlow, C. L. (2014). APOE associations with severe CAA-associated vasculopathic changes: Collaborative meta-analysis. *Journal of Neurology, Neurosurgery, and Psychiatry, 85*(3), 300–305.

Ridker, P. M., Danielson, E., Fonseca, F. A., Genest, J., Gotto, A. M., Jr., Kastelein, J. J., ... JUPITER Study Group. (2008). Rosuvastatin to prevent vascular events in men and women with elevated C-reactive protein. *New England Journal of Medicine, 35*(21), 2159–2207.

Rodgers, H., Bond, S., & Curless, R. (2001). Inadequacies in the provision of information to stroke patients and their families. *Age and Ageing, 30*, 129–133.

Roldán, V., Marín, F., Fernández, H., Manzano-Fernandez, S., Gallego, P., Valdés, M., ... Lip, G. Y. (2013). Predictive value of the HAS-BLED and ATRIA bleeding scores for the risk of serious bleeding in a real-world population with atrial fibrillation receiving anticoagulant therapy. *Chest, 143*(1), 79–84.

Romero, J. R., Morris, J., & Pikula, A. (2008). Stroke prevention: Modifying risk factors. *Therapeutic Advances in Cardiovascular Disease, 2*(4), 287–303.

Rossouw, J. E., Anderson, G. L., Prentice, R. L., LaCroix, A. Z., Kooperberg, C., Stefanick, M. L., ... Writing Group for the Women's Health Initiative Investigators. (2002). Risks and benefits of estrogen plus progestin in healthy postmenopausal women: Principal results from the women's health initiative randomized controlled trial. *JAMA, 288*, 321–333.

Ruppar, T. M., & Conn, V. S. (2010). Interventions to promote physical activity in chronically Ill adults. *American Journal of Nursing, 110*(7), 30–37.

Sacco, R. L., Gan, R., Boden-Albala, B., Lin, I. F., Kargman, D. E., Hauser, W. A., ... Paik, M. C. (1998). Leisure-time physical activity and ischemic stroke risk: The Northern Manhattan Stroke Study. *Stroke, 29*, 380–387.

Sacks, F. M., Svetkey, L. P., Vollmer, W. M., Appel, L. J., Bray, G. A., Harsha, D., ... DASH-Sodium Collaborative Research Group. (2001). Effects on blood pressure of reduced dietary sodium and the Dietary Approaches to Stop Hypertension (DASH) diet. *New England Journal of Medicine, 344*, 3–10.

Sauvaget, C., Nagano, J., Allen, N., & Kodama, K. (2003). Vegetable and fruit intake and stroke mortality in the Hiroshima/Nagasaki Life Span Study. *Stroke, 34*, 2355–2360.

Sever, P. S., Dahlöf, B., Poulter, N. R., Wedel, H., Beevers, G., Caulfield, M., ... ASCOT investigators. (2003). Prevention of coronary and stroke events with atorvastatin in hypertensive patients who have average or lower-than-average cholesterol concentrations, in the Anglo-Scandinavian Cardiac Outcomes Trial–Lipid Lowering Arm (ASCOT-LLA): A multicentre randomised controlled trial. *Lancet, 361*, 1149–1158.

Simon, J. A., Hsia, J., Cauley, J. A., Richards, C., Harris, F., Fong, J., ... Hulley, S. B. (2001). Postmenopausal hormone therapy and risk of stroke: The Heart and Estrogen-Progestin Replacement Study (HERS). *Circulation, 103*, 638–642.

Sowers, J. R. (2003). Recommendations for special populations: Diabetes mellitus and the metabolic syndrome. *American Journal of Hypertension, 16*(11 Pt 2), 41S–45S.

Standridge, J. B., Zylstra, R. G., & Adams, S, M. (2004). Alcohol consumption: An overview of benefits and risks. *Southern Medical Journal, 97*(7), 664–672.

Subhi Ali, Y. (2014). Lipoprotein(a). *Medscape*. Retrieved March 17, 2014 from http://emedicine.medscape.com/article/2088118-overview#showall.

Suk, S. H., Sacco, R. L., Boden-Albala, B., Cheun, J. F., Pittman, J. G., Elkind, M. S., ... Northern Manhattan Stroke Study. (2003). Abdominal obesity and risk of ischemic stroke: The Northern Manhattan Stroke Study. *Stroke, 34*, 1586–1592.

Sztriha, L. K., Sas, K., and Vecsei, L. (2005). Aspirin resistance in stroke: 2004. *Journal of Neurological Science, 229-230*, 163–169.

Teunissen, L. L., Rinkel, G. J., Algra, A., & van Gijn, J. (1996). Risk factors for subarachnoid hemorrhage: A systematic review. *Stroke, 27*, 544–549.

Threapleton, D. E., Greenwood, D. C., Evans, C. E., Cleghorn, C. L., Nykjaer, C., Woodhead, C., ... Burley, V. J. (2013). Dietary fiber intake and risk of first stroke: A systematic review and meta-analysis. *Stroke, 44*(5), 1360–1368.

Torres Duarte, A. P., Dong, Q. S., Young, J., Abi-Younes, S., & Myers, A. K. (1995). Inhibition of platelet aggregation in whole blood by alcohol. *Thrombosis Research, 78*, 107–115.

Tuomilehto, J., & Rastenyte, D. (1999). Diabetes and Glucose Intolerance as Risk Factors for Stroke. *Journal of Cardiovascular Risk, 6*, 241–249.

University of Iowa Hospitals and Clinic. (2006). Options for smoking cessation. Retrieved August 7, 2006 from www.uihealthcare.com/topics/smoking/smokingcessation.html.

University of Minnesota, Boynton Health Service. (2013). Alcohol, tobacco and other drugs. Retrieved April 1, 2013 fromwww.bhs.umn.edu/alcohol-drugs/index.htm.

U.S. Department of Health and Human Services. (2001). *ATP III Guidelines At-A-Glance Quick Desk Reference*. (NIH Publication No. 01-3305). Bethesda, MD: National Institutes of Health/National Heart, Lung, and Blood Institute. Retrieved from www.nhlbi.nih.gov/guidelines/cholesterol/atglance.pdf.

U.S. Department of Health and Human Services. (2004). *The Seventh Report of the Joint National Committee on Prevention, Detection, Evaluation and Treatment of High Blood Pressure*. (NIH Publication No. 04-5230). Bethesda, MD: National Heart, Lung, and Blood Institute. National High Blood Pressure Education Program. http://www.nhlbi.nih.gov/guidelines/hypertension/jnc7full.pdf.

U.S. Department of Health and Human Services. (2006). *Your guide to lowering your blood pressure with DASH*. (NIH Publication No. 06-4082). Bethesda, MD: National Heart, Lung, and Blood Institute. Retrieved from http://www.nhlbi.nih.gov/health/public/heart/hbp/dash/new_dash.pdf.

U.S. Department of Health and Human Services. (2008). *2008 Physical Activity Guidelines for Americans*. Retrieved from www.health.gov/paguidelines/.

van Gijn, J., & Rinkel, G. J. E. (2001). Subarachnoid Haemorrhage: Diagnosis, Causes and Management. *Brain, 124*, 249–278.

van Walraven, C., Hart, R. G., Singer, D. E., Laupacis, A., Connolly, S., Petersen, P., ... Hellemons B. (2002). Oral anticoagulants vs aspirin in nonvalvular atrial fibrillation: an individual patient meta-analysis. *JAMA, 288*(19), 2441–2448.

Vecchione, M. (2011). Primary stroke prevention and community education. *Medicine and Health, Rhode Island, 94*(12), 369–371.

Wiebers, D. O., Whisnant, J. P., Huston, J., III, Meissner, I., Brown, R. D., Jr., Piepgras, D. G., ... International Study of Unruptured Intracranial Aneurysms Investigators. (2003). Unruptured intracranial aneurysms: Natural history, clinical outcome and risks of surgical and endovascular treatment. *Lancet, 362*, 103–110.

Wolff, T., Guirguis-Blake, J., Miller, T., Gillespie, M., & Harris, R. (2007). Screening for asymptomatic carotid artery stenosis. Evidence synthesis No. 50. (AHRQ Publication No. 08-05102-EF-1.) Rockville, MD: Agency for Healthcare Research and Quality, December 2007.

Yaggi, H., & Mohsenin, V. (2003). Sleep-disordered breathing and stroke. *Clinics in Chest Medicine, 24*, 223–237.

Yantis, M. A., & Neatherlin, J. (2005). Obstructive sleep apnea in neurological patients. *Journal of Neuroscience Nursing, 37*(3), 150–155.

You, S. H., Kong, D. S., Kim, J. S., Jeon, P., Kim, K. H., Roh, H. K., ... Hong, S. C. (2010). Characteristic features of unruptured aneurysms: Predictive risk. *Journal of Neurology, Neurosurgery, and Psychiatry, 81*(5), 479–484.

Zhang, X., Patel, A., Horibe, H., Wu, Z., Barzi, F., Rodgers, A., ... Asia Pacific Cohort Studies Collaboration. (2003). Cholesterol, coronary heart disease, and stroke in the Asia Pacific region. *International Journal of Epidemiology, 32*(4), 563–572.

Zhang, Y., Galloway, J. M., Welty, T. K., Wiebers, D. O., Whisnant, J. P., Devereux, R. B., ... Lee, E. T. (2008). Incidence and risk factors for stroke in American Indians: The Strong Heart Study. *Circulation, 118*, 1577–1584.

Zuber, M., Toulon, P., Marnet, L., & Mas, J. L. (1996). Factor V Leiden mutation in cerebral venous thrombosis. *Stroke, 27*, 1721–1723.

Chapter

3

Hyperacute Care

JJ Baumann, MS RN C-CNS

The nurse plays an integral role in the hyperacute phase of stroke care. Through effective communication with prehospital providers, rapid physical and neurological evaluation, facilitation of the stroke work-up, and assistance with expedited treatment, nurses can help prevent further neurological injury. A stroke-savvy nurse understands his or her part in timely delivery of stroke care, and effectively executing the nursing plan of care significantly improves neurological outcomes.

Objectives

1. Understand the importance of rapid identification and intervention of the acute stroke patient.
2. Identify the symptoms of stroke.
3. Describe the initial care of the acute stroke patient.
4. Recognize the implications of the various stroke scales.
5. Discuss administration of thrombolytic and other mechanical interventions used in acute ischemic stroke treatment.
6. Describe interventions for hemorrhagic stroke.
7. Articulate a nursing plan of care for the management of the acute stroke patient.

Initial Stroke Triage and Arrival to the Emergency Department

A. Initial triage
   1. Prehospital personnel and staff at the receiving hospital need to effectively communicate.
      a. When a stroke victim activates emergency medical services (EMS) instead of accessing the emergency department directly, the time to acquisition of brain imaging, evaluation by an emergency physician, and completion of a neurologic evaluation is shorter (Jauch et al., 2013).
      b. Activating EMS should be emphasized in community outreach as the key to improving patient outcomes and preventing disability.
      c. A lack of stroke symptom recognition, a poor understanding of the urgent need for medical care, and any delay in activating EMS lead to delays in the stroke patient arriving at an emergency department.

d. The greatest time delay is from symptom onset to the arrival at the emergency department. This time delay is often the reason acute reperfusion treatment is not immediately instigated (Higashida et al., 2013).

2. Primary goals of EMS assessment and management (Jauch et al., 2010; Summers et al., 2009)
   a. Rapid evaluation
      (1) Obtain the time of symptom onset, or the last time the patient appeared normal.
      (2) Obtain glucose, if possible, and treat per protocol.
   b. Early stabilization
      (1) Support the cardiopulmonary system.
         (a) Obtain vital signs.
         (b) Monitor cardiac function.
      (2) Provide oxygen if needed.
         (a) Keep SaO_2 >94%.
         (b) If pulse oximetry is not available, provide oxygen at a rate of 2–3 L/min.
   c. Neurologic evaluation
      (1) Cincinnati Prehospital Stroke Scale (Kothari, Pancioli, Liu, Brott, & Broderick, 1999)
         (a) Based on physical findings only
         (b) Observe for facial drooping, arm weakness, or speech difficulties.
         (c) Assessment most likely to identify anterior circulation ischemic stroke
      (2) Los Angeles Prehospital Stroke Screen (Kidwell, Starkman, Eckstein, Weems, & Saver, 2000)
         (a) Consists of screening criteria and physical findings
         (b) Screening includes age, baseline status, history of seizure activity, blood glucose, and onset of neurologic symptoms.
         (c) Physical findings include asymmetry of smile or grimace, hand grip strength, and arm strength.
   d. Triage to a stroke-ready hospital
3. EMS should alert the receiving hospital about a stroke patient's impending arrival to the hospital.
   a. Allow for the mobilization of resources for the care of the acute stroke patient (Jauch et al., 2013).
   b. Advance notification by EMS has been shown to increase the use of intravenous tissue plasminogen activator (IV tPA; Abdullah, Smith, Biddinger, Kalenderian, & Schwamm, 2008).
4. EMS personnel should receive continuing stroke education to ensure the proper identification and treatment of stroke patients, including transporting patients to appropriate facilities (Summers et al., 2009).

B. Arrival or presentation to the emergency department
   1. Recognize the need for rapid evaluation and assessment in the emergency department (Jauch et al., 2013). A stroke patient who has had or who is undergoing a large vessel stroke loses an estimated 1.9 million neurons every minute (Saver, 2006).
      a. Notifying the emergency department and stroke team of a suspected stroke en route to the hospital is associated with faster treatment once the patient arrives to the emergency department.

b. Triage is a high priority (equivalent to a serious trauma or acute myocardial infarction; Summers et al., 2009).
  (1) Nurses should recognize stroke symptoms.
  (2) Obtain the last known time the patient was well.
  (3) Use protocols and procedures to mobilize the acute stroke team.
  (4) Recognize that the goal door-to-needle time is 60 minutes.
    (a) This goal should be met in more than 80% of IV tPA cases (Jauch et al., 2013).
    (b) Decreased time to treatment improves stroke patient outcomes at 90 days (Hacke et al., 2004).
    (c) Goal action times (Bock, 1996)
      1) Hospital door to physician: ≤10 minutes
      2) Hospital door to stroke team: ≤15 minutes
      3) Hospital door to computed tomography (CT) initiation: ≤25 minutes
      4) Hospital door to CT interpretation: ≤45 minutes
      5) Hospital door to drug administration: ≤60 minutes

2. Support cardiopulmonary functioning (ABCs)

a. Airway
  (1) Maintaining a proper airway is important to the prevention of hypoxia, common causes of which include
    (a) Partial airway obstruction
    (b) Aspiration
    (c) Decreased consciousness
      1) Hemorrhagic stroke patients have a high rate of early deterioration. Emergent treatment may include intubation (Morgenstern et al., 2010).
    (d) Impaired oropharyngeal mobility or loss of protective reflex, more of a concern with posterior strokes
  (2) Proper positioning is important to maintain the airway and prevent hypoxia.
    (a) Some nonhypoxic ischemic stroke patients who are able to tolerate lying flat may benefit from supine positioning.
    (b) For patients at risk for airway obstruction, aspiration, or elevated intracranial pressure (ICP), positioning the head of the bed at 15°–30° is recommended.
    (c) The patient's neck should be kept straight regardless of positioning to facilitate venous drainage from the brain to systemic circulation. Slumped sitting should be avoided (Jauch et al., 2013; Summers et al., 2009; Wojner-Alexander, Garami, Chernyshev, & Alexandrov, 2005).

b. Breathing
  (1) Supplemental oxygen is not always needed (Summers et al., 2009).
  (2) Supplemental oxygen should be delivered using the least invasive means available to keep SaO_2 >94% (Jauch et al., 2013).

c. Circulation
  (1) Continuous cardiac monitoring is recommended for at least the first 24 hours after a stroke.
    (a) Monitor for consistent or intermittent arrhythmia, which may be a risk factor for or contribute to the stroke or symptoms.
  (2) Ensure the placement and patency of 2–3 IV lines.

(3) Isotonic IV fluid boluses can be administered if the stroke patient is hypovolemic with resulting hypotension and cerebral hypoperfusion. Avoid solutions containing dextrose.

(4) Tests, including a metabolic panel, platelet count, and coagulation studies, should be sent to the laboratory immediately. A finger stick blood glucose test also should be obtained. Obtain a troponin test, although awaiting results should not delay treatment (Jauch et al., 2013; Summers et al., 2009).

3. Differentiate between anterior and posterior circulation signs and symptoms (Lindsay & Bone, 2004; Searls, Pazdera, Korbel, Vysata, & Caplan, 2012; Tocco, 2011). Refer to chapter 1 for additional information regarding localizing stroke syndromes.
   a. Anterior strokes
      (1) Middle cerebral artery (MCA)
         (a) Hemiplegia for the contralateral side
            1) Affects lower face, arm, and hand
            2) Leg often spared
         (b) Contralateral sensory loss
         (c) If left (dominant) side is affected
            1) Expressive aphasia
            2) Receptive aphasia
         (d) If right (nondominant) side is affected
            1) Neglect of the affected side
            2) Neglect or unawareness of deficits
      (2) Anterior cerebral artery
         (a) Contralateral leg weakness and sensory loss
         (b) Behavioral abnormalities may occur.
         (c) Incontinence may occur.
      (3) Internal carotid artery (ICA)
         (a) Contralateral face, arm, leg weakness occur
         (b) Contralateral sensory loss
         (c) Gaze palsy (away from affected side, to the side of the brain lesion)
         (d) If left (dominant) side is affected, complete aphasia occurs.
         (e) If right (nondominant) side is affected, neglect.
         (f) Contralateral visual-field deficit
   b. Posterior strokes
      (1) Ataxia, nausea or vomiting, nystagmus, vertigo, and diplopia are relatively good indicators of posterior, rather than anterior, stroke.
      (2) Vertebral artery
         (a) Ataxia
         (b) Vertigo
         (c) Nausea or vomiting
         (d) Headache
         (e) Nystagmus
         (f) Dysarthria
      (3) Basilar artery
         (a) Quadriplegia or "locked-in" syndrome
         (b) Sensory loss
         (c) Weakness of facial, lingual, and pharyngeal muscles

(d) Dysconjugate gaze
(e) Abnormal respirations
(4) Posterior cerebral artery
(a) Contralateral visual-field deficit
(b) Impaired depth perception
(c) Chorea
(d) Ipsilateral third nerve palsy with contralateral hemiplegia (Weber's syndrome)

c. Specific to hemorrhagic strokes (Greenberg, 2000)
(1) Focal deficits are the same as ischemic deficits and also may include
(a) Headache: In subarachnoid hemorrhage, this is often described as the "worst headache of my life" or a "thunderclap" headache.
(b) Nausea and vomiting
(c) Decreased level of consciousness: Rapid loss of consciousness over minutes to hours usually is indicative of intracranial hemorrhage (Morgenstern et al., 2010).
(d) Light intolerance
(e) Neck pain
1) Nuchal rigidity is more often associated with aneurysmal subarachnoid hemorrhage (aSAH).
2) Meningeal irritation usually appears 4–8 hours after aSAH.

4. Facilitate urgent diagnostics
a. Obtain CT or magnetic resonance imaging tests (Summers et al., 2009).
(1) Explain the test to the patient.
(2) Facilitate his or her safe transport to the scan.
(3) Pre-alert the radiology technician about the acute stroke patient to ensure the scanner is ready upon the patient's arrival.

b. Noncontrast head CT often is preferred (Jauch et al., 2013; Summers et al., 2009).
(1) Quickly determines if there is intracranial hemorrhaging.
(2) Readily available at more institutions
(3) Allows for fast acquisition of images
(4) Size, severity, and duration of time from infarct can be determined using structured scoring systems such as the Alberta Stroke Program Early CT Score (ASPECTS Score; Jauch et al., 2013; Pexman et al., 2001).

c. Noninvasive vessel imaging is recommended if intra-arterial (IA) thrombolysis or mechanical thrombectomy are being considered. Advance imaging should not delay IV fibrinolysis treatment.

d. Perfusion imaging can be obtained if treatment outside the time window for IV fibrinolysis is being considered.

e. Telemedicine or telestroke
(1) Through computer-based technology, remote audio and visual assessment of the stroke patient can be performed. Electronic medical information, clinical assessment tools, neuroradiology, laboratory data, and clinical pathways also can be shared (Hess et al., 2006; Levine & Gorman, 1999).
(2) Patients can be diagnosed, treated locally, and then transferred to a stroke facility. This often is referred to as drip and ship treatment of the patient. Drip and ship has been shown to be a safe means of treating the acute stroke patient (Pervez et al., 2010).

5. Perform baseline assessment
   a. Patient history
      (1) The most important information to obtain in the history is the time of symptom onset. If the onset was not witnessed, the last known time the patient was well, at baseline, or symptom free should be determined. If the patient awoke with symptoms, try to ascertain when the patient went to sleep (Jauch et al., 2013; Summers et al., 2009).
      (2) Additional history can provide information regarding the stroke diagnosis, possible stroke mimics, and the patient's eligibility for acute treatment.
         (a) Risk factors of cardiovascular disease include hypertension, diabetes, smoking, and atrial fibrillation.
         (b) Possible stroke mimics—seizure, migraine, hypoglycemia, and infection (Fernandes, Whiteley, Hart, & Al-Shahi Salman, 2013)
         (c) Data related to eligibility for therapeutic treatment or risk for hemorrhage expansion in intracerebral hemorrhage (ICH) or aSAH
            1) Recent events—stroke, myocardial infarction, trauma, seizures
            2) Medications—anticoagulants, antithrombotics
   b. Physiologic exam
      (1) Vital signs, including blood pressure, heart rate, oxygen saturation, and temperature, should be obtained.
      (2) A thorough, but brief, medical exam should be done to help determine whether the event is a stroke, the possible etiology of the stroke, comorbidities, and other factors that may impact treatment.
   c. Neurologic exam
      (1) The neurological exam should be performed and documented efficiently. Obtaining the necessary information and communicating the results of the exam to other providers is essential (Spilker et al., 1997).
      (2) The National Institutes of Health Stroke Scale (NIHSS) is the preferred assessment tool. The NIHSS is the evidence-based standard for detecting changes, determining severity, and measuring neurologic function over time. Highly standardized, it allows for the communication of deficits across various providers (Brott et al., 1989; Jauch et al., 2013; Summers et al., 2009).
6. Various stroke scores—measure utility and function. Tests include the NIHSS, Hunt and Hess Stroke Scale, Glasgow Coma Scale (GCS), ABCD^2 score, ICH score, and Fisher Grade
   a. NIHSS (**Table 3-1**)
      (1) The scale was designed to standardize the neurologic exam used in acute stroke trials and has high reliability and validity. It assesses 15 components, with total scores ranging between 0 and 42. Higher numbers are associated with poorer neurological outcomes (Brott et al., 1989; Spilker et al., 1997).
      (2) To ensure reliability, formal training on or certification in the NIHSS is recommended (Summers et al., 2009).
   b. ABCD^2 Score (**Table 3-2**; Johnston et al., 2007)
      (1) Used to predict 2-day stroke risk following transient ischemic attack (TIA)
      (2) Scores range from 0 to 7. A score of 0–3 is correlated with a 1% chance of the TIA patient having a stroke in the next 2 days.
      (3) Patients with a higher ABCD^2 score are at high risk and need immediate evaluation to optimize stroke prevention after TIA.
      (4) Score calculated from five criteria

Table 3-1. National Institutes of Health Stroke Scale

Instructions	Scale Definition
1a. Level of Consciousness: The investigator must choose a response if a full evaluation is prevented by such obstacles as an endotracheal tube, language barrier, orotracheal trauma or bandages. A 3 is scored only if the patient makes no movement (other than reflexive posturing) in response to noxious stimulation.	0 = **Alert**; keenly responsive. 1 = **Not alert**; but arousable by minor stimulation to obey, answer, or respond. 2 = **Not alert**; requires repeated stimulation to attend, or is obtunded and requires strong or painful stimulation to make movements (not stereotyped). 3 = Responds only with reflex motor or autonomic effects or totally unresponsive, flaccid, and areflexic.
1b. LOC Questions: The patient is asked the month and his/her age. The answer must be correct - there is no partial credit for being close. Aphasic and stuporous patients who do not comprehend the questions will score 2. Patients unable to speak because of endotracheal intubation, orotracheal trauma, severe dysarthria from any cause, language barrier, or any other problem not secondary to aphasia are given a 1. It is important that only the initial answer be graded and that the examiner not "help" the patient with verbal or non-verbal cues.	0 = **Answers** both questions correctly. 1 = **Answers** one question correctly. 2 = **Answers** neither question correctly.
1c. LOC Commands: The patient is asked to open and close the eyes and then to grip and release the non-paretic hand. Substitute another one step command if the hands cannot be used. Credit is given if an unequivocal attempt is made but not completed due to weakness. If the patient does not respond to command, the task should be demonstrated to him or her (pantomime), and the result scored (e.g., follows none, one or two commands). Patients with trauma, amputation, or other physical impediments should be given suitable one-step commands. Only the first attempt is scored.	0 = **Performs** both tasks correctly. 1 = **Performs** one task correctly. 2 = **Performs** neither task correctly.
2. Best Gaze: Only horizontal eye movements will be tested. Voluntary or reflexive (oculocephalic) eye movements will be scored, but caloric testing is not done. If the patient has a conjugate deviation of the eyes that can be overcome by voluntary or reflexive activity, the score will be 1. If a patient has an isolated peripheral nerve paresis (CN III, IV or VI), score a 1. Gaze is testable in all aphasic patients. Patients with ocular trauma, bandages, pre-existing blindness, or other disorder of visual acuity or fields should be tested with reflexive movements, and a choice made by the investigator. Establishing eye contact and then moving about the patient from side to side will occasionally clarify the presence of a partial gaze palsy.	0 = **Normal**. 1 = **Partial gaze palsy**; gaze is abnormal in one or both eyes, but forced deviation or total gaze paresis is not present. 2 = **Forced deviation**, or total gaze paresis not overcome by the oculocephalic maneuver.

continued

Table 3-1. National Institutes of Health Stroke Scale continued

Instructions	Scale Definition
3. Visual: Visual fields (upper and lower quadrants) are tested by confrontation, using finger counting or visual threat, as appropriate. Patients may be encouraged, but if they look at the side of the moving fingers appropriately, this can be scored as normal. If there is unilateral blindness or enucleation, visual fields in the remaining eye are scored. Score 1 only if a clear-cut asymmetry, including quadrantanopia, is found. If patient is blind from any cause, score 3. Double simultaneous stimulation is performed at this point. If there is extinction, patient receives a 1, and the results are used to respond to item 11.	0 = **No visual loss**. 1 = **Partial hemianopia**. 2 = **Complete hemianopia**. 3 = **Bilateral hemianopia** (blind including cortical blindness).
4. Facial Palsy: Ask—or use pantomime to encourage—the patient to show teeth or raise eyebrows and close eyes. Score symmetry of grimace in response to noxious stimuli in the poorly responsive or non-comprehending patient. If facial trauma/bandages, orotracheal tube, tape or other physical barriers obscure the face, these should be removed to the extent possible.	0 = **Normal** symmetrical movements. 1 = **Minor paralysis** (flattened nasolabial fold, asymmetry on smiling). 2 = **Partial paralysis** (total or near-total paralysis of lower face). 3 = **Complete paralysis** of one or both sides (absence of facial movement in the upper and lower face).
5. Motor Arm: The limb is placed in the appropriate position: extend the arms (palms down) 90 degrees (if sitting) or 45 degrees (if supine). Drift is scored if the arm falls before 10 seconds. The aphasic patient is encouraged using urgency in the voice and pantomime, but not noxious stimulation. Each limb is tested in turn, beginning with the non-paretic arm. Only in the case of amputation or joint fusion at the shoulder, the examiner should record the score as untestable (UN), and clearly write the explanation for this choice.	0 = **No drift**; limb holds 90 (or 45) degrees for full 10 seconds. 1 = **Drift**; limb holds 90 (or 45) degrees, but drifts down before full 10 seconds; does not hit bed or other support. 2 = **Some effort against gravity**; limb cannot get to or maintain (if cued) 90 (or 45) degrees, drifts down to bed, but has some effort against gravity. 3 = **No effort against gravity**; limb falls. 4 = **No movement**. UN = **Amputation** or joint fusion **5a. Left Arm** **5b. Right Arm**
6. Motor Leg: The limb is placed in the appropriate position: hold the leg at 30 degrees (always tested supine). Drift is scored if the leg falls before 5 seconds. The aphasic patient is encouraged using urgency in the voice and pantomime, but not noxious stimulation. Each limb is tested in turn, beginning with the non-paretic leg. Only in the case of amputation or joint fusion at the hip, the examiner should record the score as untestable (UN), and clearly write the explanation for this choice.	0 = **No drift**; leg holds 30-degree position for full 5 seconds. 1 = **Drift**; leg falls by the end of the 5-second period but does not hit bed. 2 = **Some effort against gravity**; leg falls to bed by 5 seconds, but has some effort against gravity. 3 = **No effort against gravity**; leg falls to bed immediately. 4 = **No movement**. UN = **Amputation** or joint fusion **6a. Left Leg** **6b. Right Leg**

continued

Table 3-1. National Institutes of Health Stroke Scale continued

Instructions	Scale Definition
7. Limb Ataxia: This item is aimed at finding evidence of a unilateral cerebellar lesion. Test with eyes open. In case of visual defect, ensure testing is done in intact visual field. The finger-nose-finger and heel-shin tests are performed on both sides, and ataxia is scored only if present out of proportion to weakness. Ataxia is absent in the patient who cannot understand or is paralyzed. Only in the case of amputation or joint fusion, the examiner should record the score as untestable (UN), and clearly write the explanation for this choice. In case of blindness, test by having the patient touch nose from extended arm position.	0 = **Absent**. 1 = **Present in one limb**. 2 = **Present in two limbs**. UN = **Amputation** or joint fusion
8. Sensory: Sensation or grimace to pinprick when tested, or withdrawal from noxious stimulus in the obtunded or aphasic patient. Only sensory loss attributed to stroke is scored as abnormal and the examiner should test as many body areas (arms [not hands], legs, trunk, face) as needed to accurately check for hemisensory loss. A score of 2, "severe or total sensory loss," should only be given when a severe or total loss of sensation can be clearly demonstrated. Stuporous and aphasic patients will, therefore, probably score 1 or 0. The patient with brainstem stroke who has bilateral loss of sensation is scored 2. If the patient does not respond and is quadriplegic, score 2. Patients in a coma (item 1a=3) are automatically given a 2 on this item.	0 = **Normal**; no sensory loss. 1 = **Mild-to-moderate sensory loss**; patient feels pinprick is less sharp or is dull on the affected side; or there is a loss of superficial pain with pinprick, but patient is aware of being touched. 2 = **Severe to total sensory loss**; patient is not aware of being touched in the face, arm, and leg.
9. Best Language: A great deal of information about comprehension will be obtained during the preceding sections of the examination. For this scale item, the patient is asked to describe what is happening in the attached picture, to name the items on the attached naming sheet and to read from the attached list of sentences. Comprehension is judged from responses here, as well as to all of the commands in the preceding general neurological exam. If visual loss interferes with the tests, ask the patient to identify objects placed in the hand, repeat, and produce speech. The intubated patient should be asked to write. The patient in a coma (item 1a=3) will automatically score 3 on this item. The examiner must choose a score for the patient with stupor or limited cooperation, but a score of 3 should be used only if the patient is mute and follows no one-step commands.	0 = **No aphasia**; normal. 1 = **Mild-to-moderate aphasia**; some obvious loss of fluency or facility of comprehension, without significant limitation on ideas expressed or form of expression. Reduction of speech and/or comprehension, however, makes conversation about provided materials difficult or impossible. For example, in conversation about provided materials, examiner can identify picture or naming card content from patient's response. 2 = **Severe aphasia**; all communication is through fragmentary expression; great need for inference, questioning, and guessing by the listener. Range of information that can be exchanged is limited; listener carries burden of communication. Examiner cannot identify materials provided from patient response. 3 = **Mute, global aphasia**; no usable speech or auditory comprehension.

continued

Table 3-1. National Institutes of Health Stroke Scale continued

Instructions	Scale Definition
10. Dysarthria: If patient is thought to be normal, an adequate sample of speech must be obtained by asking patient to read or repeat words from the attached list. If the patient has severe aphasia, the clarity of articulation of spontaneous speech can be rated. Only if the patient is intubated or has other physical barriers to producing speech, the examiner should record the score as untestable (UN), and clearly write an explanation for this choice. Do not tell the patient why he or she is being tested.	0 = **Normal**. 1 = **Mild-to-moderate dysarthria**; patient slurs at least some words and, at worst, can be understood with some difficulty. 2 = **Severe dysarthria**; patient's speech is so slurred as to be unintelligible in the absence of or out of proportion to any dysphasia, or is mute/anarthric. UN = **Intubated** or other physical barrier
11. Extinction and Inattention (formerly Neglect): Sufficient information to identify neglect may be obtained during the prior testing. If the patient has a severe visual loss preventing visual double simultaneous stimulation, and the cutaneous stimuli are normal, the score is normal. If the patient has aphasia but does appear to attend to both sides, the score is normal. The presence of visual spatial neglect or anosagnosia may also be taken as evidence of abnormality. Since the abnormality is scored only if present, the item is never untestable.	0 = **No abnormality**. 1 = **Visual, tactile, auditory, spatial, or personal inattention** or extinction to bilateral simultaneous stimulation in one of the sensory modalities. 2 = **Profound hemi-inattention or extinction to more than one modality**; does not recognize own hand or orients to only one side of space.

Table 3-2. ABCD^2 Score (Johnston et al., 2007)

Risk Factor	Score
A: Age	
> = 60	1
B: Blood pressure	
> = 140/90 mmHg	1
C: Clinical features of the TIA	
Unilateral weakness	2
Speech disturbance without weakness	1
D(1): Duration of symptoms	
> = 60 min	2
10–59 min	1
<10 min	0
D(2): Patient diagnosed with diabetes?	
Yes	1
No	0

c. GCS (**Table 3-3**; Teasdale & Jennett, 1974)
   (1) Developed to assess level of consciousness
   (2) Designed to be used by various providers in various locations
   (3) Three components—eye opening, best verbal response, and best motor response
   (4) Highest score is 15, lowest is 3

Table 3-3. Comparison of the Full Outline of UnResponsiveness Score (FOUR Score) with the Glascow Coma Scale

FOUR Score	Glasgow Coma Scale
Eye response 4 = eyelids open or opened, tracking, or blinking to command 3 = eyelids open but not tracking 2 = eyelids closed but open to loud voice 1 = eyelids closed but open to pain 0 = eyelids remain closed with pain	Eye response 4 = eyes open spontaneously 3 = eye opening to verbal command 2 = eye opening to pain 1 = no eye opening
Motor response 4 = thumbs-up, fist, or peace sign 3 = localizing to pain 2 = flexion response to pain 1 = extension response to pain 0 = no response to pain or generalized myoclonus status	Motor response 6 = obeys commands 5 = localizing pain 4 = withdrawal from pain 3 = flexion response to pain 2 = extension response to pain 1 = no motor response
Brainstem reflexes 4 = pupil and corneal reflexes present 3 = one pupil wide and fixed 2 = pupil or corneal reflexes absent 1 = pupil and corneal reflexes absent 0 = absent pupil, corneal, and cough reflex	Verbal response 5 = oriented 4 = confused 3 = inappropriate words 2 = incomprehensible sounds 1 = no verbal response
Respiration 4 = not intubated, regular breathing pattern 3 = not intubated, Cheyne–Stokes breathing pattern 2 = not intubated, irregular breathing 1 = breathes above ventilator rate 0 = breathes at ventilator rate or apnea	

Reprinted from "Validation of a New Coma Scale: The FOUR Score," by E. F. Wijdicks, W. R. Bamlet, B. V. Maramattom, E. M. Manno, and R. L. McClelland, 2005, Annals of Neurology, 58*(4), pp. 585–589. © 2005 by Wiley. Reprinted with permission.*

d. Full Outline of UnResponsiveness Score (FOUR Score; Table 3-3; Wijdicks, Bamlet, Maramattom, Manno, & McClelland, 2005)
   (1) Four components— eye, motor, brain stem, and respiration
   (2) Each component is scored 0–4, with 16 being the best score.

e. Hunt and Hess Stroke Scale
   (1) Score is based on the clinical presentation of a patient with a subarachnoid hemorrhage.
   (2) Higher scores correlate to poorer outcomes.
   (3) Grades
      (a) Grade I—asymptomatic, or minimal headache and slight nuchal rigidity
      (b) Grade II—moderate to severe headache, nuchal rigidity, and no neurological deficit other than cranial nerve palsy
      (c) Grade III—drowsiness, confusion, or mild focal deficit
      (d) Grade IV—stupor, moderate to severe hemiparesis, possibly early decerebrate rigidity, and vegetative disturbances
      (e) Grade V—deep coma, decerebrate rigidity, moribund appearance (Hunt & Hess, 1968)

f. Fisher Grade
   (1) Designed to predict vasospasm after subarachnoid hemorrhage
   (2) Based on location of blood on CT scan
   (3) Grades
      (a) 1 = No hemorrhage evident
      (b) 2 = SAH less than 1 mm thick
      (c) 3 = SAH more than 1 mm thick
      (d) 4 = SAH of any thickness with intraventricular hemorrhage (IVH) or parenchymal extension (Fisher, Kistler, & Davis, 1980).

g. ICH Score (**Table 3-4**)
   (1) Score is designed to predict 30-day mortality risk for a patient with intracerebral hemorrhage.
   (2) Score range is 0–6. Higher ICH scores are correlated with higher mortality rates.

h. Spetzler-Martin grading system (Iancu-Gontard et al., 2007; Spetzler & Martin, 1986)
   (1) Used to calculate the surgical risk of an arteriovenous malformation (AVM)
   (2) Scale is based on the size of the AVM, the eloquence of the brain tissue, and the pattern of venous drainage.

Table 3-4. Determination of the Intracerebral Hemorrhage Score

Component	ICH Score Points
GCS score	
3–4	2
5–12	1
13–15	0
ICH volume, cm^3	
≥30	1
<30	0
IVH	
Yes	1
No	0
Infratentorial origin of ICH	
Yes	1
No	0
Age, years	
≥80	1
<80	0
Total ICH Score	0–6

GCS score indicates GCS score on initial presentation (or after resuscitation); ICH volume, volume on initial CT calculated using ABC/2 method; IVH, presence of any IVH on initial CT.

Reprinted from "The ICH Score: A Simple, Reliable Grading Scale for Intracerebral Hemorrhage," by J. C Hemphill, 3rd, D. C. Bonovich, L. Bermertis, G. T. Manley, and S. C. Johnston, 2001, Stroke, *32(4), pp. 891–897. © 2001 by the American Heart Association/American Stroke Association. Reprinted with permission.*

(3) Size of AVM (the larger the AVM, the more technically difficult to remove)
  (a) Small (<3 cm): 1
  (b) Medium (3–6 cm): 2
  (c) Large (>6 cm): 3
  (d) Location
    1) Noneloquent site: 0
    2) Eloquent site: 1 (*eloquent* is defined as areas controlling speech and noticeable neurologic function)
(4) Venous drainage (deep veins reflect more difficult accessibility)
  (a) Superficial: 0
  (b) Deep: 1

Acute Treatment and Interventions

A. Acute treatment for ischemic stroke
  1. IV tPA
    a. IV tPA is the only U.S. Food and Drug Administration (FDA)–approved drug for the treatment of acute stroke. Currently, it is only approved for use within 3 hours of the time the patient was last seen normal. Use of the drug has been shown to improve neurologic outcomes in stroke patients (Jauch et al., 2013).
    b. IV tPA has been shown to have better outcomes when given closer to the stroke's onset (Lansberg, Schrooten, Bluhmki, Thijs, & Saver, 2009); therefore, efforts should be made to administer tPA as quickly as possible. The nurse is responsible for administering tPA once the patient's eligibility has been determined (Summers et al., 2009).
    c. IV tPA has been shown to be beneficial in the extended 3–4.5-hour time window, and this usage is endorsed by the American Stroke Association (Bluhmki et al., 2009; Hacke et al., 2008; Lees et al., 2010). However, additional exclusion criteria apply:
      (1) Age >80 years
      (2) Severe stroke (NIHSS >25)
      (3) Taking an oral anticoagulant regardless of international normalized ratio
      (4) History of both diabetes and prior ischemic stroke
    d. Identify inclusion and exclusion criteria (from package insert; **Table 3-5**)
    e. Calculate dosing
      (1) Alteplase (also, tPA) is a weight-based drug. The dose is 0.9 mg/kg, not to exceed a dose of 90 mg. The first 10% is given as a bolus over 1 minute. The remainder (90%) is given over an hour.
      (2) It is recommended that the excess drug amount (i.e., the portion of the drug not being delivered) be removed from the main bottle and discarded. This is to prevent the administration of excess medication to the patient.
    f. Know delivery method
      (1) The medication needs to be reconstituted prior to delivery. Sterile water is used to reconstitute the crystals for a total drug amount of 100 mg.
      (2) Alteplase should be given intravenously through a dedicated line; a peripheral or central line is acceptable.
      (3) Delivering alteplase through an interosseous line is not recommended at this time.
      (4) Drug administration should not be delayed while waiting for laboratory values, provided the patient does not indicate the use of anticoagulant medication or risk factors associated with bleeding.

Table 3-5. Inclusion and Exclusion Characteristics of Patients with Ischemic Stroke Who Could Be Treated with IV rtPA Within 3 Hours from Symptom Onset

Inclusion criteria

Diagnosis of ischemic stroke causing measurable neurological deficit
Onset of symptoms <3 hours before beginning treatment
Aged ≥18 years

Exclusion criteria

Significant head trauma or stroke in prior 3 months
Symptoms suggesting subarachnoid hemorrhage
Arterial puncture at noncompressible site in prior 7 days
History of previous intracranial hemorrhage
Intracranial neoplasm, arteriovenous malformation, or aneurysm
Recent intracranial or intraspinal surgery
Elevated blood pressure (systolic >185 mmHg or diastolic >110 mmHg)
Active internal bleeding
Acute bleeding diathesis, including but not limited to
Platelet count <100000/mm^3
Heparin received within 48 hours, resulting in abnormally elevated aPTT higher than the upper limit of normal
Current use of anticoagulant with INR >1.7 or PT >15 seconds
Current use of direct thrombin inhibitors or direct factor Xa inhibitors with elevated sensitive laboratory tests (such as aPTT, INR, platelet count, and ECT; TT; or appropriate factor Xa activity assays)
Blood glucose concentration <50 mg/dL (2.7 mmol/L)
CT demonstrates multilobar infarction (hypodensity >1/3 cerebral hemisphere)

Relative exclusion criteria

Recent experience suggests that under some circumstances—with careful consideration and weighing of risk to benefit—patients may receive fibrinolytic therapy despite one or more relative contraindications. Consider risk to benefit of IVrtPA administration carefully if any of these relative contraindications are present:
Only minor or rapidly improving stroke symptoms (clearing spontaneously)
Pregnancy
Seizure at onset with postictal residual neurological impairments
Major surgery or serious trauma within prior 14 days
Recent gastrointestinal or urinary tract hemorrhage (within prior 21 days)
Recent acute myocardial infarction (within prior 3 months)

The checklist includes some FDA-approved indications and contraindications for administration of IVrtPA for acute ischemic stroke. Recent guideline revisions have modified the original FDA-approved indications. A physician with expertise in acute stroke care may modify this list.

Onset time is defined as either the witnessed onset of symptoms or the time the patient was last known to be acting normally if the symptom onset was not witnessed.

In patients who have not recently used oral anticoagulants or heparin, treatment with IVrtPA can be initiated before the availability of coagulation test results but should be discontinued if INR is >1.7 or PT is abnormally elevated by local laboratory standards.

In patients without a history of thrombocytopenia, treatment with IVrtPA can be initiated before the availability of a platelet count but should be discontinued if the platelet count is <100 000/mm^3.

aPTT indicates activated partial thromboplastin time; CT, computed tomography; ECT, ecarin clotting time; FDA, Food and Drug Administration; INR, international normalized ratio; IV, intravenous; PT, partial thromboplastin time; rtPA, recombinant tissue plasminogen activator; TT, thrombin time.

Reprinted from "Guidelines for the Early Management of Patients with Acute Ischemic Stroke: A Guideline for Healthcare Professionals from the American Heart Association/American Stroke Association" by E. D. Jauch, J. L. Saver, H. P. Adams, A. Bruno, J. T. Connors, B. M. Demaerscalk, et al., 2013, Stroke, 44, *pp. 870–974.*

g. Provide post-administration care
   (1) Vital signs and neurological status should be assessed every 15 minutes during tPA infusion, then every 15 minutes for 2 hours, every 30 minutes for 6 hours, and hourly for 16 hours.
   (2) Vital signs should include heart rate (including arrythmia, if present), blood pressure, and oxygen saturation.
   (3) Neurologic exams should be completed while checking vital signs to assess for neurologic deterioration.
   (4) If the patient has neurologic deterioration, stop the tPA infusion and obtain an emergent CT to evaluate for hemorrhage.

h. Identify post-administration complications
   (1) Symptomatic ICH
      (a) Development of a severe headache, acute hypertension, nausea or vomiting, or worsening neurological examination are concerning indications of symptomatic ICH.
      (b) Interventions
         1) If not already done, stop the alteplase infusion.
         2) Notify the physician immediately.
         3) Prepare the patient for rapid transport to obtain a CT scan.
         4) Obtain laboratory tests, including
            a) Coagulation panel (prothrombin time, partial thromboplastin time, international normalized ratio)
            b) Fibrinogen level
            c) Complete blood count with platelets
            d) Type and crossmatch.
         5) Prepare to administer
            a) Six to 8 U of cryoprecipitate containing factor VIII
            b) Six to 8 U of platelets
            c) Note: There are no standardized measures to treat symptomatic ICH after IV tPA administration.
         6) Hematology and neurosurgery teams may be consulted.
   (2) Bleeding from another site
      (a) Minor bleeding can occur from the gums, venipuncture sites, and catheters. Hematuria and hemoptysis also may occur (Braimah et al., 1997; Jauch et al., 2013; The National Institute of Neurological Disorders and Stroke rt-PA Stroke Study Group, 1995; Summers et al., 2009).
      (b) Check the patient's skin for signs of excessive bruising (Braimah et al., 1997).
   (3) Angioedema (Hill et al., 2003; Jauch et al., 2013)
      (a) Swelling of the tongue, lips, and oropharynx is rare but can occur as a reaction after IV tPA.
      (b) Often associated with angiotensin-converting enzyme inhibitor medications
      (c) Prepare the patient for treatment with histamine antagonists, such as ranitidine and diphenhydramine, and corticosteroids. Aggressive airway management may be needed depending on the extent of the swelling.

2. Interventional treatment of ischemic stroke (Jauch et al., 2013; Summers et al., 2009)
   a. This treatment requires rapid access to cerebral angiography. A trained interventionalist will place a catheter in the cerebral artery next to the occlusion. Mechanical thrombectomy or clot lysis with IA tPA generally will be used to reperfuse the vessel.

(1) As with IV tPA, treatment should be implemented without delay. The ideal time from door to IA treatment is a matter of controversy. Current consensus suggests 90–120 minutes from door arrival to IA treatment initiation is optimal.

(2) When appropriate, the stroke patient may transfer to a facility that is able to perform interventional treatment. Stabilizing and preparing the patient for transport will be a priority.

b. These options are considered for instances of stroke in which IV tPA is contraindicated, IV tPA has failed to reperfuse the vessel, or treatment outside the 4.5-hour time window is plausible.

(1) Interventional treatment is considered for patients with evidence of a large vessel occlusion based on a clinical exam or indicated by imaging or a high NIHSS score.

c. IA tPA treatment consists of injecting concentrated tPA to dissolve the clot and reperfuse the vessel. IA use of tPA is not approved by the FDA.

d. Mechanical thrombectomy devices are designed to physically remove or disrupt the clot. Thrombectomy devices are categorized by their mechanism of action and include coil retrievers, aspiration and debulking systems, and stent retriever devices. Stent retrievers have shown favor in effectiveness and improved outcomes.

3. Hemicraniectomy

a. Cerebral edema occurs from all infarcts and has a more disastrous effect in large-volume infarcts. Occlusions of the ICA and proximal MCA can lead to a large territory of ischemia. During the following 4 days, this tissue can swell, leading to herniation (Jauch et al., 2013). These large-territory strokes with significant edema often are referred to as malignant MCA strokes.

b. Hemicraniectomy allows for decompression of the brain. Surgery within the first 48 hours following stroke results in better neurologic outcomes and fewer instances of mortality than occur in medically managed malignant stroke patients (Hofmeijer et al., 2009).

B. Interventions for hemorrhagic strokes

1. Correct coagulopathies

a. Hemostatic abnormalities: For patients with severe thrombocytopenia, platelets should be given. No consensus exists to guide platelet transfusion; however, platelets generally are maintained at a level of more than 100,000 ppm. For patients with coagulation factor deficiencies, those factors may be replaced (Morgenstern et al., 2010).

b. Use of anticoagulation is known to increase the chance of ICH. When an ICH occurs, initiation of anticoagulation reversal should be expedited to prevent hematoma expansion (Frumkin, 2013; Morgenstern et al., 2010).

(1) Warfarin (Coumadin) reversal

(a) Vitamin K restores intrinsic clotting factors and maintains reversal, and comes in both an oral and IV form. The latter is faster acting and recommended for emergent reversal.

(b) Fresh frozen plasma (FFP) is given as a means to replace intrinsic clotting factors. Determination of the patient's ABO blood type is required prior to transfusion. Because of the volume of FFP needed, it is important to monitor the patient for fluid overload. There is little evidence to support the benefits of FFP use in cases of warfarin-associated ICH. Other agents are favored.

(c) Prothrombin complex concentrates (PCC) contains three to four of the intrinsic clotting factors II, VII, IX, and X. The factors come in powder form and can be reconstituted quickly. No ABO blood typing is required. The use of PCC is quickly becoming favored as a reversal agent (Frumkin, 2013; Morgenstern et al., 2010).

(2) Other anticoagulants

(a) Newer anticoagulants directly inhibit thrombin (IIa) or Xa. Unlike warfarin, no reversal agent has been identified. The half-life of these medications is much shorter than warfarin—less than 24 hours compared with 4–5 days. In the patient with renal impairments, the half-life might be longer because the medication is cleared through the kidneys. Several methods for blunting the anticoagulation effect have been suggested; for example, activated charcoal is recommended for a patient who recently has ingested the medication. Hemodialysis, FFP, or PCC also could be used (Kaatz et al., 2012).

2. Understand need for ventriculostomy

a. Ventriculostomy is used to remove fluid (cerebral spinal fluid [CSF] or blood) from the ventricles to reduce ICP.

(1) In ischemic stroke, edema may prevent the flow of CSF, causing hydrocephalus (Summers et al., 2009).

(2) In instances of intracerebral stroke, ventriculostomy is used for patients with a low GCS score (≤8), or for those who have IVH, hydrocephalus, or signs of herniation (Morgenstern et al., 2010).

(3) In instances of subarachnoid hemorrhage, it is used for patients with acute hydrocephalus. This often occurs because of the accumulation of blood in the ventricles (Connolly et al., 2012).

3. Manage ICP (Summers et al., 2009): Please refer to Chapter 5 for additional information on the management of elevated ICP.

a. Head-of-bed positioning is a key intervention for controlling increased ICP. Certain head and body alignments allow for venous drainage and prevent intrathoracic pressure. The head of the bed should be kept >30°.

b. Pain management should provide pain control without overly sedating the patient.

c. Maintain normothermia.

4. Understanding surgical options

a. Surgical options for removing blood in instances of ICH have been explored; however, the strength of the evidence supporting surgery varies depending on the location of the bleed (Morgenstern et al., 2010).

(1) Cerebellar hemorrhage clots with neurologic deterioration, brain stem compression, or hydrocephalus caused by compressing obstruction should be removed surgically.

(2) Supratentorial clots >30 mL and within 1 cm of the surface can be removed by craniectomy; this method may prove beneficial.

(3) For other supratentorial clots, there is no evidence supporting improved outcomes after surgery. Early surgery also may propagate rebleeding.

b. Minimally invasive techniques are being explored as a means to remove clots without disrupting healthy brain tissue. For example, one study showed a decrease in perihematomal edema by placing a catheter into the clot then infusing tPA to break down and drain the blood (Morgenstern et al., 2010; Mould et al., 2013).

Plan of Care

A. Develop and establish a nursing plan of care.

1. During the hyperacute phase of stroke, the focus of the nursing plan of care is to prevent complications leading to poor patient outcomes. Controlling vital signs and performing vigilant neurological examinations are integral to successful care management (AANN, 2009).
   a. Assess the patient's oxygenation level.
      (1) Supplemental oxygen should be delivered using the least invasive means available to keep SaO_2 >94% (Jauch et al., 2013). If unable to maintain oxygen saturation with supplemental oxygen, a chest radiograph or arterial blood gas should be obtained (Summers et al., 2009).
      (2) A decreased level of consciousness, atelectasis, and aspiration can compromise oxygenation. Nursing assessment should include monitoring for impaired swallow and auscultation of lungs (Summers et al., 2009).
   b. Assess the patient's hydration level.
      (1) Fluid balance is important for the stroke patient. Care should be taken to ensure the patient does not become fluid overloaded or dehydrated. Altered mental status or dysphagia can increase the risk of dehydration (Jauch et al., 2013).
      (2) Normal saline, administered at a rate of approximately 75–100 mL/hr, is used to maintain euvolemia as needed. In stroke patients who may be relatively hypovolemic, careful administration of normal intravenous saline boluses may be appropriate (Summers et al., 2009).
      (3) Hypotonic IV fluids, such as those containing dextrose, should be avoided in the patient with a brain injury (Connolly et al., 2012; Summers et al., 2009),
   c. Assess the patient's oral intake and swallowing ability.
      (1) The acute stroke patient should have nothing by mouth until his or her ability to swallow safely has been evaluated. This includes restricting the consumption of oral medications, ice chips, or water until the assessment has been made (Summers et al., 2009).
      (2) Using a validated dysphagia tool, the nurse can screen the stroke patient to determine if oral intake is safe. This screening often starts in the hyperacute setting, emergency department, or admitting unit (Lees, Sharpe, & Edwards, 2006).
      (3) The recommendations of the speech pathologist should be used (Summers et al., 2009).
      (4) Stroke patients also can experience silent aspiration, meaning they may aspirate without any outward signs of difficulty such as coughing (Ramsey, Smithard, & Kalra, 2005). See chapter 5 for additional information.
   d. Manage the patient's blood pressure.
      (1) Blood pressure can rise during acute stroke as a compensatory mechanism, allowing increased cerebral perfusion and enhancing collateral circulation. Blood pressure is not treated prior to the determination of the stroke type unless there are signs of hypertensive encephalopathy or it is >220/120 mmHg.
      (2) Blood pressure goals
         (a) Ischemic stroke (Jauch et al., 2013)
            1) If the patient is eligible for acute ischemic stroke treatment, his or her blood pressure should be lowered prior to treatment to <185/110 mmHg.

2) During the initiation of treatment and for 24 hours posttreatment—<180/105 mmHg

3) If there will be no treatment, withhold blood pressure medication unless the pressure is >220/120 mmHg. Blood pressure should be lowered by 15% during the next 24 hours.

(b) ICH without evidence of increased ICP—gentle blood pressure management to target 160/90 mmHg, with a mean arterial pressure of 110 mmHg (Morgenstern et al., 2010)

(c) Ruptured aSAH before aneurysm obliteration—systolic blood pressure <160 mmHg. A titratable agent is recommended. A delicate balance is kept between hypertension-related rebleeding and the maintenance of cerebral perfusion pressure (Connolly et al., 2012).

e. Manage blood glucose (Connolly et al., 2012; Diringer et al., 2011; Jauch et al., 2013; Morgenstern et al., 2010; Summers et al., 2009).

(1) Hypoglycemia should be avoided. Blood glucose levels <60 mg/dl in instances of acute ischemic stroke should be treated immediately. Hypoglycemia can mimic a stroke.

(2) Hyperglycemia has been correlated with poor outcomes. However, aggressive, tight blood glucose control may not be favorable. In one study, a tight blood glucose regime (goal, 80–110 mg/dl) was shown to have poorer outcomes than those for a moderate glucose regime (Diringer et al., 2011; Schlenk, Vajkoczy, & Sarrafzadeh, 2009).

f. Prevent hyperthermia (Connolly et al., 2012; Diringer et al., 2011; Jauch et al., 2013; Morgenstern et al., 2010; Summers et al., 2009).

(1) Normothermia should be maintained.

(2) Hyperthermia is associated with poor outcomes in instances of ischemic and hemorrhagic stroke.

(a) An infectious cause for the fever should be evaluated and treated. However, the fever may be the result of a systemic inflammatory reaction, not an infectious cause, as in subarachnoid hemorrhage patients with poor Hunt and Hess Grade scores.

(b) Antipyretic agents (acetaminophen, ibuprofen) often are used to control fever.

(c) Surface or endovascular cooling also are effective, but shivering should be prevented (Diringer et al., 2011).

References

Abdullah, A. R., Smith, E. E., Biddinger, P. D., Kalenderian, D., & Schwamm, L. H. (2008). Advance hospital notification by EMS in acute stroke is associated with shorter door-to-computed tomography time and increased likelihood of administration of tissue-plasminogen activator. *Prehospital Emergency Care, 12*(4), 426–431. doi: 10.1080/10903120802290828

American Association of Neuroscience Nurses. (2009). *Guide to the care of the hospitalized patient with ischemic stroke* (2nd ed.). Chicago, IL: Author.

Bluhmki, E., Chamorro, Á., Dávalos, A., Machnig, T., Sauce, C., Wahlgren, N., ... Hacke, W. (2009). Stroke treatment with alteplase given 3.0–4.5 h after onset of acute ischaemic stroke (ECASS III): Additional outcomes and subgroup analysis of a randomised controlled trial. *The Lancet Neurology, 8*(12), 1095–1102.

Bock, B. F. (1996, December). *Response system for patients presenting with acute stroke.* Paper presented at the National Symposium on Rapid Identification and Treatment of Acute Stroke, Washington, DC. Abstract retrieved from http://www.ninds.nih.gov/news_and_events/proceedings/stroke_proceedings/bock.htm

Braimah, J., Kongable, G., Rapp, K., Daley, S., Bratina, P., Sailor, S., ... Spilker, J. (1997). Nursing care of acute stroke patients after receiving rt-PA therapy. The NINDS rt-PA Stroke Study Group. *Journal of Neuroscience Nursing, 29*(6), 373–383.

Brott, T., Adams, H. P., Jr., Olinger, C. P., Marler, J. R., Barsan, W. G., Biller, J., ... Hertzberg, V. (1989). Measurements of acute cerebral infarction: A clinical examination scale. *Stroke, 20*(7), 864–870.

Connolly, E. S., Jr., Rabinstein, A. A., Carhuapoma, J. R., Derdeyn, C. P., Dion, J., Higashida, R. T., ... Council on Clinical Cardiology. (2012). Guidelines for the management of aneurysmal subarachnoid hemorrhage: A guideline for healthcare professionals from the American Heart Association/American Stroke Association. *Stroke, 43*(6), 1711–1737. doi: 10.1161/STR.0b013e3182587839

Diringer, M. N., Bleck, T. P., Claude Hemphill, J., 3rd, Menon, D., Shutter, L., Vespa, P., ... Neurocritical Care Society. (2011). Critical care management of patients following aneurysmal subarachnoid hemorrhage: Recommendations from the Neurocritical Care Society's Multidisciplinary Consensus Conference. *Neurocritical Care, 15*(2), 211–240. doi: 10.1007/s12028-011-9605-9

Fernandes, P. M., Whiteley, W. N., Hart, S. R., & Al-Shahi Salman, R. (2013). Strokes: Mimics and chameleons. *Practical Neurology, 13*(1), 21–28. doi: 10.1136/practneurol-2012-000465

Fisher, C. M., Kistler, J. P., & Davis, J. M. (1980). Relation of cerebral vasospasm to subarachnoid hemorrhage visualized by computerized tomographic scanning. *Neurosurgery, 6*(1), 1–9.

Frumkin, K. (2013). Rapid reversal of warfarin-associated hemorrhage in the emergency department by prothrombin complex concentrates. *Annals of Emergency Medicine, 62*(6), 616–626. doi: 10.1016/j.annemergmed.2013.05.026

Greenberg, M. S. (2000). SAH and aneurysms. In *Handbook of neurosurgery* (5 ed., pp. 754–803). New York, NY: Thieme Medical.

Hacke, W., Donnan, G., Fieschi, C., Kaste, M., von Kummer, R., Broderick, J. P., ... NINDS rt-PA Study Group Investigators. (2004). Association of outcome with early stroke treatment: Pooled analysis of ATLANTIS, ECASS, and NINDS rt-PA stroke trials. *Lancet, 363*(9411), 768–774. doi: 10.1016/s0140-6736(04)15692-4

Hacke, W., Kaste, M., Bluhmki, E., Brozman, M., Davalos, A., Guidetti, D., ... ECASS Investigators. (2008). Thrombolysis with alteplase 3 to 4.5 hours after acute ischemic stroke. *New England Journal of Medicine, 359*(13), 1317–1329. doi: 10.1056/NEJMoa0804656

Hemphill, J. C., 3rd, Bonovich, D. C., Besmertis, L., Manley, G. T., & Johnston, S. C. (2001). The ICH score: A simple, reliable grading scale for intracerebral hemorrhage. *Stroke, 32*(4), 891–897.

Hess, D. C., Wang, S., Gross, H., Nichols, F. T., Hall, C. E., & Adams, R. J. (2006). Telestroke: Extending stroke expertise into underserved areas. *Lancet Neurology, 5*(3), 275–278. doi: 10.1016/s1474-4422(06)70377-5

Higashida, R., Alberts, M. J., Alexander, D. N., Crocco, T. J., Demaerschalk, B. M., Derdeyn, C. P., ... American Heart Association Advocacy Coordinating Committee. (2013). Interactions within stroke systems of care: A policy statement from the american heart association/american stroke association. *Stroke, 44*(10), 2961–2984. doi: 10.1161/STR.0b013e3182a6d2b2

Hill, M. D., Lye, T., Moss, H., Barber, P. A., Demchuk, A. M., Newcommon, N. J., ... Buchan, A. M. (2003). Hemi-orolingual angioedema and ACE inhibition after alteplase treatment of stroke. *Neurology, 60*(9), 1525–1527. doi: 10.1212/01.wnl.0000058840.66596.1a

Hofmeijer, J., Kappelle, L. J., Algra, A., Amelink, G. J., van Gijn, J., & van der Worp, H. B. (2009). Surgical decompression for space-occupying cerebral infarction (the Hemicraniectomy After Middle Cerebral Artery infarction with Life-threatening Edema Trial [HAMLET]): A multicentre, open, randomised trial. *Lancet Neurology, 8*(4), 326–333. doi: 10.1016/s1474-4422(09)70047-x

Hunt, W. E., & Hess, R. M. (1968). Surgical risk as related to time of intervention in the repair of intracranial aneurysms. *Journal of Neurosurgery, 28*(1), 14–20. doi: 10.3171/jns.1968.28.1.0014

Iancu-Gontard, D., Weill, A., Guilbert, F., Nguyen, T., Raymond, J., & Roy, D. (2007). Inter- and intraobserver variability in the assessment of brain arteriovenous malformation angioarchitecture and endovascular treatment results. *American Journal of Neuroradiology, 28*(3), 524–527.

Jauch, E. C., Cucchiara, B., Adeoye, O., Meurer, W., Brice, J., Chan, Y. Y., ... Hazinski, M. F. (2010). Part 11: Adult stroke: 2010 American Heart Association Guidelines for Cardiopulmonary Resuscitation and Emergency Cardiovascular Care. *Circulation, 122*(18 Suppl 3), S818–828. doi: 10.1161/circulationaha.110.971044

Jauch, E. C., Saver, J. L., Adams, H. P., Jr., Bruno, A., Connors, J. J., Demaerschalk, B. M., ... Council on Clinical Cardiology. (2013). Guidelines for the early management of patients with acute ischemic stroke: A guideline for healthcare professionals from the American Heart Association/American Stroke Association. *Stroke, 44*(3), 870–947. doi: 10.1161/STR.0b013e318284056a

Johnston, S. C., Rothwell, P. M., Nguyen-Huynh, M. N., Giles, M. F., Elkins, J. S., Bernstein, A. L., & Sidney, S. (2007). Validation and refinement of scores to predict very early stroke risk after transient ischaemic attack. *Lancet, 369*(9558), 283–292. doi: 10.1016/s0140-6736(07)60150-0

Kaatz, S., Kouides, P. A., Garcia, D. A., Spyropolous, A. C., Crowther, M., Douketis, J. D., ... Ansell, J. (2012). Guidance on the emergent reversal of oral thrombin and factor Xa inhibitors. *American Journal of Hematology,* 87 Suppl 1, S141–145. doi: 10.1002/ajh.23202

Kidwell, C. S., Starkman, S., Eckstein, M., Weems, K., & Saver, J. L. (2000). Identifying stroke in the field. Prospective validation of the Los Angeles prehospital stroke screen (LAPSS). *Stroke, 31*(1), 71–76.

Kothari, R. U., Pancioli, A., Liu, T., Brott, T., & Broderick, J. (1999). Cincinnati Prehospital Stroke Scale: Reproducibility and validity. *Annals of Emergency Medicine, 33*(4), 373–378.

Lansberg, M. G., Schrooten, M., Bluhmki, E., Thijs, V. N., & Saver, J. L. (2009). Treatment time-specific number needed to treat estimates for tissue plasminogen activator therapy in acute stroke based on shifts over the entire range of the modified Rankin Scale. *Stroke, 40*(6), 2079–2084. doi: 10.1161/strokeaha.108.540708

Lees, K. R., Bluhmki, E., von Kummer, R., Brott, T. G., Toni, D., Grotta, J. C., ... Byrnes, G. (2010). Time to treatment with intravenous alteplase and outcome in stroke: An updated pooled analysis of ECASS, ATLANTIS, NINDS, and EPITHET trials. *Lancet, 375*(9727), 1695–1703. doi: 10.1016/s0140-6736(10)60491-6

Lees, L., Sharpe, L., & Edwards, A. (2006). Nurse-led dysphagia screening in acute stroke patients. *Nursing Standard, 21*(6), 35–42. doi: 10.7748/ns2006.10.21.6.35.c6373

Levine, S. R., & Gorman, M. (1999). "Telestroke": The application of telemedicine for stroke. *Stroke, 30*(2), 464–469.

Lindsay, K. W., & Bone, I. (2004). *Neurology and neurosurgery illustrated* (4th ed.). London, England: Elsevier.

Morgenstern, L. B., Hemphill, J. C., 3rd, Anderson, C., Becker, K., Broderick, J. P., Connolly, E. S., Jr., ... American Heart Association Stroke Council and Council on Cardiovascular Nursing. (2010). Guidelines for the management of spontaneous intracerebral hemorrhage: A guideline for healthcare professionals from the American Heart Association/American Stroke Association. *Stroke, 41*(9), 2108–2129. doi: 10.1161/STR.0b013e3181ec611b

Mould, W. A., Carhuapoma, J. R., Muschelli, J., Lane, K., Morgan, T. C., McBee, N. A., ... MISTIE Investigators. (2013). Minimally invasive surgery plus recombinant tissue-type plasminogen activator for intracerebral hemorrhage evacuation decreases perihematomal edema. *Stroke, 44*(3), 627–634. doi: 10.1161/strokeaha.111.000411

Pervez, M. A., Silva, G., Masrur, S., Betensky, R. A., Furie, K. L., Hidalgo, R., ... Schwamm, L. H. (2010). Remote supervision of IV-tPA for acute ischemic stroke by telemedicine or telephone before transfer to a regional stroke center is feasible and safe. *Stroke, 41*(1), e18–24. doi: 10.1161/strokeaha.109.560169

Pexman, J. H., Barber, P. A., Hill, M. D., Sevick, R. J., Demchuk, A. M., Hudon, M. E., ... Buchan, A. M. (2001). Use of the Alberta Stroke Program Early CT Score (ASPECTS) for assessing CT scans in patients with acute stroke. *American Journal of Neuroradiology, 22*(8), 1534–1542.

Ramsey, D., Smithard, D., & Kalra, L. (2005). Silent aspiration: What do we know? *Dysphagia, 20*(3), 218–225. doi: 10.1007/s00455-005-0018-9

Saver, J. L. (2006). Time is brain—quantified. *Stroke, 37*(1), 263–266. doi: 10.1161/01.STR.0000196957.55928.ab

Schlenk, F., Vajkoczy, P., & Sarrafzadeh, A. (2009). Inpatient hyperglycemia following aneurysmal subarachnoid hemorrhage: relation to cerebral metabolism and outcome. *Neurocritical Care, 11*(1), 56–63. doi: 10.1007/s12028-009-9222-z

Searls, D. E., Pazdera, L., Korbel, E., Vysata, O., & Caplan, L. R. (2012). Symptoms and signs of posterior circulation ischemia in the new England medical center posterior circulation registry. *Archives of Neurology, 69*(3), 346–351. doi: 10.1001/archneurol.2011.2083

Spetzler, R. F., & Martin, N. A. (1986). A proposed grading system for arteriovenous malformations. *Journal of Neurosurgery, 65*(4), 476–483. doi: 10.3171/jns.1986.65.4.0476

Spilker, J., Kongable, G., Barch, C., Braimah, J., Brattina, P., Daley, S., ... Sailor, S. (1997). Using the NIH Stroke Scale to assess stroke patients. The NINDS rt-PA Stroke Study Group. *Journal of Neuroscience Nursing, 29*(6), 384–392.

Summers, D., Leonard, A., Wentworth, D., Saver, J. L., Simpson, J., Spilker, J. A., ... American Heart Association Council on Cardiovascular Nursing and the Stroke Council. (2009). Comprehensive overview of nursing and interdisciplinary care of the acute ischemic stroke patient: A scientific statement from the American Heart Association. *Stroke, 40*(8), 2911–2944. doi: 10.1161/strokeaha.109.192362

Teasdale, G., & Jennett, B. (1974). Assessment of coma and impaired consciousness. A practical scale. *Lancet, 2*(7872), 81–84.

The National Institute of Neurological Disorders and Stroke rt-PA Stroke Study Group. (1995). Tissue plasminogen activator for acute ischemic stroke. *New England Journal of Medicine, 333*(24), 1581–1588. doi: 10.1056/nejm199512143332401

Tocco, S. (2011). Identify the vessel, recognize the stroke . *American Nurse Today, 6*(9), 8–11.

Wijdicks, E. F., Bamlet, W. R., Maramattom, B. V., Manno, E. M., & McClelland, R. L. (2005). Validation of a new coma scale: The FOUR score. *Annals of Neurology, 58*(4), 585–593. doi: 10.1002/ana.20611

Wojner-Alexander, A. W., Garami, Z., Chernyshev, O. Y., & Alexandrov, A. V. (2005). Heads down: Flat positioning improves blood flow velocity in acute ischemic stroke. *Neurology, 64*(8), 1354–1357. doi: 10.1212/01.wnl.0000158284.41705.a5

Chapter

4

Stroke Diagnostics

Millie Hepburn, MPhil MSN RN ACNS-BC SCRN

Patients with ischemic stroke, intracerebral hemorrhage (ICH), or subarachnoid hemorrhage (SAH) will undergo multiple diagnostic tests through the acute diagnosis and treatment of their stroke events. The Stroke Certified Registered Nurse (SCRN) demonstrates expertise in anticipating, facilitating, and mitigating complications associated with diagnostic testing of stroke patients. This chapter focuses on the indications for diagnostic testing and the posttest monitoring of stroke patients who have undergone diagnostic testing.

Objectives

1. Describe radiological studies used in the diagnosis and treatment of stroke patients.
2. Identify the indications, procedures, and clinical implications for diagnostic tests for the stroke patient.
3. Describe the laboratory tests used to diagnose and treat stroke.
4. Describe nursing interventions related to specific diagnostic exams.

Patient Education and Preparedness

A. Preprocedure care
  1. Ensure patient and family understanding of diagnostic procedures and laboratory tests that represent informed decision making.
  2. Use teach-back techniques to validate the patient and family learning process.
  3. Use patient-oriented handouts, videos, slide presentations, or other audiovisual educational tools.
  4. Encourage the patient and family to ask questions.
     a. Carry out preprocedural preparations.
     b. Explain the specific procedure or test to the patient and family to assist understanding of the test and to ensure an informed decision-making process.
     c. Verify informed consent.
  5. For all invasive procedures, conduct a preprocedure neurological and vitals assessment.
  6. Adhere to unit and facility protocols and specific patient-oriented physician or licensed provider orders to prepare the patient for procedures.
  7. Apply department's universal protocol, or time-out process, prior to all invasive procedures.

B. Management during test or procedure
   1. If accompanying the patient to a procedure or if the procedure is performed at the bedside, provide supportive care, such as comfort, positioning, emotional support, and toileting.

C. Preprocedure care
   1. Adhere to unit or facility protocols and documented orders by licensed provider.
   2. Special considerations
      a. Radiation exposure and pregnancy
         (1) For any procedure that involves radiation exposure, such as a computed tomography (CT) scan, determine the possibility of pregnancy in women of childbearing age and ensure appropriate precautions are met.
      b. Magnetic exposure
         (1) Screen patient and environment for the presence of implanted metal or external metal objects such as jewelry or hair accessories to ensure removal prior to magnetic exposure.
         (2) Recognize that credit cards will be deactivated in a magnetic environment and should be removed prior to magnetic exposure.
      c. Allergies
         (1) Check for allergies to shellfish, iodine, or contrast dyes and notify licensed provider prior to any administration.
      d. Renal and liver function and contrast media
         (1) Check baseline liver and kidney function laboratory tests before administering any form of contrast media to ensure appropriate metabolism will take place.
            (a) Seek renal consultation for patients with suspected renal impairment.
         (2) Hydration
            (a) Assess for and ensure adequate hydration before and after administration of any contrast medium.

Immediate Diagnostic Studies for the Evaluation of a Patient with Suspected Acute Ischemic Stroke (Adams et al., 2007; European Stroke Organisation [ESO], 2008; Hacke et al., 1995, 2008; Jauch et al., 2013; Patel et al., 2001)

A. All patients
   1. Non-enhanced computed tomography (NECT) or brain magnetic resonance imaging (MRI)
   2. Blood glucose
   3. Oxygen saturation
   4. Serum electrolytes/renal function tests
   5. Complete blood count, including platelet count
   6. Markers of cardiac ischemia
   7. Prothrombin time (PT)/international normalized ratio (INR)
   8. Activated partial thromboplastin time (aPTT)
   9. Electrocardiogram (EKG)

B. Selected patients
   1. Thromboplastin time and Ecarin clotting time if it is suspected the patient is taking direct thrombin inhibitors or factor Xa inhibitors
   2. Hepatic function tests
   3. Toxicology screen
   4. Blood alcohol level

5. Pregnancy test
6. Arterial blood gas tests (if hypoxia is suspected)
7. Chest radiography (if lung disorder or disease is suspected)
8. Lumbar puncture (if SAH is suspected and CT scan is negative for blood)
9. Electroencephalogram

C. Early diagnosis
1. Timely brain imaging and interpretation are critical to rapid evaluation and diagnosis of patients with suspected stroke. Although hemorrhage is visible on NECT within moments of occurring, infarcted tissue is not visible for several hours after initial vessel occlusion. Brain imaging findings that are critical to treatment include those that identify the size, location, and distribution of the cerebral infarction, as well as the presence of bleeding, severity of stroke, and presence of large-vessel occlusion, affecting immediate and long-term treatment decisions.
2. NECT remains the most available diagnostic imaging to identify contraindications to fibrinolysis, thereby allowing patients with ischemic stroke to receive timely fibrinolytic therapy. The ideal timeframe for performing NECT is within 25 min of the patient's arrival in the emergency department, and the brain imaging study should be interpreted within 45 min of arrival by a physician with expertise in reading CT and MRI studies of the brain parenchyma.

Detail of Neuroradiological Studies in Stroke Patients

A. CT (Demchuk et al., 2005; Dzialowski et al., 2006; von Kummer et al., 2001)
1. Parenchymal brain imaging—NECT and contrast-enhanced CT scans of the brain
2. Description of CT
   a. These images utilize computer-processed X rays obtained in multiple directions to produce tomographic images, or slices, of specific areas of the head. These cross-sectional images are used for diagnostic and therapeutic purposes.
      (1) Noninvasive
      (2) Computer assisted
      (3) Ionized radiological means of examining anatomic structures; forms 2-dimensional (2D) or 3-dimensional (3D) pictures
   b. Different tissues have different densities to X-ray penetration and are reported as hypo-, iso-, and hyperdense. The NECT is able to identify subtle, early signs of ischemic brain injury or arterial occlusion that might affect decisions regarding treatment.
   c. Iodine-based contrast medium is used to enhance areas of increased blood flow or capillary leakage. The areas appear dense because they have an increased load of radioactive medium. Contrast medium is contraindicated in renal failure and may cause diuresis.
3. Purpose of CT
   a. Head CT scanning is conducted to detect cerebral infarction, tumors, hemorrhage, calcifications, and bone trauma. Hypodense (dark) structures can indicate infarction and brain edema, and hyperdense (bright) structures indicate calcifications and hemorrhage, while bone trauma can be seen as disjunction in bone windows. Detailed imaging of specific areas of the head assists clinicians to diagnose stroke and rule out other etiologies of neurologic changes.
   b. Head CT scan can depict the location and extent of SAH and the pattern of hemorrhage, as well as hydrocephalus and midline shift.

c. Detection of vascular changes within the brain tissue and spaces
d. These images detect edema, shift from midline or compartment, hydrocephalus, and swelling of the gyri.
(1) The more rapidly these signs become evident, the more profound the degree of ischemia.
(2) The ability of the observers to detect these early infarct signs is variable.
(3) Detection is influenced by the infarct size, degree of ischemia, and the time lapse between symptom onset and imaging.

4. Procedure
a. CT imaging involves circular gantry with X-ray tubes and detectors. Detectors measure penetration of tissue radiation. Tissues with various densities result in differing gradations of white to black. These gradations of color apply both to CT and MRI.
(1) Methods to increase detection include use of a structured scoring system such as the Alberta Stroke Program Early CT score (ASPECTS) or the CT Summit Criteria as well as the use of CT "windowing and leveling" to differentiate between normal and abnormal tissues.

5. Significance of gradations from white to black
a. White (hyperdense)
(1) Bone
(2) Calcium deposit
(3) Blood (during acute period)
b. Cerebral tissue
(1) Blood (during subacute period)
c. Dark gray appearance (hypodense)
(1) Cerebrospinal fluid (CSF)
(2) Cerebral edema
(3) Fat
(4) Blood (chronic)
d. Black
(1) Air

6. Significance of findings
a. Early signs of ischemia seen on NECT
b. Decreased attenuation of grey matter in area of ischemia, often referred to as the loss of insular or cortical ribbon, or loss of grey and white matter differentiation
c. Hypodensity of cerebral tissue
d. Reflect early ionic edema formation at the site of ischemia or infarction and may not be visible for 6 or more hours after the event, depending on the size of ischemia and infarct
e. Increased density within the occluded artery, such as the hyperdense middle cerebral artery (MCA) or basilar artery sign indicates large-vessel occlusion.
(1) Large-vessel occlusion typically causes severe stroke and may independently predict neurological deterioration.
f. Frank hypodensity on NECT may increase the risk of hemorrhage with fibrinolysis and should be considered in treatment decisions. If frank hypodensity involves more than one-third of the MCA territory, intravenous (IV) treatment of rtPA should be withheld.

(1) Frank hypodensity on the NECT may increase the risk of hemorrhage with fibrinolysis and should be considered in treatment.

7. Nursing considerations in patient preparation
   a. Head of bed must be flat for CT. If possible, gradually lower head of bed in increments prior to placing patient in scanner to prevent an inadvertent rise in intracranial pressure.
   b. Assess for allergies to shellfish and iodine and assess renal impairment prior to procedure in the event that a CT with contrast medium is considered following a NECT.
8. Advantages and disadvantages
   a. CT offers visualization of bony definition and involves a relatively short scan time. This is helpful when rapid diagnosis is necessary.
   b. CT is superior to MRI for diagnosing SAH.
   c. There are no known risks of CT scan to a fetus during pregnancy; however, abdominal shielding is advised.
   d. In patients with a history of iodine allergy, steroid preparation is required for contrast CT films.

B. CT perfusion studies (Bammer & Moseley, 2005; Christensen et al., 2008; Schellinger et al., 2010)

1. Description: *Perfusion* refers to the passage of fluid through the lymphatic system or blood vessels to an organ or a tissue. *CT perfusion scanning* is the process by which cerebral perfusion can be observed, recorded, and quantified.
2. Purpose
   a. Useful in the selection of patients for acute reperfusion therapy beyond the time window for IV fibrinolysis, because it measures cerebral blood flow and ischemic tissue that has not yet infarcted
   b. CT perfusion studies can demonstrate hypoperfusion states in various brain regions and can distinguish tissue at risk for infarction from previously infarcted tissue.
   c. CT perfusion provides additional information that may improve diagnosis, mechanism, and severity of ischemic stroke and allow for informed decision making. However, although information obtained from a CT angiography (CTA) such as distinguishing areas of hypoperfusion and cerebral blood flow measurement is extremely valuable, the time required to complete the test may delay the administration of IV rt-PA in ischemic stroke patients.
3. Procedure—uses CT procedure with iodinated contrast IV bolus via antecubital IV
4. Significance of findings: Perfusion is calculated in different areas of the brain by the flow of contrast media.
   a. Recommended diagnostic to exclude the presence of proximal intracranial stenosis or occlusion and should be obtained when knowledge of intracranial stenoocclusive disease will alter management
   b. Provides reliability in the diagnosis in potential presence and degree of intracranial stenosis
5. Nursing considerations
   a. Assess patient for allergy to shellfish and iodine. Ensure epinephrine is available in the event of an allergic reaction or anaphylaxis.
   b. Ensure adequacy of IV access via antecubital vein with PowerPort to allow rapid infusion of IV contrast medium.

6. Advantages and disadvantages
   a. Low cost and noninvasive
   b. No known disadvantages

C. Cerebral angiography (Jauch et al., 2013; Wahlgren et al., 2008)
   1. Description—creates detailed images of the veins (venogram) or arteries (arteriogram) through the injection of dye into a large vessel, generally the femoral artery
   2. Purpose—rapid evaluation of intracranial and extracranial vasculature for relevant information regarding the presence of vessel occlusions or stenosis to assist in diagnosis of a narrowing or obstruction of the arteries or presence of an aneurysm, deep vein thrombosis, pulmonary embolism, or another vascular condition; has a high accuracy (specificity 92%–100%)
   3. Significance of findings—useful to determine abnormal circulation, assess collateral circulation, and identify the presence of space-occupying lesions
      a. Can be used to assess carotid arteries for stenosis
      b. Can be used to exclude the presence of proximal intracranial stenosis or occlusion
      c. Can be used to detect aneurysm, arteriovenous malformation (AVM), fistula, and angioma
   4. Procedure
      a. Baseline labs (PT, aPTT, blood urea nitrogen, creatinine) and peripheral IV
      b. Prepare patient, obtain informed consent, and obtain neurological and vital signs (maintain nothing by mouth [NPO] for 4–6 hours prior to procedure).
      c. Following site preparation, catheter insertion, and catheter threading to the target site, radiopaque contrast medium is injected into the carotid or vertebral arteries via catheter placement into the femoral or brachial artery.
      d. Radiographs of the cerebral vasculature are performed.
         (1) Radiographic images detect the movement of the medium through the artery and cerebral blood vessels and detect blockages in blood flow.
   5. Nursing considerations
      a. Ensure that the procedure is adequately explained and informed consent is obtained from the patient and family prior to the procedure.
      b. Verify any allergies to shellfish or iodine prior to the procedure.
      c. During procedure: Observe patient for neurological changes, anaphylaxis, bleeding, or impaired circulation.
      d. Postprocedure: Instruct patient to lie flat with a pressure dressing for 6 hours unless a collagen plug device is used, in which case manufacturer instructions should be followed.
      e. The procedure may cause damage to vessels. Therefore, the patient must be closely observed for bleeding, hematoma, or impaired circulation. The peripheral pulses in the affected extremity must be closely monitored in the hours after the procedure.
         (1) Assess vital signs, the catheterization site (for bleeding or hematoma), peripheral pulses, and neurovascular status every 15 minutes for the first hour, every 30 minutes for the next hour, and then hourly for 4 hours or until discharge.
         (2) Maintain bed rest as ordered, usually for 6 hours.
         (3) The head of the bed may be raised to 30°.
         (4) Keep a pressure dressing or sandbag in place over the arterial access site. Check frequently for bleeding. If the arterial access site is in the groin, check for bleeding under the buttocks as well as around the puncture site.

(5) Instruct patient to avoid flexing or hyperextending the affected extremity for 12–24 hours.
(6) Unless contraindicated, encourage liberal fluid intake.
(7) Promptly report diminished peripheral pulses, formation of a new hematoma or enlargement of an existing one, severe pain at the insertion site or in the affected extremity, chest pain, or dyspnea.

6. Advantages and disadvantages
   a. Angiography is the long-standing standard for the diagnosis for cerebral aneurysms, AVMs, arterial dissections, and fistulas.
   b. Because of the invasive nature of the procedure, serious complications may result.

D. CTA (Jauch et al., 2013; Kidwell, Villablanca, & Saver, 2000; Strayer, Prendergast, & Henwood, 2010)

1. Description: *CTA* is the 3D rendering of vessel anatomy offered by newer-generation helical CT machines. A bolus of iodinated contrast is administered, and images are obtained as the contrast bolus passes through the cerebral vasculature. CTA is a fast and easily applied method to determine the presence of cerebral aneurysms and large-vessel thrombus associated with ischemic stroke. CTA is a noninvasive procedure that is accurate for both large and small aneurysms and is accurate with calcified vessels.
2. Purpose: CTA is performed to quantify vessel abnormalities such as occlusion, AVM, and aneurysm and to confirm abnormalities detected with noninvasive testing to determine appropriate management.
   a. CTA is also used to assess collateral circulation and to detect space-occupying lesions, aneurysms, or cerebral venous thrombosis.
   b. High sensitivity for surgical lesions
   c. CTA may also be used to detect the presence of vasospasm.
3. Procedure: High-speed CT is obtained with peripheral IV power injection of contrast material with the use of 2D and 3D reformations.
   a. This technique provides high-quality anatomic detail of both deep and superficial intracranial venous system defects.
4. Nursing considerations
   a. Assess patient for allergy to shellfish and iodine. Ensure epinephrine is available in the event of an allergic reaction or anaphylaxis.
   b. Ensure adequacy of IV access via antecubital vein with PowerPort to allow rapid infusion of IV contrast medium.
5. Advantages and disadvantages
   a. Fast and reliable, not operator dependent, and often used in emergency situations
   b. Less expensive and less invasive with fewer complications than cerebral angiography
   c. Renal clearance is a vital component of preprocedure assessment and postprocedure evaluation, as acute kidney injury (AKI) and contrast-induced nephropathy may be a disadvantage of the use of contrast medium.

E. MRI (Christensen et al., 2008; Jauch et al., 2013; Kidwell et al., 2000; Mohr et al., 1995; Strayer et al., 2010; Wessels et al., 2005)

1. Description: MRI technology involves a powerful magnet that surrounds the patient. The magnetic field is used to align magnetized nuclei of atoms in the body, and radio frequency magnetic fields are applied to systematically alter the alignment of this magnetization. Nuclei then produce a rotating magnetic field detectable by the scanner. This information is recorded to construct an image of the scanned area of the body.

a. Magnetic field gradients cause nuclei at different locations to process at different speeds, allowing spatial information to be recovered using 2D images or 3D volumes. Using this technology, MRI provides contrast between the different soft tissues, rendering it especially useful in brain, muscle, and heart imaging, as compared to other technologies.
b. MRI does not emit ionizing radiation and may be recommended as an alternative to CT prior to IV rtPA administration to exclude ICH and to determine if MRI hyperintensity of ischemia is present.

2. Purpose: MRI is used to diagnose structural and biochemical abnormalities of the brain and nervous system and can detect necrotic tissue, oxygen-deprived tissue, and degenerative diseases of the central nervous system.
   a. Can demonstrate white matter changes and provide visualization of brain stem and posterior fossa structures
   b. The artery susceptibility sign correlates with the hyperdense MCA seen on NECT.
3. Nursing considerations
   a. Use of MRI preprocedure checklist ensures patient safety.
      (1) Ensure that all contraindications to MRI technology are reviewed with the patient and family.
      (2) Abbreviated sequence of magnetic resonance images is offered in some institutions to assist with rapid identification of ischemic stroke candidates who may benefit from reperfusion procedures. In these instances, testing must be expedited from the emergency department.
4. Advantages and disadvantages
   a. Conventional MRI is more sensitive than NECT in identifying new and preexisting ischemic lesions in patients with 24-hour time-defined transient ischemic attacks (TIAs).
   b. Not ideal for depicting SAH acutely, but it is helpful in determining the age of bleeding (acute versus subacute) and delineating characteristics of an AVM.
   c. Helpful in determining the presence of hemorrhage in the past through gradient recalled echo (GRE) sequence, useful in diagnosing previous microhemorrhages in suspected amaloyd angiopathy
   d. Not suitable for unstable patients because of the length of the test
   e. Measures infarct core and penumbra and may be considered for the selection of patients for acute reperfusion therapy beyond the time windows for IV fibrinolysis
      (1) These techniques provide additional information that may improve the patient's diagnosis, improve the mechanism and lessen the severity of ischemic stroke, and allow more informed clinical decision making.
   f. May be contraindicated with certain metal implants secondary to the presence of magnetic fields
   g. May not be used with Medtronic and Advanced Neuromodulation Systems spinal cord stimulator systems because they are not MRI compatible
   h. Claustrophobic patients may not be able to tolerate MRI.

F. Magnetic resonance spectroscopy (MRS; Jauch et al., 2013; Strayer et al., 2010)
1. Description—a specialized technique established as a complement to MRI that investigates metabolic changes in brain disorders
2. Purpose—allows a noninvasive method to obtain biochemical information regarding neurochemical data to detect altered tissue. Most useful to detect cancers, epilepsy,

Alzheimer's disease, Parkinson's disease, Huntington's chorea, and pituitary tuberculosis.

G. Digital subtraction angiography (DSA; Jauch et al., 2013; Strayer et al., 2010)
   1. Description—a fluoroscopy technique used to visualize vascular lesions and atherosclerotic disease in a bony or dense soft-tissue environment to detect the presence of cerebral aneurysms and AVM. Has been used in the postoperative evaluation of endarterectomy patients, aneurysm clipping, or post AVM repair
      a. Once known as the standard for arterial imaging, this technique is being utilized less frequently than CTA, because CTA can produce 3D images and is less invasive.
   2. Procedure—images created using a contrast medium by subtracting a precontrast image after the contrast medium has been introduced
   3. Purpose—used to visualize cranial vessels and lesions
      a. Arterial and venous occlusions, such as carotid artery stenosis, cerebral aneurysms, and AVM
   4. Nursing considerations
      a. Ensure adequate clearance and informed consent has been obtained for procedure.
      b. Assess patient for allergy to shellfish and iodine. Ensure epinephrine is available in the event of an allergic reaction or anaphylaxis.
   5. Advantages and disadvantages
      a. DSA is less expensive than cerebral angiography and there is less exposure to radiation, but the field of view is also much smaller.
      b. DSA is most accurate in detection of a very high-grade stenosis.
      c. DSA may not be suitable for patients with diabetes or renal insufficiency because the dye load is higher than that used in arteriography.

H. Magnetic resonance angiography (MRA; Jauch et al., 2013; Strayer et al., 2010)
   1. Description
      a. This technology uses a magnetic field and pulses of radio wave energy to visualize blood flow through the blood vessels. Much of this information is unobtainable from other types of films.
      b. Performed in combination with brain MRI in the setting of acute stroke to guide decision making. Use of two concordant noninvasive techniques to assess treatment candidacy has the advantage of avoiding catheterization risks.
   2. Purpose—to guide therapeutic decision making regarding reduced blood flow in conditions of the blood vessel walls, such as aneurysms, calcium deposits, and dissections.
   3. Technology: Time-of-flight or inflow angiography uses short echo time and flow compensation (2D or 3D) to make flowing blood bright compared to stationary tissue. Areas with slow flow (aneurysms or flow that is in the plane of the image) may not be well visualized. Sensitivity ranges from 60%–85% for stenosis and 80%–90% for occlusions compared with CTA or DSA. Useful in identifying acute proximal large-vessel occlusions
      a. Recommended to exclude the presence of proximal intracranial stenosis or occlusion and should be obtained when knowledge of intracranial stenoocclusive disease will alter management. Reliable diagnosis of the presence and degree of intracranial stenosis requires the performance of catheter angiography to confirm abnormalities detected with noninvasive testing.

b. Useful in the detection of cerebral aneurysms, AVM, fistulas and narrowing of vessels, sacular aneurysms, and vessel narrowing and can evaluate cerebral vessels intracranially

4. Nursing considerations
   a. Utilize checklist for MRI to avoid use if contraindicated.
   b. Assess patient for history of claustrophobia prior to proceeding with test.
5. Advantages and disadvantages
   a. Noninvasive
   b. More costly than NECT
   c. May have limited availability
   d. Long duration of the test
   e. More vulnerable to motion than NECT. Approximately 10% of patients have an inability to remain motionless.
   f. Two studies report that MRI was as accurate as NECT in detecting hyperacute intraparenchymal hemorrhage in symptomatic stroke patients within 6 hr of onset.
   g. Provides pictures of cerebral vasculature and may be the sole initial imaging modality to evaluate acute stroke patients
      (1) May have advantages over NECT for distinguishing small cortical posterior fossa infarcts
   h. Inadequate for patients with metallic implants or claustrophobia
   i. Technology and use in clinical practice is still evolving.
   j. Can detect sacular aneurysms not seen on cerebral angiography

I. Magnetic resonance perfusion studies (Arakawa et al., 2006; Barber et al., 1999; Fiebach et al., 2002; Jauch et al., 2013; Kidwell et al., 2000; Keir, Wardlaw, Bastin, & Dennis, 2004; Schellinger et al., 2010; Seifert et al., 2005; Strayer et al., 2010)
   1. Description—measures cerebral perfusion via assessment of various hemodynamic measurements such as cerebral blood volume, cerebral blood flow, and mean transit time
   2. Purpose: Magnetic resonance perfusion studies are clinically useful in the assessment of cerebral ischemia, especially in combination with diffusion imaging to detect viable cerebral tissue at risk following stroke (ischemic penumbra).
      a. Diffusion weighted imaging (DWI) has emerged as the most sensitive (sensitivity 88%–100%) and specific (specificity 95%–100%) imaging technique for acute infarct.
         (1) Allows identification of the lesion size, site, and age and can detect relatively small cortical lesions, including those in brain stem or cerebellum, as well as subclinical satellite ischemic lesions
         (2) DWI positivity in TIA patients is associated with a higher risk of recurrent ischemic events.
   3. Significance of findings
      a. Magnetic resonance perfusion imaging has been shown to be more sensitive in defining the extent of gliomas than anatomic MRI.
      b. Measures serial concentration of a tracer agent, such as iced saline, iodinated radiographic contrast, and radionuclides
      c. Increased specificity is increased when perfusion imaging is combined with MRS.

J. Transcranial Doppler (TCD; Jauch et al., 2013; Strayer et al., 2010)
   1. Description—ultrasound 2D imaging to measure blood flow velocities over time. Through use of a Doppler effect probe, velocities are graphed over time.

a. Application of a transducer capable of converting electrical energy to ultrasound waves in frequencies of 5–20 kHz. Blood flow rate is measured and recorded by a high-pitched sound wave from the ultrasound probe through the intact skull into the brain.
b. The bones of the skull are too thick to transmit ultrasound; therefore, regions with thinner walls are used, such as the cheekbone, the zygomatic arch, the back of the head, and through the eyes and under the jaw.
c. The speed of the blood flow in relation to the probe causes a shift, and the frequency is increased or decreased, directly correlating with the speed of the blood, and is electronically recorded for analysis.

2. Purpose: TCD identifies intracranial vessel abnormalities, occlusions, and stenosis.
3. Significance of findings
   a. TCD has been shown to be an effective tool in monitoring vasospasm in SAH and has been shown in some cases to predict and enhance IV rtPA outcomes. It is also useful in the monitoring of occlusions and stenosis in intracranial vessels.
   b. Detection and identification of AVM blood supply
   c. Preoperative evaluation of collateral capacity of the Circle of Willis
   d. Clinical utility in the assessment of patients with intracranial stenosis, collateral circulation, SAH, and brain death
   e. Provides continuous real-time imaging and can determine the timing of recanalization and reocclusion of vessels capable of visualization by sonography
   f. Used to monitor the response of cerebral vessels to fibrinolytic therapy over time through detecting changes in blood flow and to augment such therapy using ultrasonic energy to enhance clot lysis
   g. Doppler effect
      (1) Reflected or scattered sound waves are shifted to a frequency higher or lower than the incidence frequency if the reflector is moving toward or away from the transducer.
      (2) Frequency is increased toward the transducer, and the frequency shift describes the difference between transmitted and reflected or scattered frequencies.
4. Nursing considerations
   a. Noninvasive, low-risk diagnostic test; no preparation required
5. Advantages and disadvantages
   a. Less accurate than CTA or MRA for stenoocclusive disease
   b. Able to monitor cerebral vessels' response to fibrinolytic therapy over time via continuous, real-time imaging and can predict post-rtPA outcomes
   c. Is not helpful in posterior circulation stroke, has limited use in patients with poor bony windows, and its overall accuracy is dependent on the patient's vascular anatomy and the experience of the technician and interpreter

K. Transthoracic echocardiogram (TTE; Jauch et al., 2013; Strayer et al., 2010)
   1. Description—also known as a cardiac ultrasound. During this noninvasive procedure, an echocardiography transducer or probe is placed on the chest, and images are obtained through the chest wall.
   2. Purpose—assesses heart valves and the degree of heart muscle contraction in all four heart chambers and can determine the strength, condition, and lining of the heart, and the aorta

3. TTE is highly accurate in the identification of cardiac vegetation such as bacteria and blood clots but has up to 20% reduced accuracy in patients who are obese or who have chronic obstructive pulmonary disease or chest wall deformities.
4. Significance: TTE may also have limited use in examining structures at the back of the heart. Bubble contrast TTE involves the injection of agitated saline into a vein, and the bubbles produced by agitation are detected as they enter the right side of the heart. If they directly enter the left side of the heart, this may indicate a patent foramen ovale, atrial or ventricular septal defect, or pulmonary AVMs in the lungs, any of which may have resulted in clot formation, potentially related to a stroke event.
5. Nursing considerations
    a. Patient requires IV access; no other patient preparation is required.
    b. Low-risk procedure
6. Advantages and disadvantages
    a. Noninvasive and highly accurate but may not be useful in some patients
    b. Not useful for detecting posterior cardiac abnormalities
    c. Obesity and body habitus may decrease sensitivity of the exam.

L. Transesophageal echocardiogram (Jauch et al., 2013; Strayer et al., 2010)
1. Description and purpose: A type of echocardiography that utilizes ultrasound waves to assess the size and shape of the heart and the presence of a patent foramen ovale, fluid in the pericardium, or blood clots within the myocardium
2. Procedure: Using mild to moderate sedation, an ultrasound probe is inserted into the esophagus to detect information regarding myocardial function.
3. Nursing considerations
    a. Patient must be kept NPO 6 hours prior to procedure
    b. Adhere to organizational protocol for moderate sedation and monitor patient's recovery; respiratory status assessment should be performed every 15 minutes for 1 hour following procedure.
    c. Patient must be deemed able to swallow.
    d. Patient's informed consent is required because of the invasiveness of the procedure.
    e. Patient will not be able to participate in physical or occupational therapy following procedure.
4. Advantages and disadvantages
    a. Provides clearer images than TTE because there is not attenuation of the ultrasound signal through the chest wall
    b. Takes longer to perform than TTE and is more invasive, requiring sedation in most cases

M. Electroencephalogram (EEG; Hirsch, 2010)
1. Description—uses up to 24 noninvasive scalp electrodes to capture and record electrical fluctuations that occur within the cerebral neurons. Digital racings recorded from each electrode are evaluated for abnormalities in waveform. Electrodes are placed on the scalp with conductive gel or paste.
    a. Each channel represents the difference between two adjacent electrodes.
    b. EEG activity is typically described in terms of rhythmic activity and transients. Rhythmic activity is divided into bands by frequency.
    c. EEG testing is most commonly performed with 20 minutes of EEG waveform recording. Continuous EEG (cEEG) represents ongoing monitoring of EEG waveform for at least 4 hours and often is offered in 24-hour increments.

2. Purpose: The main application of EEG is for the diagnosis and analysis of convulsive and nonconvulsive seizure; however, other uses include the diagnosis of various encephalopathies, sleep disorders, tumors, stroke and other focal brain disorders, and recording of brain activity as a confirmatory exam to determine brain death.
   a. Use of the EEG facilitates correlation of cerebral injury with abnormal EEG patterns in patients with cerebrovascular disease, tumors, and other brain lesions and can facilitate appropriate identification of subclinical seizures in patients with brain injury.
   b. Some evidence indicates that cEEG may detect delayed ischemia associated with vasospasm.
3. Clinical significance
   a. EEG with simultaneous video recording can be diagnostic of epilepsy.
   b. EEG recordings can detect changes that occur in milliseconds, making EEG a suitable choice in the investigation of the action potential across a single neuron, which takes approximately 0.5–130 milliseconds.
4. Nursing considerations
   a. Ensure patient safety if the patient is ambulatory. Institute fall precautions because the patient will be connected to EEG recording via cable, creating fall risk.
   b. If a patient is undergoing cEEG in the ICU
      (1) Work with EEG technicians to maintain integrity of EEG lead contact with scalp, EEG machine operation, and camera recording of the patient.
      (2) Annotate in the EEG and medical record relevant patient motions (e.g., shivering) and care maneuvers (e.g., bathing, cardiopulmonary resuscitation, and dialysis) that may be mistaken for abnormal EEG waveforms.
      (3) Annotate in the EEG and medical record any assessment findings suggestive of seizure activity for correlation to EEG waveform.
      (4) Monitor skin under electrodes for breakdown each shift.
      (5) Communicate with team if significant changes in EEG waveform are noted.
5. Advantages and disadvantages
   a. EEG measures the brain electrical activity directly, while other methods record indirect changes in blood flow or metabolic activity.
   b. EEG recording is inexpensive and noninvasive and may be used in a wide variety of settings, such as in surgery, or may also be used to monitor a comatose patient as well as a cooperative awake patient.
      (1) *Evoked potentials*, or the electrical signals associated with neuron transmission, are generated in response to sensory stimulation and may be used as a diagnostic tool for detecting the presence of cerebral cortex lesions and spinal cord ascending or descending pathways and may also be used in the operating room.
         (a) Types include brain stem auditory evoked responses (BAER), visual evoked potential (VEP), or somatosensory evoked potential (SSEP)
   c. EEG monitoring may be used simultaneously with other methods of looking at brain activity, such as functional MRI and functional near-infrared spectroscopy, to detect changes in blood flow or metabolic activity, which are indirect markers of electrical activity.

N. Electrocardiogram (ECG; Christensen, Fogh Christensen, & Boysen, 2005; Jauch et al., 2013; Strayer et al., 2010)
   1. Description—a painless test used to get snapshot information regarding the electrical activity of the heart, such as the rate and regularity of the heartbeat
   2. Purpose: Cardiac irregularities such as atrial fibrillation that lead to the forming of blood clots are the causative agents for ischemic stroke. ECG abnormalities in acute stroke may predict 6-month mortality. The ECG evaluation of patients with acute stroke provides relevant information regarding an interaction of underlying hypertensive or atherosclerotic cardiovascular disease that may cause ECG changes and contribute to the advent of stroke.
   3. Nursing considerations
      a. Ensure appropriate lead placement to ensure accuracy of ECG tracing.
   4. Advantages
      a. Low cost
      b. Noninvasive
      c. Accessible

O. Carotid Doppler ultrasound
   1. Description—application of noninvasive ultrasound transducer capable of detecting a degree of stenosis at the origin of the internal carotid artery
   2. Purpose—superior method for measuring stenosis or vasospasm of the cervical carotid, vertebral and temporal arteries, and the Circle of Willis; can monitor progression and response to treatment
   3. Indications
      a. Intermittent and follow-up monitoring for stroke and migraine, possible recanalization of occluded vessels, and identification of collateral pathways after occluding interventions or occlusive disease during anticoagulation or fibrinolytic therapies
         (1) Evaluation of the effects of intra- or extracranial occlusive disease on intracranial flow
         (2) Carotid stenosis: Doppler ultrasonography of carotid bifurcation
         (3) Evaluation and characterization of carotid plaque
         (4) Functional tests to obtain response to vasoactive drugs, neuropsychological tests, neurosonography, congenital brain pathology, lesions and anomalies, neoplasias, histogenesis, or neurotubular disorders
         (5) Carotid artery peak systolic velocity and end-diastolic velocity as well as ratios of internal carotid artery and common artery peak systolic velocity have been correlated with angiographic stenosis. Carotid ultrasound sensitivity and specificity for detecting lesions >70% are less than for other modalities (83%–86% for sensitivity and 87%–99% for specificity).
   4. Nursing considerations
      a. No patient preparation required, noninvasive
   5. Advantages and disadvantages
      a. Is safe, inexpensive, reliable, and painless; can be performed at bedside; and can be conducted in both conscious and unconscious patients
      b. Limited ability to image the extracranial vasculature proximal or distal to the bifurcation

P. Chest radiography (Goldstein, 2007)

1. Purpose—used to diagnose pneumonia and gross cardiac abnormalities in selected stroke patients, or as a screening test if lung disease is suspected
2. Indications: The utility of routine chest radiography is debatable in the absence of underlying pulmonary, cardiac, or vascular disease and should not delay the administration of IV rtPA unless there are specific concerns about intrathoracic pathology, including aortic dissection.
3. Nursing considerations: Thorough evaluation of patient's respiratory assessment provides guidance for the exam.

Q. Lumbar puncture (Jauch et al., 2013; Strayer et al., 2010)

1. Description—the insertion of a hollow needle in the subarachnoid space of the lumbar region of the spine at a level between L3/L4 and L4/L5
2. Purpose and indications: Lumbar punctures are performed to withdraw fluid for diagnostic purposes, in cases where elevated intracranial pressure is suspected, or to administer medication.
   a. Diagnostic indications
      (1) Measurement of CSF pressure
      (2) Collection of CSF samples for laboratory analysis
      (3) Determination of the presence of blood in CSF is a confirmatory diagnostic test for SAH.
   b. Therapeutic indications
      (1) Removal of CSF to reduce intracranial pressure
3. Preprocedure: Explain procedure to patient, including positioning, verify informed consent, obtain baseline vital signs, and have patient empty bladder. Review coagulation studies.
4. Procedure: Place patient in lateral position with neck bent in full flexion and knees bent in full flexion to the chest (fetal position). Lower back is prepared using aseptic technique, and after appropriate location is palpated, the physician instills local anesthetic under the skin along the intended path of the spinal needle.
   a. A spinal needle is advanced between the lumbar vertebrae at the level of L3/L4 or L4/L5 until a change in needle pressure signifies that the needle is past the ligamentum flavum. The needle is advanced once more until a second puncture or change in needle pressure is evidenced, indicating that the needle is past the Dura mater. The stylet of the needle is subsequently removed, and drops of CSF are collected. The opening pressure of the CSF is relevant and is monitored using a column manometer.
   b. Pressure may be decreased in dehydration, hyperosmolality or circulatory collapse, subarachnoid blockage, or leakage of spinal fluid.
5. Significance of findings: The presence of white blood cells may indicate meningitis, reactions to prior injections of medicine or dyes, prior hemorrhage, recent seizure, leukemia, or metastatic tumor.
   a. CSF is measured for the presence of chloride, glucose, glutamine, lactate, and various bacterial pathogens.
6. Pressure may be elevated in patients with congestive heart failure, cerebral edema, SAH, hypo-osmolality, meningeal inflammation, meningitis, and hydrocephalus or pseudotumor cerebri.

7. Nursing considerations
   a. Sedation may be required. Utilize moderate sedation protocol if indicated.
   b. The patient's informed consent is required.
   c. Assess the patient for presence of back deformity and ability to maintain proper positioning during procedure.
   d. Observe the patient carefully—opening pressure can be elevated by patient anxiety, especially if the patient is tensing muscles or flexing knees too tightly against the chest.
   e. Keeping the patient as calm as possible during this time is important to identify the rationale for opening pressure.
   f. Postprocedure: Keep patient lying flat for 6 hours or per protocol to prevent headache and to monitor neurologic and vital signs every 15 minutes for 1 hour and respiratory status if sedation was required. Ensure adequate fluid intake, and administer analgesia for headache.

R. Diagnostic laboratory studies (Cucchiara, Jackson, Weiner, & Messe, 2007; Jauch et al., 2013; Rost, Masrur, Pervez, Viswanathan, & Schwamm, 2009)
   1. All patients
      a. Blood glucose
         (1) Low blood sugar can mimic stroke symptoms.
         (2) Hypoglycemia is associated with unfavorable outcomes following stroke.
   2. Although it is desirable to know the results of these laboratory tests before giving IV recombinant tissue type plasminogen activator, fibrinolytic therapy should not be delayed while awaiting the results unless there is a clinical suspicion of bleeding abnormality or thrombocytopenia, the patient has received heparin or warfarin, or the patient has received other anticoagulants.
      a. Serum electrolytes
      b. Complete blood count including platelets
         (1) Should be greater than 100,000 cells/ml
      c. Renal function tests
      d. Markers of cardiac ischemia
         (1) Cardiac markers are elevated in ischemic stroke in up to 34% of cases. This elevation may signify the presence of myocardial infarction in conjunction with or preceding the ischemic stroke event. Cardiac markers are also elevated in some patients with ICH and SAH.
            (a) Troponin T is associated with increased stroke severity and mortality as well as poor outcomes.
      e. PT, aPTT, INR
         (1) Fibrinolytic therapy should not be delayed while awaiting the results of PT, aPTT, or platelet count unless bleeding abnormality or thrombocytopenia is suspected.
            (a) These tests are helpful if warfarin or heparin has recently been administered.
            (b) These tests are not helpful if dabigatran was administered to the patient.
      f. Thrombin time is a sensitive indicator to presence of dabigatran.
      g. Ecarin clotting time excludes a significant direct thrombin inhibitor effect.
   3. Examination of the CSF has a limited role in the acute evaluation of patients with suspected stroke, unless there is a strong suspicion for SAH or an acute central nervous system infection.

References

Adams, H., del Zoppo, G., Alberts, M., Bhatt, D., Brass L., Furlan, A., ...Wijdicks, E. (2007). Guidelines for the early management of adults with ischemic stroke: A guideline from the American Heart Association/American Stroke Association Stroke Council, Clinical Cardiology Council, Cardiovascular Radiology and Intervention Council, and the Atherosclerotic Peripheral Vascular Disease and Quality of Care Outcomes in Research Interdisciplinary Working Groups. *Stroke, 38*(6), 1655–1711.

Arakawa, S., Wright, P., Koga, M, Phan, T., Reutens, D., Lim, I., ... Donnan, G. (2006). Ischemic thresholds for gray and white matter: A diffusion and perfusion magnetic resonance study. *Stroke, 37*(5), 1211–1216.

Bammer, R., & Moseley, M. (2005). Perfusion magnetic resonance and the perfusion/diffusion mismatch in stroke. In R. E. Latchaw, J. Kucharczyk, & M. E. Moseley (Eds.), *Imaging of the nervous system: Diagnostic and therapeutic applications* (pp. 227–248). Philadelphia, PA: Elsevier Mosby.

Barber, P., Darby, D., Desmond, P., Gerraty, R., Yang, Q., Li,T., ... Davis, S. (1999). Identification of major ischemic change: Diffusion-weighted imaging versus computed tomography. *Stroke, 30*(10), 2059–2065.

Christensen, H., Fogh Christensen, A., & Boysen, G. (2005). Abnormalities on ECG and telemetry predict stroke outcome at 3 months. *Journal of Neurological Sciences, 234*(1–2), 99–103.

Christensen, S., Parsons, M., De Silva, D., Ebinger, M., Butcher, K., Fink, J., & Davis, S. (2008). Optimal mismatch definitions for detecting treatment response in acute stroke. *Cerebrovascular Diseases, 25*(suppl 2), 33.

Cucchiara, B., Jackson, B., Weiner, M., & Messe, S. (2007). Usefulness of checking platelet count before thrombolysis in acute ischemic stroke. *Stroke, 38*(5), 1639–1640.

Demchuk, A., Hill, M., Barber, P., Silver, B., Patel, S., Levine, S., & NINDS rtPA Stroke Study Group, NIH. (2005). Importance of early ischemic computed tomography changes using ASPECTS in NINDS rtPA Stroke Study. *Stroke, 36*(10), 2110–2115.

Dzialowski, I., Hill, M., Coutts, S., Demchuk, A., Kent, D., Wunderlich, O., & von Kummer, R. (2006). Extent of early ischemic changes on computed tomography (CT) before thrombolysis: Prognostic value of the Alberta Stroke Program Early CT Score in ECASS II. *Stroke, 37*(4), 973–978.

European Stroke Organisation (ESO) Executive Committee & ESO Writing Committee. (2008). Guidelines for management of ischaemic stroke and transient ischaemic attack 2008. *Cerebrovascular Diseases, 25*(5), 457–507.

Fiebach, J., Schellinger, P., Jansen, O., Meyer, M., Wilde, P., Bender, J., ... Sartor, K. (2002). CT and diffusion-weighted MRI in randomized order: Diffusion-weighted imaging results in higher accuracy and lower interrater variability in the diagnosis of hyperacute ischemic stroke. *Stroke, 33*(9), 2206–2210.

Goldstein, L. (2007). Stroke code chest radiographs are not useful. *Cerebrovascular Diseases, 24*(5), 460–462.

Hacke, W., Kaste, M., Fieschi, C., Toni, D., Lesaffre, E., von Kummer, R., . . . Hennerici, M. (1995). Intravenous thrombolysis with recombinant tissue plasminogen activator for acute hemispheric stroke: The European Cooperative Acute Stroke Study (ECASS). *Journal of the American Medical Association, 274*(13), 1017–1025.

Hacke, W., Kaste, M., Bluhmki, E., Brozman, M., Dávalos, A., Guidetti, D., . . . Toni, D. (2008). Thrombolysis with alteplase 3 to 4.5 hours after acute ischemic stroke. *New England Journal of Medicine, 359*, 1317–1329.

Hirsch, L. (2010). Urgent continuous EEG (cEEG) monitoring leads to changes in treatment in half of cases. *Epilepsy Currents, 10*(4), 82–85.

Jauch, E., Saver, J., Adams, H., Bruno, A., Connors, J., Demaerschalk, B., ...Yonas, H. (2013). Guidelines for the early management of patients with acute ischemic stroke. *Stroke, 44,* 870–947.

Keir, S., Wardlaw, J., Bastin, M., & Dennis, M. (2004). In which patients is diffusion weighted magnetic resonance imaging most useful in routine stroke care? *Journal of Neuroimaging, 14*(2), 118–122.

Kidwell, C., Villablanca, J., & Saver, J. (2000). Advances in neuroimaging of acute stroke. *Current Atherosclerosis Reports, 2*(2),126–135.

Mohr, J., Biller, J., Hilal, S., Yuh, W., Tatemichi, T., Hedges, S., . . . Marler, J. (1995). Magnetic resonance versus computed tomographic imaging in acute stroke. *Stroke, 26*(5), 807–812

Patel, S., Levine, S., Tilley, B., Grotta, J., Lu, M., Frankel, M., ...Welch, K. (2001). Lack of clinical significance of early ischemic changes on computed tomography in acute stroke. *Journal of the American Medical Association, 286*(22), 2830–2838.

Rost, S., Masrur, S., Pervez, M., Viswanathan, A., & Schwamm, L. (2009). Unsuspected coagulopathy rarely prevents IV thrombolysis in acute ischemic stroke. *Neurology, 73*(23), 1957–1962.

Schellinger, P., Bryan, R., Caplan, L., Detre, J., Edelman, R., Jaigobin, C., … Warach, S. (2010). Evidence-based guideline: The role of diffusion and perfusion MRI for the diagnosis of acute ischemic stroke: Report of the Therapeutics and Technology Assessment Subcommittee of the American Academy of Neurology. *Neurology, 75*(2), 177–185.

Seifert, T., Enzinger, C., Storch, M., Pichler, G., Niederkorn, K., & Fazekas, F. (2005). Acute small subcortical infarctions on diffusion weighted MRI: Clinical presentation and aetiology. *Journal of Neurological Neurosurgical Psychiatry, 76*(11), 1520–1524.

Strayer, A., Prendergast, V., & Henwood, A. (2010). Spine disorders. In M. Bader & L. Littlejohns (Eds.), *AANN core curriculum for neuroscience nursing* (pp. 458–492). Glenview, IL: American Association of Neuroscience Nurses.

von Kummer, R., Bourquain, H., Bastianello, S., Bozzao, L., Manelfe, C., Meier, D., & Hack, W. (2001). Early prediction of irreversible brain damage after ischemic stroke at CT. *Radiology, 219*(1), 95–100.

Wahlgren, N., Ahmed, N., Eriksson, N., Aichner, F., Bluhmki, E., Dávalos, A., … Vanhooren, G. (2008). Multivariable analysis of outcome predictors and adjustment of main outcome results to baseline data profile in randomized controlled trials: Safe Implementation of Thrombolysis in Stroke-Monitoring STudy (SITS-MOST). *Stroke, 39*(12), 3316–3322.

Wessels, T., Röttger, C., Jauss, M., Kaps, M., Traupe, H., & Stolz, E. (2005). Identification of embolic stroke patterns by diffusion-weighted MRI in clinically defined lacunar stroke syndromes. *Stroke, 36*(4), 757–761.

Chapter

5

Acute Care

Sarah Livesay, DNP RN ACNP-BC CNS-BC SCRN

With contributions by Angela West, MSN RN CCRN CNRN, and Susan Wilson, MSN RN C-ANP

The hours and days after an acute ischemic stroke, intracerebral hemorrhage (ICH), or subarachnoid hemorrhage (SAH) follow a generally predictable trajectory of stroke evolution, development of complications, and recovery. The immediate care of the patient with ischemic stroke, ICH, and SAH, including recognition of the event, stabilization, and immediate interventions, are covered in chapter 3. This chapter will focus on the acute care of stroke patients.

Objectives

1. Understand and implement general acute stroke care and acute care specific to ischemic stroke, ICH, and SAH.
2. Collaborate with other healthcare teams, using a holistic approach to provide quality nursing care.
3. Identify disorders that commonly and uncommonly lead to stroke syndromes.

Defining the Stroke Timeline

A. The exact moment of transition from hyperacute to acute care is difficult to define, particularly in the care of ICH and SAH patients, and many interventions initiated in the hyperacute phase of care carry through to the acute phase of care (Summers et al., 2009).
   1. Ischemic stroke: Acute ischemic stroke care is often divided into two phases.
      a. Phase 1 of stroke care is defined as hyperacute and spans the prehospital care of the stroke patient in the first hours of stroke through the first 24 hours of care.
      b. Phase 1 includes emergency department (ED) protocols to triage the suspected stroke patient, identify a stroke, initiate thrombolytics and intra-arterial therapies as appropriate, and admit the patient to the appropriate level of care in the hospital.
      c. The acute phase, or phase 2 of stroke care, generally describes the 24–72-hour period after stroke ictus or until hospital discharge.
   2. ICH: The acute phase of ICH care generally begins as the patient is admitted to a hospital unit, generally the intensive care unit (ICU), from the ED and continues through hospital discharge.

3. SAH: The acute phase of SAH care generally begins as the patient is admitted to a hospital unit, generally the ICU, from the ED and continues through hospital discharge.

Implementing Generalized Acute Stroke Care: Stroke-Focused Health Assessment

A. During the first hours and days after ischemic stroke, ICH, or SAH, patients are at risk for rapid decline in their neurologic status and stroke-related complications (Summers et al., 2009).

 1. The stroke nurse must have expertise in conducting a neurologic exam and understand how the exam findings correlate to the anatomical location and pathophysiology of the stroke syndrome. The stroke nurse then can identify the patient's needs and prioritize appropriate interventions.

B. A number of scales are frequently used in the care of stroke patients.

 1. Function of stroke scales
  a. Facilitating clinical research
  b. Assessment of stroke deficit or clinical severity
  c. Estimating prognosis and functional recovery after stroke
  d. Estimating the patients' likelihood of experiencing certain common complications associated with their stroke syndrome
  e. Many patients will require assessment with multiple scales throughout their course of care.
 2. Stroke scales applied in the in-patient setting after the hyperacute phase of care
  a. Coma assessment scores
   (1) Glasgow Coma Scale (GCS): The GCS is the most widely studied coma score; it was initially developed in the mid 1970s to assess the patient's level of consciousness after traumatic brain injury (TBI).
    (a) Three assessment parameters: eye opening, verbal response, and motor response, with patients scoring between a minimum score of 3 and a maximum score of 15. The GCS is widely used outside of TBI because of its ease and speed of administration (McNett et al., 2014).
    (b) The GCS poses significant limitations when used as the primary assessment of stroke patients. Studies on the GCS demonstrate only moderate interrater reliability. Intubated patients and patients with aphasia are difficult to assess using the scale. Patients with stroke may worsen or improve significantly before registering a change on the GCS scale (Kornbluth & Bhardwaj, 2011).
   (2) FOUR score—A newer coma assessment scale, incorporating brain stem reflex assessment and intubation whereas the GCS does not include these assessment parameters. The FOUR score assesses eye reaction, motor function, brain stem reflexes, and respiratory pattern. The score exceeds the GCS in 30-day outcome prediction power (Chen, Grothe, & Schaller, 2013).
  b. Ischemic stroke scores
   (1) National Institutes of Health Stroke Scales (NIHSS)—quantitatively measures 15 neurological assessment items, including level of consciousness, extraocular movement, visual fields, facial muscle function, extremity strength, sensory function, coordination, language, speech, and hemi-inattention (Kasner, 2006)
    (a) Originally designed for clinical trials, validity is established in predicting long-term outcomes as well (Kasner, 2006)

(b) Stroke score correlates with infarct volume, with a higher score correlating with a larger infarct volume.

(c) Score is predictive of outcome at 7 days and 2 months, with excellent outcomes associated with a score of 3 or less and few patients with a score of 15 or more having excellent outcomes after 3 months. It may also be useful in predicting hospital discharge status, with a score of 5 or less predictive of discharge home, a score of 7–13 associated with inpatient rehabilitation, and a score of 14 or more generally requiring care in a long-term acute care facility or nursing facility.

(d) Allows for comparison of the stroke exam between clinicians and trending of the stroke exam over time, particularly in the hyperacute and acute settings

(e) A change in NIHSS of 2–4 points or more is associated with a clinically relevant change in neurologic status.

(2) Modified NIHSS (mNIHSS): The mNIHSS is an abbreviated version of the NIHSS. Several items of the NIHSS that were shown in multiple studies to have poor reliability and redundancy were removed. The mNIHSS has demonstrated greater reliability in multiple cohorts than the NIHSS and has been studied in multiple settings, including telemedicine, for acute stroke management. The scale removes level of consciousness, facial palsy, and dysarthria, and simplifies the sensory item. The scale quantifies the degree of stroke deficit, with a higher number indicating a larger stroke and more significant deficit. The mNIHSS is often used in ongoing assessment of patients when they are admitted to the hospital (Meyer & Lyden, 2009). The full NIHSS may be more appropriate during the acute intervention of administering thrombolytics, and the mNIHSS may be used for ongoing neurologic assessment in the days following hospital admission (Summers et al., 2009).

(3) Israeli Vertebrobasilar Stroke Scale (IVBSS): The IVBSS is an 11-item scale that incorporates posterior circulation signs and symptoms missing in the NIHSS, including diplopia, dysphagia, and gait assessment. A significant limitation to the NIHSS is the absence of several posterior circulation stroke symptoms and the lack of adequate weighting of posterior circulation stroke symptoms. The maximum score on the IVBSS is 44. The score may be used to assess ischemic and hemorrhagic stroke patients. Interrater reliability and concurrent validity is adequate, and the scale may better represent posterior circulation strokes compared with the NIHSS (Gur et al., 2007).

c. Hemorrhagic stroke scores

(1) ICH score: Developed and published in 2001, the score is an outcome prediction tool conducted during initial ICH presentation. The score has been validated for a 30-day mortality, 12-month functional outcome (Hemphill, Bonovich, Besmertis, Manley, & Johnston, 2001).

(a) Patients are graded according to admission GCS, initial hematoma volume, presence of intraventricular hemorrhage, infratentorial location of bleed, and age. Patients may receive a score of 1–6.

(b) A score of 1 is associated with a 13% 30-day mortality. A score of 2 is associated with a 26% chance of 30-day mortality. A score of 3 is associated with a 72% chance of 30-day mortality. A score of 4 is associated with

97% chance of 30-day mortality. A score of 5 or 6 is associated with a 100% chance of 30-day mortality.

(2) Hunt and Hess Score: Originally developed in 1968 as a tool to identify ideal timing of surgical intervention, the score has also been shown to correlate with outcome after SAH (Rosen & Macdonald, 2005).

(a) Score is graded 1–5 and incorporates three clinical axes.

(b) The score has been modified over the years and now includes a score of 0 for unruptured aneurysms and 1a for fixed neurologic deficit in the absence of other signs of SAH.

(c) Criticisms of the score include vague definitions of level of consciousness and the presence of three clinical axes, which occasionally forces the clinician to choose between classes.

(d) Another score modification occasionally employed is the addition of one grade level if the patient has severe systemic disease or severe vasospasm.

(e) Outcomes for patients in grades 4 and 5 are worse than for patients in grades 1, 2, or 3. However, the scale's ambiguity has called into question data that correlate score with outcome.

(3) World Federation of Neurological Surgeons Scale—developed in the late 1980s to clarify terminology and includes elements of the GCS and focal neurologic deficits (Rosen & Macdonald, 2005)

(a) Score is graded 1–5 and is based on GCS and presence of motor deficit.

(b) Studies generally report a step-wise association between increasing scores and worsening outcomes. However, data are mixed, with some studies showing no significant difference in outcomes between adjacent grades.

(4) Fisher Scale—originally developed to predict cerebral vasospasm (Rosen & Macdonald, 2005)

(a) Assigns patients a score of 1–4 based on assessment of blood volume during the initial computed tomography (CT) scan. A higher score is associated with a higher likelihood of cerebral vasospasm.

(b) Score has since been studied and correlated to clinical outcomes, particularly in combination with the Hunt and Hess Score.

(c) Score was developed before recent advances in imaging and does not take into account clot density or clearing rate.

d. Transient ischemic attack (TIA) scores

(1) $ABCD^2$ score—risk assessment tool used with TIA patients to assess their risk of stroke immediately following and up to 90 days after the stroke. The nurse who provides acute care for the TIA patient must understand the relevance of this score, because a high-risk patient may be admitted to the hospital for several days to complete his or her diagnostic evaluation and implement secondary stroke prevention.

(2) Score includes five factors: age of 60 years or older, elevated systolic or diastolic blood pressure, presence of unilateral weakness or speech impairment during TIA event, TIA duration more or less than 60 minutes, and the presence of diabetes at the time of the TIA (Johnston et al., 2007).

(3) The score may range from 0 to 7. Higher scores are associated with a greater risk of stroke at 2, 7, 30, and 90 days.

(4) The score is often used to risk stratify patients to determine the need for immediate hospitalization or follow up at an outpatient clinic (Johnston, et al., 2007).

(a) Generally, patients with a score of 0–3 have a 1% 2-day stroke risk and a 0%–3.5% 90-day stroke risk. These patients are often discharged and followed in the outpatient setting.
(b) Patients with a score of 4–5 have a 4.1% 2-day stroke risk and an 8%–12% 90-day stroke risk, therefore justifying hospital admission for observation, diagnostic work-up, and immediate initiation of stroke prevention measures.
(c) Patients with a score of 6–7 have an 8.1% 2-day stroke risk and a 17%–22% 90-day stroke risk, warranting hospital admission for observation, diagnostic work-up, and immediate initiation of stroke prevention measures.

e. Stroke outcome scales
(1) Modified Rankin Scale (mRS): The mRS was modified in the late 1980s to achieve a comprehensive stroke-outcomes scale (Wilson et al., 2002). The score measures functional independence in the areas of body function, activity, and participation. The score ranges from 0, measured as no symptoms, to 6, measured as clinically dead. A certification program exists to ensure the reliability of the score, particularly when used in clinical trials. Although the scale measures functional disability, it does not quantify disability such as aphasia, visual field deficits, or cognitive or emotional impairment. The mRS may be trended over time through stroke recovery (Kasner, 2006).
(2) Barthel Index (BI): The BI is a self-care and mobility measurement scale in which a normal score is 100 and the lower the score the higher the disability and dependency. The BI score generally correlates with infarct volume for ischemic stroke (Collin, Wade, Davies, & Horne, 1988). The BI has not been correlated to hemorrhagic stroke size. The score may be trended over time to assess progression of dependency. However, patients with a high degree of mobility and function but some disability may score high. The score does not adequately quantify disability in high-functioning stroke survivors (Kasner, 2006).
(3) Functional Independence Measure (FIM): The FIM measures 18 activities of daily living (ADLs), including self-care, sphincter control, transfers, locomotion, communication, and social cognition, to estimate the level of assistance needed (Cavanagh, Hogan, Gordon, & Fairfax, 2000). Patients are ranked on a scale of 1–7, in which 1 indicates total assistance and 7 complete independence. The FIM score is often used to measure inpatient rehabilitation progress (Kasner, 2006).

3. Use of scores as an ongoing measure of neurologic status and stroke progression
   a. Many patients will require the use of multiple scores to assist with care planning during the course of their stroke.
   b. Scores may be used to enroll patients in clinical trials, quantify assessment parameters, guide interventions, trend progress, and plan discharge care.
   c. Multiple scores are often used to trend neurologic nursing assessments over hours, shift-to-shift, or at specific time points during hospital admission and discharge. No one model for assessment utilizing scales is identified in the literature as superior. Use of stroke scales is generally guided by stroke program policy and procedure.
4. Ongoing neurologic assessment
   a. Frequency: The frequency of assessment is dictated by patient acuity and the risk for complication or decline.

(1) Patients with acute ischemic stroke are at risk for decline after thrombolytic administration, other emergent interventions, and in the first few hours after stroke. Neurologic assessment must be frequent in these settings. See chapter 3.

(2) Assessment is generally dictated by the risk for decline and level of care. Frequent neurologic assessments, generally defined as occurring every 15 minutes or sooner, are necessary in an acute situation in which the patient is fluctuating or deteriorating. Otherwise, the frequency of assessment is generally dictated by the level of care, hospital policy and procedure, and practitioner orders.

b. Contents

(1) Trending of the neurologic assessment in a stroke patient should include all pertinent assessment parameters that are necessary to detect improvement or deterioration in patient status.

(2) Although a coma scale may be used in the assessment of stroke patients, a coma scale alone generally is not specific enough to identify subtle changes in neurologic exam and should be combined with additional assessment parameters.

(3) The NIHSS is often used to trend neurologic assessment in stroke patients and is generally recommended with any decline in patient status (Summers et al., 2009). The NIHSS is often used to assess hemorrhagic stroke patients as well; however, clear parameters for the use of the NIHSS to trend the neurologic exam in patients with ICH and SAH have not been developed.

(4) Ongoing neurologic assessment should include the assessment of any parameters that are likely to be affected by ischemic and hemorrhagic stroke, including level of consciousness, cognition, movement and sensory function, speech and language function, neglect, and inattention.

C. Conduct comprehensive assessment

1. History of present illness

a. The history of present illness is usually obtained during the hyperacute phase of ischemic and hemorrhagic stroke care. During the acute phase of care, the Stroke Certified Registered Nurse (SCRN) should be knowledgeable about the history of stroke onset to guide continued care.

2. Head-to-toe assessment

a. The first priority when stabilizing the stroke patient is always to address the ABCs: airway, breathing, and circulation.

(1) Initial stabilization and the first few hours of acute stroke management are addressed in chapter 3.

b. Stroke-related head-to-toe assessment

(1) When a patient is admitted to the hospital for an ischemic or hemorrhagic stroke, the SCRN should conduct a head-to-toe exam with a focus on clinical information related to stroke (Jauch et al., 2013).

(a) Head, eyes, ears, nose, and throat assessment: Evaluate the patient who has any sign of cranial or peripheral trauma that might suggest trauma or seizure as the origin of his or her symptoms. Assess the patient's neck for carotid bruit that might suggest carotid disease or jugular venous distension that might suggest heart failure or fluid overload; both findings may suggest cardiovascular illness contributing to stroke development (Jauch et al., 2013).

(b) Chest and lung assessment: Evaluate the patient for the presence of cardiac dysrhythmia, murmur, or rales, because this suggests that cardiovascular illness is potentially contributing to stroke development (Jauch et al., 2013).

(c) Musculoskeletal assessment: Evaluate the patient for signs of coagulopathy, embolic disease, or trauma, including ecchymosis, Janeway lesions, or Osler nodes. *Janeway lesions* are small, non-painful, erythematous lesions on the palms or soles that suggest infectious endocarditis. *Osler's nodes* are painful erythematous lesions on the hands and feet that also suggest infectious endocarditis (Jauch et al., 2013).

(d) The patient's history should correlate with his or her signs and symptoms. If a discrepancy is noted, further investigation is warranted.

Acute Care Diagnostic Testing

A. SCRN role

1. Facilitate diagnostic tests according to stroke guidelines and research.
2. Understand the indications, contraindications, and pre- and posttest care for the diagnostic test.
3. Facilitate patient and family education regarding the testing.
4. Please refer to chapter 4 for more details on each test.

B. CT imaging

1. Noncontrast CT imaging of the brain and neck allows for rapid identification of hemorrhage and other abnormalities, such as cerebral edema, mass effect, and structural pathology that may mimic stroke, such as trauma (Siddiqui, Bekker, & Qureshi, 2011; Tong, Hou, Fiebach, & Wintermark, 2014).
   a. Ischemic stroke will not be apparent on noncontrast CT for several hours. Advanced CT imaging, such as CT angiography and CT perfusion, may be helpful in identifying vascular malformations or a blood clot in the brain vasculature.
   b. ICH and SAH are generally visible on CT imaging within moments of bleeding occurring.
   c. CT imaging usually is conducted in the emergent workup of stroke to identify the stroke syndrome.
   d. CT imaging is often conducted throughout the hospital stay to monitor for stroke, hemorrhage progression, or new stroke, or to evaluate the progression of edema, shift, or brain herniation.

C. Magnetic resonance imaging (MRI)

1. MRI of the brain and neck consists of several sequences including T1 weighted, T2 weighted, fluid-attenuated inversion recovery, diffusion weighted imaging, and gradient echo (Siddiqui et al., 2011; Tong et al., 2014).
   a. MRI may be helpful for identifying acute ischemia, hemorrhage, or old ischemia, and structural abnormalities such as tumor, infection, or vascular malformations.
   b. Most poststroke MRI is completed without contrast unless there is clinical concern that there may be a tumor or infection, which would necessitate contrast administration.
   c. Most stroke patients undergo an MRI during their hospital admission to evaluate their stroke and help identify the underlying pathophysiology contributing to their stroke.

D. Additional vascular imaging including angiography
   1. Certain ischemic stroke and ICH patients and nearly all SAH patients may require further vascular imaging beyond CT and MRI (Siddiqui et al., 2011; Tong et al., 2014).
      a. Catheter angiography is generally accepted as the most sensitive test for assessing cerebral vasculature and is helpful in diagnosing cerebral aneurysms, arteriovenous malformation (AVM), dissection, and other vascular abnormalities.
      b. Occasionally, the clinical team may determine the presence of a vascular malformation from a CT or MRI.
      c. Most often, patients with vascular lesions causing the ischemic stroke, ICH, or SAH undergo diagnostic catheter angiography.
      d. Several therapeutic treatments are often provided at the time of diagnostic angiography, including coil embolization of an aneurysm; embolization of AVM; angioplasty and stenting of a narrowed artery; administration of medication directly into the cerebral arterial vasculature, such as tissue plasminogen activator (tPA) into a large vessel thrombus or nicardipine into an artery with vasospasm; and mechanical thrombectomy to remove a thrombus in a large artery.
   2. Carotid doppler ultrasound may be indicated to assess the carotid arteries in a patient who did not receive neck vessel imaging from a CT or MRI.
      a. Carotid doppler ultrasound may show evidence of atherosclerosis in the neck that might be the source of ischemic stroke. The evaluation of neck vessels as a possible source of stroke is often completed using CT or MR angiography imaging. Studies continue to evaluate the role of carotid artery plaque in stroke (Bayer-Karpinska et al., 2013).
   3. Transcranial doppler (TCD) is an ultrasound of cranial arteries to determine the presence of vessel occlusion or vessel narrowing, such as in ischemic stroke and vasospasm in SAH (Purkayastha & Sorond, 2012).
      a. TCD velocities are trended over time and may indicate the presence of cerebral vasospasm before the patient exhibits clinical signs and symptoms.
      b. TCD may be trended in patients with SAH undergoing treatment for cerebral vasospasm.

E. Cardiac imaging
   1. Echocardiogram is often performed during the care of patients with all stroke subtypes.
      a. Echocardiography in an ischemic stroke patient may reveal potential sources of cardioembolic ischemic stroke, including the presence of blood clots in the heart, valve dysfunction, and decreased ejection fraction.
      b. For patients with ICH and SAH, echocardiogram assessment of ejection fraction and systolic or diastolic dysfunction may support the diagnosis of chronic hypertension and may change patient management if the patient has heart failure (Connolly et al., 2012; Jauch et al., 2013; Morgenstern et al., 2010).
      c. Echocardiogram is available via several approaches, including transthoracic and transesophageal.

F. Additional lab work
   1. A variety of additional lab work may be ordered to monitor the effect of new or titrated medications and for further stroke work-up after hospital admission.

G. All testing requires monitoring of patient safety before, during, and after diagnostic and therapeutic procedures. Please refer to chapter 4 for additional information.

Acute Stroke Care

A. Admission to a specialized unit

1. The role of the stroke unit

a. Approximately 25% of patients with ischemic stroke will deteriorate clinically during the first 1–2 days, and patients with ICH and SAH are at risk for deterioration from hemorrhage expansion, edema progression, and herniation (Jauch et al., 2013).

b. Specialized monitoring by an interdisciplinary team with stroke expertise is central to the prevention and early recognition of complications, initiation of early rehabilitation activities, and overall improved outcomes in stroke patients.

c. Specialized care administered in a stroke unit is associated with lower morbidity and mortality in patients with ischemic stroke.

d. Centers that care for higher volumes of stroke patients, particularly hemorrhagic stroke patients, generally have patients with better outcomes (Connolly et al., 2012).

e. Interdisciplinary coordination of care and regular communication between team members is a hallmark of stroke units (Jauch et al., 2013).

B. Patient monitoring

1. The SCRN must collaborate with other healthcare teams and use a holistic approach that is based on the patient's identified needs when providing quality nursing care.

a. Implement emergency nursing measures if needed.

(1) If the stroke patient deteriorates clinically, indicating worsening or a new stroke, or experiences a complication from a stroke, proper response to the emergency is paramount.

(a) Stroke patients are at risk for further stroke, a new stroke, or a stroke complication.

1) Neurologic stroke complications include cerebral edema, herniation, secondary brain injury after a hemorrhage, and seizure.

2) Systemic complications include venous thromboembolism, pulmonary embolism (PE), aspiration pneumonia, and other infections.

b. Nursing care includes monitoring, reporting any abnormal findings, and documentation.

(1) Neuroassessment and vital signs

(a) Frequency of neurologic assessment and vital sign monitoring during the acute phase of care should be tailored to the patient's level of care and likelihood of deterioration, as well as hospital standards.

(2) Cardiac rate and rhythm

(a) Continuous cardiac monitoring is recommended for the first 24 hours after an ischemic stroke (Jauch et al., 2013).

(b) Cardiac monitoring is necessary to screen for atrial fibrillation and other cardiac arrhythmias that contribute to the cause of the stroke.

(c) Most patients with an ICH or SAH are admitted to the neurocritical care unit, where they undergo continuous cardiac and blood pressure monitoring.

(d) Blood pressure monitoring

1) Ischemic stroke patient

a) Blood pressure monitoring in the first 24 hours according to thrombolytic status is covered in chapter 3.

b) After the first 24 hours of care, frequency of blood pressure monitoring and blood pressure targets will depend on the patient's clinical course. Generally, permissive hypertension is allowed for patients with ischemic stroke as discussed later in this chapter. However, the goal blood pressure must be individualized to the patient according to their clinical course.

2) ICH and SAH

a) Patients with ICH and SAH require frequent blood pressure monitoring in the hours and days following their stroke. Specific targets are discussed later in this chapter.

(3) Proper oxygenation and ventilation

(a) During the first several days after a stroke, hypoxia frequently occurs for several reasons, including airway obstruction, hypoventilation, aspiration, atelectasis, and pneumonia (Jauch et al., 2013).

(b) Patients may also exhibit abnormal breathing patterns, such as central periodic breathing, particularly in patients with middle cerebral artery or brain stem stroke.

(c) Hypoxia should be corrected with supplemental oxygen to maintain oxygen saturation >94%. The cause of hypoxia should be investigated (Jauch et al., 2013).

(d) Routine supplemental use of oxygen in the absence of hypoxia should be avoided.

(4) Readiness for activity

(a) Stroke patients should participate in early mobilization and rehabilitation. Patients should be assessed for stability before participating in activity (Jauch et al., 2013).

(5) Pain assessment and management

(a) Pain occurs for various reasons during hospitalization for all types of stroke (Connolly et al., 2012; Jauch et al., 2013; Morgenstern et al., 2010)

1) Pain may be related to the initial stroke event, particularly in ICH and SAH patients.

2) Pain may be related to the management of stroke, including mechanical ventilation, testing, or other interventions initiated during the acute phase of stroke recovery.

3) Pain may be related to positioning, particularly in patients with paretic limbs (Lin et al., 2013).

4) Chronic pain is a well-known complication for stroke survivors.

(b) Pain should be assessed frequently, and pharmacologic and nonpharmacologic interventions should be provided to achieve adequate pain control.

C. Blood and glucose management (Godoy, Di Napoli, & Rabinstein, 2010)

1. Brain cells require a constant source of glucose for metabolism. Even only seconds without adequate glucose for metabolism results in cell injury and subsequent death.
2. Even a single episode of hypoglycemia is associated with increased morbidity and mortality in brain-injured patients.
3. The brain consumes 20%–25% of the body's total glucose at any given time when in a steady, healthy state.
4. Injured brain cells do not tolerate hyperglycemia. Hyperglycemia elicits an inflammatory and an oxidative stress response, impacting overall metabolism, cerebral perfusion, and the injured cell's ability to repair itself. Hyperglycemia is associated with increased morbidity and mortality in all types of stroke.

D. Ischemic stroke-associated hyperglycemia
  1. Occurs in 30%–40% of patients with acute ischemic stroke, most without a known history of diabetes mellitus (Luitse, Biessels, Rutten, & Kappelle, 2012)
  2. Hyperglycemia after stroke results from a neuroendocrine stress response as well as an inflammatory response to injury. Therefore, stroke patients may be hyperglycemic even if they have no history of diabetes mellitus or being prediabetic (Radermecker & Scheen, 2010).
  3. Hypergycemia after stroke may also exacerbate known or unknown diabetes.
  4. The degree of hyperglycemia after stroke often correlates with the size of the stroke (Radermecker & Scheen, 2010).
  5. Patients with hyperglycemia after stroke have worse outcomes, and those without an underlying history of diabetes have worse outcomes in particular (Radermecker & Scheen, 2010).
  6. Management
    a. Measurement: Glucose should be routinely measured upon hospital admission and frequently thereafter. No standard exists that states the recommended frequency of measurement. However, most facilities monitor glucose every 4–8 hours and more frequently when necessary.
    b. Hourly glucose measurement is necessary for patients with marked hyperglycemia that needs an insulin infusion for adequate management.
    c. The ideal target glucose range for managing hyperglycemia is a matter of debate and ongoing study. Current consensus is to treat glucose to a range of 140–180 mm/dL. When patients require insulin infusions, great care should be taken to titrate the infusion to avoid hypoglycemia.
    d. Glucose-lowering treatment options include intravenous (IV) and subcutaneous insulin as well as oral antihyperglycemic medication.
  7. Hypoglycemia in ischemic stroke
    a. Hypoglycemia should be avoided as previously discussed. Hypoglycemia should be rapidly corrected with slow IV push of 25 mL of 50% dextrose (Jauch et al., 2013).

E. Hyperglycemia in SAH
  1. Hyperglycemia is associated with higher grade SAH and age older than 54 years. Prolonged glucose higher than 105 mm/dL during the first 10 days of an SAH is associated with significant multi-organ complications and is an independent predictor of death (Frontera et al., 2006; Godoy et al., 2010).
  2. Research is needed to identify the ideal target blood glucose range for SAH patients.

F. Hyperglycemia in ICH
  1. Hyperglycemia during the first 72 hours after an ICH is associated with increased mortality. Elevated glucose is also associated with hematoma expansion after initial ICH (Godoy et al., 2010).
  2. Measurement: Glucose should be routinely measured upon admission to the hospital and frequently thereafter. No standard exists stating the recommended frequency of measurement. However, most facilities monitor glucose every 4–8 hours and more frequently when necessary.
  3. Hourly glucose measurement is necessary for patients with marked hyperglycemia who need an insulin infusion for adequate management.
  4. The ideal target glucose range for managing hyperglycemia is a matter of debate and ongoing study. Current consensus is to achieve a glucose range of 140–180 mm/dL. When

patients require insulin infusions, great care should be taken to titrate the infusion to avoid hypoglycemia.

G. Neuroprotective properties of insulin
   1. Several studies demonstrate that insulin may confer neuroprotective properties by limiting free radicle formation and inflammation after brain injury (Godoy et al., 2010).
   2. Trials evaluating the role of intensive insulin control for stroke patients are inconclusive.

H. Targeted temperature management
   1. Incidence of fever in stroke
      a. Fever is common in patients with all types of stroke. Seventy percent of brain-injured patients experience fever, yet only half of the fever episodes are related to infection. *Central fever* is defined as a spontaneous increase in temperature that is not related to infection and that occurs in brain-injured patients (Badjatia, 2009a, 2009b).
   2. Cause of poststroke fever
      a. An inflammatory response to injury may result from damage to the thermoregulatory centers (hypothalamus and pons) and is also associated with blood in the intraventricular space (Badjatia, 2009b).
      b. Results in exacerbation of inflammatory cascade, elevated cytokines, and neutrophils in damaged tissue. Increases neuronal excitotoxicity, free-radical production, and intracellular glutamate concentration.
      c. Fever may also induce nervous system injury (Badjatia, 2009b).
   3. Normothermia in brain-injured patients is associated with stabilization of the blood-brain barrier, decreased cerebral metabolism, and decreased ischemic depolarizations in patients with ischemic stroke (Badjatia, 2009b).
   4. Association with outcomes in ischemic stroke: Fever is more common in patients with large territory ischemic stroke and independently contributes to death and disability at 30 days (Badjatia, 2009b).
   5. Association with outcomes in ICH: Development of fever during the first 72 hours of ICH is associated with death and disability at 30 days (Badjatia, 2009b).
   6. Association with outcomes in SAH: Fever is very common in patients with SAH, particularly if they have significant intraventricular blood. The presence of fever seems to be involved in the development of vasospasm. Fever independently contributes to death and disability at 30 days (Badjatia, 2009b).
   7. Management of fever
      a. Infection surveillance: Because stroke patients are prone to central fever, fever episodes may or may not be related to an infectious process. The presence of infection should be monitored through cultures and blood-count monitoring to identify and treat any infection early (Badjatia, 2009b).
      b. Pharmacologic interventions with antipyretics (Badjatia, 2009b)
         (1) Acetaminophen, with attention to total dose per day and liver function
         (2) Ibuprofen, with attention to renal function and potential impact on platelet function
      c. External cooling: Several external cooling modalities exist, from water blankets placed underneath the patient to blankets that adhere to the patient's body using gel. Some blankets have an automatic feedback system that monitors and controls the water temperature. Other blankets offer cold water circulation only and require

the nurse to monitor and turn the blanket on and off as needed (Linares & Mayer, 2009).

(1) Skin surveillance is important for any patient who has cold water circulating next to his or her skin. Skin should be routinely monitored to prevent breakdown or blistering from the cold contact.

(2) Patients should be routinely assessed for shivering. When shivering is identified, the team must institute interventions to eliminate it. Shivering is associated with discomfort, increased metabolic demand, increased oxygen consumption, and worse outcomes.

d. Intravascular cooling: Several intravascular cooling devices exist, providing central venous access and cooling through cold metal conduction or intravascular balloons filled with cold water (Linares & Mayer, 2009).

(1) Patients receiving intravascular cooling should be monitored for infection and venous thrombosis due to the invasive access.

(2) Patients should be routinely assessed for shivering as noted previously.

e. Management of shivering (Linares & Mayer, 2009)

(1) Assessment: Shivering should be assessed every hour for any patient receiving cooling measures. The Bedside Shivering Assessment Scale allows for the objective measurement of shivering and can be administered and documented by nursing staff (**Table 5-1**).

Table 5-1. Bedside Shivering Assessment Scale

Score	Term	Description
0	No	Absence of shivering on palpation of neck and pectoralis muscles
1	Mild	Localized to the neck or thorax. May be present only on palpation
2	Moderate	Involvement of the upper extremities with or without neck or pectoralis muscles
3	Severe	Generalized, whole-body involvement

Reprinted from "Metabolic Impact of Shivering During Therapeutic Temperature Modulation: The Bedside Shivering Assessment Scale," by N. Badjatia, E. Strongilis, E. Gordon, M. Prescutti, M., L. Fernandez, A. Fernandez, et al., 2008, Stroke, *39(12), pp. 3242–3247. © 2008 by the American Heart Association. Reprinted with permission.*

(2) Pharmacologic interventions (Linares & Mayer, 2009)

(a) Buspirone—partial serotonin agonist with antishivering properties that activate hypothalamic heat-loss mechanisms

(b) Magnesium—promotes cutaneous vasodilation and mild muscle relaxation. In addition, magnesium may have neuroprotective properties, and mild elevation in serum magnesium is generally well tolerated. Generally, magnesium is administered to maintain levels between 3–4 mg/dL.

(c) Dantrolene—decreases the amplitude of shivering response

(d) Meperidine—the only opiate with antishivering characteristics that are caused by a reaction with K-receptors

(3) Skin counter warming: Patients may benefit from having warm blankets on their extremities and around their face to combat the cold sensation caused by surface or intravascular cooling modalities.

(4) Sedation and paralysis: When other methods are not effective, sedation or paralysis may be considered to minimize shivering.

Safety Measures for the Stroke Patient

A. Aspiration precautions
1. Swallow dysfunction is a frequent complication of stroke.
2. Patients who have or are suspected of having had a stroke should take nothing by mouth (NPO) until a swallow screen is conducted (Jauch et al., 2013).
3. The nurse should assess the patient for swallow function (Eisenstadt, 2010).
   a. Signs and symptoms of possible aspiration include
      (1) Respiratory—dyspnea, tachycardia, cough, wet vocal quality, wheeze, rales, rhonchi, and hypoxia
      (2) Systemic—fever, delirium or confusion, poor feeding, decline in functional status
   b. Swallow function assessment may be performed as a screening by the nurse or as a formal clinical swallow evaluation by a speech and language pathologist. Many bedside swallow-assessment tools are available, and no one tool has emerged as a best practice. The SCRN or stroke program may choose a swallow tool to help guide bedside assessment (Donovan et al., 2013).
      (1) Toronto Bedside Swallow Screening Test
      (2) 3-oz Water Swallow Test
      (3) Any 2 Test
      (4) Bedside Swallow Assessment
      (5) Standardized Swallow Assessment
      (6) Gugging Swallow Screen
      (7) Acute Stroke Dysphagia Screening
      (8) Emergency Physician Dysphagia Screen
      (9) Modified Mann Assessment of Swallowing Ability
4. The nurse may institute evidence-based swallow safety strategies including (Eisenstadt, 2010)
   a. Provide oral feeding only when patient is awake and alert.
   b. Supervise feeding with inspection of oral cavity.
   c. Elevate head of bed with oral feeding.
   d. Flex head to neutral position or slightly downward with swallow.
   e. Avoid rushed or forced feeding.
   f. Provide thickened liquid or a pureed diet.
   g. Provide frequent oral care.
5. A formal clinical evaluation of swallow function should be provided by a speech and language therapist for any stroke patient with signs of altered swallow and aspiration risk (Jauch et al., 2013).

B. Fall precautions
1. Patients with stroke are at a higher risk for fall due to paretic limbs, alteration in sensation, and alteration in cognition.
2. Many factors in addition to stroke affect fall risk, including nurse staffing levels, the patient's history of falls, continence status, medications, medical comorbidities, and procedures (Titler, Shever, Kanak, Picone, & Qin, 2011).
3. Patients should be assessed for fall risk factors and provided with interventions tailored to address fall risk. Several fall assessment tools are available for use (Agency for Healthcare Research and Quality, 2013)
   a. STRATIFY Scale for Identifying Fall Risk Factor
   b. Morse Fall Scale

4. Universal fall precaution interventions include (Agency for Healthcare Research and Quality, 2013)
   a. Familiarize the patient with the environment.
   b. Educate the patient on call light use and keep controls within the patient's reach.
   c. Place the hospital bed in low position, keep brakes locked.
   d. Keep nonslip, comfortable, well-fitting footwear on the patient.
   e. Keep floor surfaces dry and clean.
   f. Keep patient-care areas uncluttered.
   g. Follow safe patient handling practices.
5. Additional fall precaution interventions (Rowe et al., 2013; Summers et al., 2009)
   a. Bed or chair alarms
   b. Special equipment
   c. Supervision

C. Seizure precautions
1. Seizure precautions include pharmacologic and nonpharmacologic interventions to decrease the seizure rate after stroke and increase the likelihood of seizure recognition (Rowe et al., 2013).
2. Data suggest that routine seizure prophylaxis, particularly phenytoin, is associated with worse patient outcomes in rehabilitation and the chronic stages of stroke recovery. Therefore, routine use of seizure prophylaxis after stroke is questioned and represents an ongoing area of debate and research (Rowe et al., 2013).
3. Ischemic stroke (Rowe et al., 2013)
   a. Ischemic stroke is one of the highest causes of epilepsy in the elderly population.
   b. The pathophysiology of seizure in acute stroke includes the presence of edema and excitotoxicity during the acute phase after ischemic stroke and scar tissue and chronic neuronal deformities during the chronic phase.
   c. However, the incidence of seizure in the acute phase of ischemic stroke treatment is generally low and does not warrant prophylactic administration of anticonvulsants. If the patient exhibits signs of seizure, the seizures should be treated with anticonvulsant medication.
4. ICH (Rowe et al., 2013)
   a. Patients with ICH are at highest risk for seizure activity in the first 24 hours after initial hemorrhage because of the metabolic and physical disturbances within the brain.
   b. The location of the hemorrhage may affect the likelihood of a seizure occurring; hematomas in the temporal lobe or those affecting the cerebral cortex have a higher risk of seizure.
   c. Prophylactic anticonvulsants should not be routinely used for patients with ICH. If clinical signs and symptoms of seizure are present, seizures should be treated with anticonvulsant medication.
5. SAH (Rowe et al., 2013)
   a. The exact rate of seizure after SAH is reported to be as high as 20%. However, this figure likely includes posturing and shaking that are associated with increased intracranial pressure (ICP) during an aneurysm rupture rather than a true seizure.
   b. Seizures occurring before an aneurysm is secured with either a clip or coil are associated with increased ICP and rebleeding.
   c. Current guidelines state seizure prophylaxis with anticonvulsant medication may be considered for a short course of 3–7 days. If patients have evidence of

seizure activity after the initial bleed event, they should receive treatment with anticonvulsant medications.

D. Skin precautions (Agency for Healthcare Research and Quality, 2014)
   1. Stroke patients are at high risk for skin breakdown as a result of immobility, paresis, and decreased sensation and cognition.
   2. Skin breakdown results from several factors, including pressure, moisture, shear, and friction.
   3. Bony prominences are at highest risk for skin damage, and moisture from incontinence increases risk.
   4. All hospitalized stroke patients should be regularly assessed for skin breakdown risk using a validated tool.
      a. The Braden Scale
   5. Skin breakdown prevention strategies include
      a. Frequent repositioning
      b. Adequate padding and mattress to prevent pressure
      c. Maximize nutrition
      d. Maintain dry and clean skin

E. Infection prevention protocols
   1. Aspiration pneumonia (Hannawi, Hannawi, Rao, Suarez, & Bershad, 2013)
      a. Reported rates of stroke-associated pneumonia (SAP) vary, with reports that as many as 50% of stroke patients in the ICU and stroke units and as many as 11% of patients in postacute care rehabilitation experience this complication.
      b. SAP is associated with increased morbidity and mortality of stroke patients.
      c. SAP is likely caused by aspiration combined with stroke-induced immunosuppression.
      d. SAP is associated with fever and hypoxia, both of which are known to have deleterious effects in stroke patients and affect outcomes.
      e. Many risk factors affect a stroke patient's risk for SAP. Higher stroke severity, dysphagia and aspiration, mechanical ventilation, brain stem infarction, large MCA infarction, and left anterior cerebral artery infarction are all associated with SAP development.
      f. A formal dysphagia screening protocol decreases pneumonia risk.
      g. Prophylactic administration of antibiotics and targeted digestive tract decontamination to prevent SAP are controversial, and data are mixed about their impact.
      h. SAP treatment follows the guidelines for management of hospital-acquired pneumonia.
   2. Urinary tract infection (UTI)
      a. Stroke patients are at higher risk than other hospitalized patients, regardless of catheterization (Poisson, Johnston, & Josephson, 2010).
         (1) Increased risk for UTI related to stroke-induced immunosuppression, bladder dysfunction, and the increased likelihood of bladder catheter placement
            (a) Urinary incontinence and retention occur in as many as 60% of stroke patients. Patients with ischemic stroke, ICH, and SAH experience urine storage and emptying disorders.
      b. Poststroke UTI is a frequent complication in stroke patients. Twenty-five percent of stroke patients experience a UTI during the first month after their stroke. Poststroke

UTI is associated with a five-fold increased odd of decline in neurologic status (Poisson, et al., 2010).

c. Methods to reduce poststroke UTI (Poisson, et al., 2010)
   (1) Prophylactic antibiotics have been studied as an intervention to decrease poststroke UTI. The role of prophylactic antibiotics is unclear and may result in more resistant organisms.
   (2) Decreased use of bladder catheters and the use of condom catheters for men in place of bladder catheters may reduce poststroke UTI risk.
   (3) When a stroke patient's bladder catheter is removed, the patient must be monitored for urinary retention and incontinence-associated dermatitis, which can occur in as many as 30% of patients with urinary incontinence.
   (4) Antibiotic-impregnated bladder catheters are understudied as a means to decrease poststroke UTI and are not routinely used.

d. Possible adverse consequences of decreasing UTI (Poisson et al., 2010)
   (1) Continued incontinence or urinary retention
   (2) Incontinence-associated dermatitis and breakdown
   (3) Renal failure associated with retention

F. Venothromboembolism (VTE) prophylaxis (Field & Hill, 2012; Guyatt et al., 2012)

1. Stroke patients are at high risk for thrombosis due to immobility, systemic inflammation, medical comorbidities, and dehydration.
   a. Sixty percent of stroke patients are immobile for a period of time after their stroke, and 33% of patients will continue to struggle with immobility 3 months after their stroke.
   b. Exact rates of deep vein thrombosis (DVT) and pulmonary embolism vary greatly. Prior to routine prophylaxis, DVT rates were reported between 25% and 75%, and pulmonary embolism rates were reported between 1% and 3%.
   c. Risk factors for VTE include older age, significant limb weakness, greater stroke severity, and severe functional impairment.
   d. Thromboprophylaxis methods include
      (1) Early mobilization: Lower DVT rates are reported on units that prioritize early mobilization.
      (2) Hydration: Dehydration is a risk factor for thrombosis and should be avoided in the acute phase after stroke.
      (3) Elastic compression stockings are no longer recommended for patients with stroke because of adverse events associated with their use, such as skin necrosis and ulcerations.
      (4) Intermittent pneumatic compression devices are recommended to prevent DVT after stroke.
      (5) Pharmacologic prophylaxis options include antiplatelets, unfractionated heparin, low molecular weight heparin, and other anticoagulants. Low-to-medium dose unfractionated heparin, low molecular weight heparin, and heparinoids all reduce VTE after stroke. The choice of one agent over another is controversial and is generally based on provider preference, the type of stroke, and the need for procedures during the initial days of hospitalization.
      (6) Timing of pharmacologic prophylaxis in patients with ICH and SAH is controversial and few studies exist that evaluate the impact of pharmacological prophylaxis. Retrospective data suggest unfractionated heparin and low molecular weight heparin are safe when started 24–48 hours after a hemorrhage, provided

the hematoma is stable and radiologic imaging shows no evidence of hematoma expansion.

G. Stress ulcer prophylaxis (Jauch et al., 2013)
   1. Critically ill stroke patients are at high risk for stress ulcer formation.
   2. Gastrointestinal bleeding from a stress ulcer increases the risk of disability and death of the stroke patient.
   3. Pharmacologic stress ulcer prophylaxis should be tailored to individual patient risk.

H. Personal care measures for the stroke patient
   1. Patient positioning (Summers et al., 2009)
      a. Stroke survivors are at risk for skin breakdown, pain, contracture, and joint damage as a result of a paretic limb.
      b. Physical and occupational therapy should be consulted early for splinting of weak or paretic limb to prevent contractures.
      c. Paretic limbs should be positioned using pillows and positioning devices to avoid pressure on shoulder and hip joints and to avoid joint subluxation.
      d. Patients should be turned frequently to prevent skin breakdown.
   2. Early mobilization (Summers et al., 2009)
      a. Early mobilization and rehabilitation is associated with decreased complications and improved functional outcomes after stroke.
         (1) Reduced risk of atelectasis, pneumonia, DVT, and PE
      b. Lack of consensus on the definition of early mobilization. Generally defined as within 24–48 hours. Patients should be mobilized when hemodynamically stable and not at risk for neurologic deterioration as a result of activity.
      c. Range of motion activities decrease joint contractures and atrophy.
   3. Elimination (Summers et al., 2009)
      a. Constipation is a frequent complication after stroke.
         (1) Decreased mobilization, use of opioid pain medication, and dehydration contribute to constipation in the stroke patient.
         (2) Routine assessment of bowel function should include the collection of the patient's bowel function history, elimination pattern, bowel sounds, and abdominal distention.
         (3) Patients may require a bowel program that includes stool softeners, laxatives, and enemas to prevent constipation and ileus after stroke.
      b. Urinary incontinence occurs in as many as 60% of stroke patients early after stroke.
         (1) Stroke patients are at risk for additional urinary dysfunction including retention, neurogenic bladder, hyperreflexia, urge incontinence, and overflow incontinence.
         (2) Bladder catheters should be discontinued when possible to avoid infection.
         (3) Patients may require intermittent straight-bladder catheterization every 4–6 hours to prevent bladder distention beyond 500 mL and if postvoid residual is more than 100 mL.
         (4) Interventions for bladder retraining should be instituted.
            (a) Offering commode, bedpan, or urinal every 2 hours when awake and every 4 hours at night.
            (b) Fluid intake should be lessened in the evening hours.

I. Therapeutic environment for the stroke patient (Summers et al., 2009)
   1. Establish appropriate levels of stimulation.
   2. Orient to time, place, and person.

3. Establish alternative means of communication if necessary.
4. Adapt environment according to patient's deficit.
5. Promote sleep hygiene, and assess patients for signs and symptoms of abnormal breathing patterns including sleep apnea.

J. Spiritual and psychosocial care of the stroke patient: Due to the acute and catastrophic nature of stroke, spiritual and psychosocial care of the stroke patient is a key role of the bedside nurse (Summers et al., 2009). The nurse should
1. Encourage the patient to verbalize his or her feelings
2. Identify positive coping mechanisms
3. Respect the patient's culture
4. Assess the patient's healthcare beliefs
5. Facilitate the patient's spiritual needs
6. Assess and manage the patient's depression, anxiety, and fatigue.

K. Facilitating care goals and decision making for the stroke patient: The SCRN and interdisciplinary team should discuss care options with the patient and family.
1. Care options may include palliative care to alleviate suffering and manage pain, hospice care to support minimizing curative treatment, and organ donation if a patient were to be declared clinically brain dead or is a candidate for donation after cardiac death (Summers et al., 2009).

L. Provide individualized education for the patient and family: The SCRN should provide ongoing education for the patient and family that addresses the etiology of the stroke including the patient's risk factors; medical, nursing, and other therapeutic interventions to manage the stroke; interventions to prevent another stroke from occurring; and how to recognize and intervene if the patient were having another stroke (Summers et al., 2009).

M. Assess the patient's capabilities to perform ADLs and provide alternative means if necessary, including adaptive devices and consultations with occupational and physical therapy (Summers et al., 2009).

N. Manage nutrition, including specialty diets, the consistency of diets, and the timing of enteral nutrition if necessary (Summers et al., 2009).
1. A registered dietician is a key member of the interdisciplinary team and should be consulted for stroke patients who are unable to maintain their nutritional needs as a result of the stroke (Summers et al., 2009).

Implementing Care Specific to Stroke Diagnosis

A. Implement care specific to ischemic stroke
1. Manage blood pressure: Overall, blood pressure management should be considered on an individualized basis for each patient; however a generalized consensus for blood pressure parameters exists (Jauch et al., 2013).
   a. Permissive hypertension: Allowing elevated blood pressure facilitates increased per fusion of the acute ischemic brain.
   b. Ischemic stroke without tPA: Blood pressure should not be treated unless it is higher than 220/120 mmHg. If blood pressure exceeds 220/120 mmHg, it is recommended to lower it by 15% in the first 24 hours after an acute ischemic stroke.
   c. Hypotension: Acute ischemic stroke patients rarely have hypotension unless it is related to another cause (e.g., cardiac arrhythmias or ischemia, aortic dissection, or shock).
   d. Orthostatic hypotension

(1) Postural (orthostatic) hypotension is diagnosed when within 2–5 minutes of quiet standing (after a 5-minute period of supine rest), one or both of the following is present: at least a 20 mmHg fall in systolic pressure and/or at least a 10 mmHg fall in diastolic pressure (Arbique, Cheek, Welliver, & Vongpatanasin, 2014).

(2) Patients with orthostatic hypotension may experience symptoms that result from cerebral hypoperfusion, including generalized weakness, dizziness or lightheadedness, visual blurring or darkening of the visual fields, and, in severe cases, loss of consciousness or syncope.

(3) Orthostatic hypotension is a frequent complication after stroke. Older patients, those with lower functional status, and patients with severe hemiparesis are more likely to experience orthostatic hypotension after stroke (Kong & Chuo, 2003).

(4) The nurse should assess for orthostatic hypotension and implement interventions such as slow mobilization from lying to standing for patients experiencing symptomatic orthostatic hypotension (Arbique et al., 2014).

2. Manage and assess patient postthrombolytic administration

a. Frequency of monitoring

(1) Monitor blood pressure, neurologic assessment, and bleeding every 15 minutes for 2 hours, then every 30 minutes for 6 hours, and then every hour for 16 hours, for a total of 24 hours (Jauch et al., 2013).

b. Blood pressure parameters

(1) If the patient is eligible for tPA, blood pressure must be treated and should be less than 185/110 mmHg before administering thrombolytics. Maintaining a blood pressure of less than 180/105 mmHg is recommended during the next 24 hours.

(a) A blood pressure of more than the parameters stated above after thrombolytic administration is associated with ICH.

(b) IV medications are used to maintain blood pressure less than than 185/110 mmHg before a patient can receive tPA.

1) Labetalol 10–20 mg IV over 1–2 minutes, may repeat one time, OR

2) Nicardipine 5 mg/hour IV, titrate up by 2.5 mg/hour to a maximum dose of 15 mg/hour

(2) During and post tPA infusion, blood pressure management goal is to maintain a level lower than 180/105 (Jauch et al., 2013).

(a) IV medications used for blood pressure control post tPA

1) If systolic blood pressure is 180–220 mmHg or diastolic blood pressure is 105–120 mmHg

a) Labetolol 10 mg IV, followed by continuous IV infusion 2–8 mg/min OR

b) Nicardipine 5 mg/hour IV, titrate up by 2.5 mg/hour to a maximum dose of 15 mg/hour.

c) If blood pressure is not controlled or diastolic blood pressure is more than 140 mmHg, consider IV sodium nitroprusside (Jauch et al., 2013).

c. Neurologic assessment

(1) A full assessment using the NIHSS should be performed before and after tPA administration. A modified NIHSS can be used to monitor the patient; however, if there is a decline in the modified version, the full NIHSS should be used (Summers et al., 2009).

d. Angioedema
   (1) Orolingual angioedema is an allergic reaction that can occur in approximately 1%–2% of patients who receive tPA.
   (2) Angioedema occurs more often in patients who are taking angiotensin converting enzyme (ACE inhibitors).
   (3) Treatment for angioedema includes stopping the tPA infusion and administering antihistamines, corticosteroids, or epinephrine, as ordered (Summers et al., 2009).

e. Hemorrhagic conversion
   (1) Approximately 6.4% of patients treated with tPA will have a symptomatic ICH after administration, which is defined as any CT-documented hemorrhage that was temporally related to deterioration in the patient's clinical condition within 36 hours of treatment (The National Institute of Neurological Disorders and Stroke rt-PA Stroke Study Group, 1995).

f. Other bleeding
   (1) Monitor for bleeding complications during every vital sign and neurological assessment for the first 24–36 hours post tPA administration. ICH is the most severe complication, but other sources of bleeding are possible (Summers et al., 2009).

3. Manage patient postinterventional procedures and assess for complications.
   a. Site and distal extremity assessment (Cox, 2008; Wiegand, 2011)
      (1) Frequent monitoring of the groin is important to assess for bleeding and hematomas.
      (2) Distal arterial pulses (e.g., posterior tibial, popliteal, and dorsalis pedis) should be examined frequently and compared bilaterally to assess for perfusion.
   b. Arterial sheath management (Cox, 2008)
      (1) The arterial sheath may be removed after the procedure, and close monitoring is essential. If the sheath is left in place, an occlusive dressing should be maintained, and frequent assessment of the insertion site and peripheral vascular checks are warranted.
   c. Complications after vascular access: Complications after femoral artery access are reported in 1%–9% of cases, depending on the case series (Cox, 2008).
      (1) Hematoma
         (a) Hematoma formation in the groin is the most common vascular complication after interventional procedures.
         (b) Occasionally, femoral nerve compression may occur.
      (2) Arterial dissection and retroperitoneal hemorrhage (Cox, 2008)
         (a) Arterial dissection may present with hemorrhage in the femoral or retroperitoneal area within approximately 12 hours of the procedure. Retroperitoneal hemorrhage occurs in less than 1% of patients.
         (b) Symptoms include abdominal pain, groin pain, back pain, diaphoresis, bradycardia, hypotension, and shock in situations with significant blood loss.
         (c) Treatment options include fluid resuscitation, administration of blood products, endovascular vessel repair, and open surgery for vessel repair.
      (3) Arterial thrombosis (Cox, 2008)
         (a) Thrombosis risk increases in females and with small femoral artery vessel lumen, peripheral artery disease, diabetes mellitus, and the use of a large diameter catheter and prolonged catheter dwell time.

(b) Distal pulses must be checked frequently to assess for occlusion.

(c) Vascular surgery or embolectomy may be needed in instances of significant arterial occlusion and ischemia.

(4) Pseudoaneurysm (Cox, 2008)

(a) Occurs in 1%–7% of patients with femoral artery access. Presentation generally includes groin pain and neuropathic symptoms if the femoral nerve is compressed. A bruit and pulsatile mass may be assessed.

(b) Inadequate compression, use of large bore sheaths, postprocedural anticoagulation, antiplatelet therapy during intervention, age older than 65 years, obesity, hypertension, peripheral artery disease, and hemodialysis all contribute to pseudoaneurysm formation.

(c) Treatment options include surgery, ultrasound-guided compression with or without a local injection of thrombin, or collagen into the pseudoaneurysm cavity.

4. Recognize signs of reperfusion syndrome

a. Hyperperfusion and reperfusion are often used interchangeably to describe the same phenomenon. After a chronic or acute vessel occlusion is removed, the brain tissue experiences normalization of blood flow in the setting of fragile or damaged tissue (Bouri et al., 2011).

b. The restoration of blood flow to fragile or damaged tissue results in an inflammatory response, cytokine release, leukocyte adhesion, and damage to the blood-brain barrier.

c. Signs and symptoms include ipsilateral headache, contralateral neurologic deficits, and seizure if the cortical areas are involved in the reperfusion.

d. Reperfusion syndrome is generally seen after carotid artery revascularization or the opening of an acutely occluded cerebral vessel with thrombolytics or mechanical reperfusion techniques.

e. Reperfusion syndrome is more common in patients with postoperative hypertension, high-grade stenosis with poor collateral flow, and acute ischemic stroke involving a large vessel territory.

f. Management and prevention (Bouri et al., 2011)

(1) Frequent neurologic assessment is important after reperfusion because neurologic deficits may recur or worsen.

(2) Blood pressure should be managed according to the guidelines for patients who receive IV thrombolysis, as discussed previously in this chapter.

(3) Management of blood pressure after carotid revascularization remains controversial. The general practice is to decrease postprocedure blood pressure using oral antihypertensives in patients who are asymptomatic and have a systolic blood pressure (SBP) less than 180 mmHg, and IV antihypertensives if SBP higher than 180 mmHg. If the patient is symptomatic, blood pressure should be reduced to less than 140 mmHg with IV agents.

5. Manage hydration (Summers et al., 2009)

a. Select proper IV solutions

(1) Acute ischemic stroke patients should be maintained in a normovolemic or euvolemic state.

(2) Avoid D5W (i.e., dextrose 5% and water) in patients with stroke. Hypotonic solutions and increased glucose levels perpetuate both cerebral injury and cerebral edema.

(3) Normal saline at an infusion rate of 75–100 mL per hour may be used to maintain a normovolemic state. Fluid rate goals should be calculated using several factors including the patient's body mass, calculation of intake and output, and clinical assessment of fluid status and cardiac status.

(4) IV boluses may be beneficial to increase cerebral perfusion.

b. Monitor oral fluid intake

(1) Swallowing is often affected after having a stroke. A nursing swallow screen and speech language pathologist dysphagia evaluation are recommended. Maintaining patients in an NPO status that includes medications until they are deemed safe to eat is important and will help prevent aspiration pneumonia (Summers et al., 2009).

(2) Approximately half of all stroke patients are or become malnourished within the first few weeks after their stroke. Monitoring nutrition status and fluid intake and supplementing when indicated is essential for healing (Summers et al., 2009).

6. Understand treatment options

a. Carotid endarterectomy (CEA)

(1) CAE is an open surgical procedure to remove carotid artery plaque. For patients with severe stenosis, CEA reduces the 2-year risk of stroke from 25% to 10%, and in moderate stenosis, it reduces the 5-year risk of stroke from 10% to 5%. CEA is generally the treatment of choice for symptomatic patients with 70% or more carotid artery stenosis.

(2) Timing of CEA is controversial. In patients with carotid stenosis who have not experienced a stroke, CEA is an elective procedure. Stroke risk that is based on the degree of stenosis is weighed against the surgical risk. Urgent or emergent CEA is occasionally performed in the acute ischemic stroke setting, particularly in patients with evolving stroke. Currently, the efficacy of CEA in the urgent or emergent setting is not well established (Jauch et al., 2013).

(3) Postop management

(a) Blood pressure monitoring, neurologic assessment including of the cranial nerve, hematoma and suture line evulsion, reperfusion injury, and myocardial infarction (MI) are all assessment priorities after a CEA (Bouri et al., 2011).

1) Blood pressure variation may occur for the first 24 hours after surgery because of the manipulation of the carotid sinus and baroreceptors.

2) SBP may need to be reduced out of concern for reperfusion injury. High blood pressure and reperfusion after surgery may cause an intracerebral hematoma, and hypotension may cause an ischemic stroke or TIA. Consensus on blood pressure parameters in the hours after surgery is lacking. General practice follows the parameters outlined in the reperfusion injury section.

3) Neurologic monitoring post-CEA is critical to detect the worsening of symptoms associated with new ischemia or reperfusion injury.

4) The facial and vagal cranial nerves may be affected due to the site of surgery.

b. Carotid stenting (CAS)

(1) CAS gained popularity in the 1990s and early 2000s because of its noninvasive approach to carotid artery revascularization. However, more recent studies

suggest patients with CAS are more likely to suffer from postoperative stroke, death, and MI. Therefore, the role of CAS in revascularization recently has been called into question. CEA is currently preferred for carotid revascularization; however, CAS may be appropriate for certain patients, such as those with advanced age or other perioperative risk factors that may favor stenting (Brott et al., 2010).

(2) Carotid surgery CEA and CAS nursing intervention
  (a) Preprocedure
    1) Reinforce provider recommendations regarding medications, particularly blood thinners and when to stop.
    2) Reinforce recommendations regarding oral intake prior to procedure.
    3) Provide information about the procedure.
    4) Check labs for any abnormalities (e.g., creatinine, platelet count, and coagulation), and notify provider.
    5) Determine baseline neurological assessment.
    6) Assess vital signs and oxygen level.
    7) Prepare groin for stent procedure.
  (b) Postprocedure—hospitalization
    1) Monitor blood pressure per provider orders or notify immediately if bradycardic or hypotensive.
    2) Neurological checks
    3) Monitor for respiratory distress: Assess respirations for edema and whether the trachea is midline and swallowing is intact.
    4) Monitor for cranial nerve impairment: Assess for facial droop, dysphagia, tongue deviation, and hoarseness.
    5) Assess incision site for bleeding, redness, and drainage.
    6) Monitor for hyperperfusion syndrome—may occur 1 hour to 1 week postprocedure
      a) Increased risk—patients with bilateral stenosis and hypertension
      b) Educate patients regarding signs and symptoms
        i. Elevated blood pressure
        ii. Severe temporal headache
        iii. Focal neurological deficits
        iv. Seizures
    7) Pain control
    8) Stent procedure
      a) Monitor sheath and keep patients leg straight.
      b) Assess groin site for bleeding.
      c) Assess peripheral pulses and color.
  (c) Postprocedure—home care
    1) Incision-care teaching per institutional policy
      a) Keep dry.
      b) Inform when the patient is allowed to shower.
      c) Provide dressing change instructions.
    2) Diet teaching—low fat, low cholesterol
    3) Increase fluids during the first 2–3 weeks
    4) No alcohol during the first 2–3 weeks
    5) Increase activity as tolerated.

a) No heavy lifting for 1 week
b) No driving for 1 week
c) Walk daily, increasing distance as tolerated
d) May return to work as tolerated, usually 1–2 weeks postprocedure

6) Reinforce provider's recommendation about restarting antiplatelet therapy.
7) Discuss signs and symptoms of stroke.
8) Discuss signs and symptoms that should prompt a call to the provider or return to the hospital.
   a) Stroke signs and symptoms
   b) Fever 101° F or higher
   c) Redness, tenderness, and drainage at incision site
   d) Swelling or bruising that worsens
   e) Severe headache

c. Patent foramen ovale (PFO) management (Kutty, Sengupta, & Khandheria, 2012)
   (1) The etiology of stroke is occasionally attributed to the presence of a PFO, an atrial septal defect, and an atrial septal aneurysm (ASA).
   (2) A PFO is an anatomical variant that is present in 25% of healthy adults. For a majority of patients with PFO, its presence is not pathological. In rare cases, a PFO may be a cause or a contributing cause of stroke. The exact relationship between a PFO and an ischemic stroke remains unclear; however, many patients with no other explainable cause for their stroke have a PFO.
   (3) The ASA is a mobile protrusion of the septum into the atrium. When combined with a PFO, the combination of an ASA and a PFO are associated with an increased stroke risk.
   (4) Emboli may be created from the abnormal blood flow as a result of these abnormalities.
   (5) Management of a PFO after an embolic stroke involves either medical therapy with antiplatelet or anticoagulation medication or surgical therapy using a percutaneous closure device to close the defect.
   (6) A recent randomized controlled trial showed that surgical closure was not superior to medical management, calling into question the role of percutaneous surgical closure (Kutty et al., 2012).

d. Atrial fibrillation management: Ischemic stroke work-up includes assessment of the patient for the presence of atrial fibrillation. When atrial fibrillation is present, secondary stroke prevention should be instituted promptly to avoid recurrent stroke. Patients with atrial fibrillation have a five-fold increased risk of ischemic stroke compared with patients without the dysrhythmia (Marmagkiolis, Nikolaidis, Politis, & Goldstein, 2008).
   (1) Telemetry monitoring: The guidelines for stroke management support at least 24 hours of telemetry monitoring in acute stroke to identify transient or sustained atrial fibrillation. For patients with known atrial fibrillation, telemetry monitoring is necessary to determine if the patient's rate is well controlled.
   (2) Generally, oral anticoagulation is the mainstay of stroke prevention in patients with atrial fibrillation (Marmagkiolis et al., 2008).
      (a) Studies show that oral anticoagulation with a goal international normalized ratio (INR) of 2.0–3.0 significantly reduces the frequency, severity, and mortality of ischemic events.
      (b) Oral anticoagulation carries risks as well, including significant cerebral and systemic bleeding. Therefore, oral anticoagulation should be carefully

considered by weighing the risks and benefits prior to the initiation of anticoagulation.

(c) The appropriate timing of oral anticoagulation initiation after an acute ischemic or hemorrhagic stroke event in a patient with atrial fibrillation remains a source of ongoing debate. General practice is to wait at least 10–14 days and longer in certain situations after a large ischemic or hemorrhagic stroke before starting oral anticoagulation. Oral anticoagulation may be considered sooner in smaller ischemic strokes.

(3) The congestive heart failure, hypertension, age, diabetes mellitus, prior stroke (CHADS) score or the $CHADS_2$ score is a risk assessment tool to determine which patients with atrial fibrillation would best benefit from oral anticoagulation (Marmagkiolis et al., 2008).

(4) Medication: Multiple oral anticoagulation medications are available for patients with atrial fibrillation. Medications are reviewed in detail in chapter 6 (Marmagkiolis et al., 2008).

(5) Patients with new onset atrial fibrillation should be referred to specialists for consideration for catheter ablation, cardioversion, and other appropriate interventions (Marmagkiolis et al., 2008).

e. Hemicraniectomy (Honeybul & Ho, 2013)

(1) Cerebral edema can be life threatening after an acute ischemic stroke.

(2) Surgical removal of a portion of the skull can allow room for swelling after a large acute ischemic stroke.

(3) Approximately 10% of acute ischemic strokes can cause cerebral edema and increased ICP. Most of these are related to an occlusion of the middle cerebral artery. However, internal carotid artery infarcts, basilar artery syndromes, and infarcts in the cerebellum may necessitate craniectomy as well.

(4) Timing of the craniectomy is both critical and controversial. The skull should be removed only when swelling is uncontrolled by other measures, including osmotherapy and ventricular drainage, and before significant herniation occurs.

(5) The nurse must monitor for complications after craniectomy (**Table 5.2**).

Table 5-2. Monitoring for Craniectomy Complications (Honeybull & Ho, 2013)

Short term (Day 0–7)	1–3 months	Long term (>3 months)	Bone flap replacement
Herniation through bone window	Infection		Infection
Infection	Infection		Infection
Contralateral hematoma			Hematoma
Ipsilateral subdural/subgial effusion	Ipsilateral/contralateral subdural effusion	Ipsilateral/contralateral subdural effusion	Hydoma
Seizure	Seizure	Seizure	
CSF leakage	Sinking skin flap/ syndrome of trephined	Hydrocephalus	Bone flap resorption
		Sinking skin flap/ syndrome of trephined	

CSF indicates cerebrospinal fluid.

Implementing Care Specific to Hemorrhagic Stroke

A. Blood pressure management: Unlike ischemic stroke, after which blood pressure is often allowed to be higher than the patient's baseline to support perfusion, hypertension after acute ICH or SAH is associated with rebleeding and worse outcomes.

1. The nurse must monitor and maintain blood pressure within identified parameters.
2. Debate currently exists regarding the ideal blood pressure parameters following ICH and SAH. Several clinical trials are currently evaluating blood pressure reduction in hemorrhagic stroke.
   a. ICH: Acute reduction of SBP to less than 140–160 mmHg is currently thought to be reasonable and safe. Clinical guidelines suggest if SBP is higher than 200 or mean arterial pressure (MAP) is more than 150, blood pressure should be reduced using continuous IV infusion, and blood pressure should be monitored every 5 minutes. If SBP is higher than 180 or MAP is more than 130 and elevated ICP is suspected, consider monitoring ICP and reducing blood pressure using intermittent or continuous infusion while maintaining cerebral perfusion pressure greater than 60. If SBP is more than 180 or MAP is more than 130, consider reduction of blood pressure to MAP of 110 or blood pressure of 160/90, and clinically reexamine the patient every 15 minutes (Morgenstern et al., 2010).
   b. SAH: After acute rupture of aneurysmal SAH (aSAH), blood pressure reduction to lower than 160/90 mmHg is reasonable (Connolly et al., 2012).

B. Hemostasis: After acute onset of ICH, assessment for coagulopathy and achievement of hemostasis is critical to prevent continued bleeding. Refer to chapter 6 for additional information on procoagulant reversal strategies.

1. Patients should be assessed for use of antiplatelet and anticoagulant medication on presentation (Morgenstern et al., 2010).
2. Clinical labs to assess coagulopathy should be obtained to assess clotting times, including prothrombin time, partial thromboplastin time, and INR. Platelet function testing may be considered if the patient reports a history of antiplatelet use (Morgenstern, et al., 2010).
3. Patients with a history of oral anticoagulant use and elevated INR should have their coagulopathy acutely reversed. Several options are available for acute reversal and may be used in various clinical situations (Morgenstern et al., 2010).
   a. Fresh frozen plasma and vitamin K
   b. Cryoprecipitate if the hemorrhage follows administration of IV tPA
   c. Prothrombin complex concentrates
   d. Recombinant factor VIIa

C. ICH management

1. In addition to blood pressure management and hemostasis, general supportive care of ICH includes prevention of complications and early rehabilitation as previously discussed.
   a. VTE prophylaxis: Patients with ICH are at risk for development of VTE and PE through mechanisms similar to patients with ischemic stroke.
      (1) Patients with ICH should receive VTE prophylaxis in the form of mechanical compression devices promptly after admission to the hospital.
      (2) Patients with ICH should be considered to receive pharmacologic VTE prophylaxis with subcutaneous heparin. The timing of heparin initiation after a hemorrhagic stroke is controversial. Several small trials showed it was safe to begin prophylactic subcutaneous heparin 24–48 hours after ICH, provided the

hematoma had not expanded and appeared to be stable on neuroimaging studies (Wu et al., 2011).

D. aSAH

1. Phases of care: The care of a patient with aSAH is generally divided into three distinct phases. The first phase includes hemorrhage ictus to secure the aneurysm, which is covered in chapter 3. The second phase is the management of the aneurysm. Options include coil embolization and surgical clipping of the aneurysm. Generally, aneurysms are secured quickly after hemorrhage to prevent rebleeding. Finally, the third phase includes a period of delayed onset ischemia, commonly referred to as vasospasm. Patients with aSAH are at risk for vasospasm between days 6 and 21 posthemorrhage (Connolly et al., 2012).
2. Aneurysm management: Aneurysms are generally treated either by surgical microvascular clipping or endovascular coil embolization.
    a. Aneurysm clipping: Surgical clipping of a ruptured cerebral aneurysm involves an open craniotomy and placement of a microsurgical clip on the outside of the vessel, obliterating blood flow to the aneurysm while maintaining blood flow in the healthy vessel.
        (1) Patients who undergo aneurysm clipping suffer from more in-hospital complications compared with patients who receive endovascular coiling. However, clipped aneurysms are less likely to undergo recurrent filling, and treatment is generally definitive.
        (2) Patients presenting with intraparenchymal hematomas may benefit from clipping because the clot may be surgically evacuated (Connolly et al., 2012).
    b. Aneurysm coiling: Coil embolization of an aneurysm is performed by a specially trained radiologist, neurologist, or neurosurgeon in an endovascular suite. The procedure is typically performed through the femoral artery, although alternate arteries may be used in certain circumstances. Small platinum coils are placed through a catheter directly into the aneurysm to stop blood flow. The aneurysm is then packed with coils. When blood flow to the aneurysm is stopped, the coils remain in the aneurysm and the microcatheter is withdrawn through the femoral artery.
        (1) Complications associated with endovascular coiling include incomplete obliteration of the aneurysm and recurrent aneurysm filling. Both may result in aneurysm rerupture (Connolly et al., 2012).
    c. Decision to clip or coil an aneurysm: A majority of aneurysms may be managed successfully by either surgical clipping or endovascular coiling. Many factors may impact why a patient is clipped or coiled.
        (1) A recent meta-analysis demonstrated that in patients who could either be clipped or coiled, coiling results in better clinical outcomes, particularly for those with good perioperative Hunt and Hess scores. Coiling is associated with higher rebleeding rates than surgical clipping. However, mortality rates were similar between both treatment groups at 1 year. The risk of vasospasm was higher in the patients who were surgically clipped; however, all other complication rates were similar between the groups (Li et al., 2013).
        (2) Location and morphology of the aneurysm may determine whether surgical clipping or endovascular coiling is the best treatment, with posterior circulation aneurysms most commonly coiled and MCA aneurysms often clipped. However, these are general trends, and institutional practices may vary (Connolly et al., 2012).

(3) Endovascular treatment of aneurysms continues to advance rapidly, with new devices providing flow diversion around the aneurysm and eliminating the need for coiling or clipping of the aneurysm. Further studies are needed to determine the safety and efficacy of this treatment modality.

(4) Determination of aneurysm treatment modality should be an interdisciplinary decision based on the patient and aneurysm's characteristics (Connolly et al., 2012).

3. Delayed cerebral ischemia (DCI) or vasospasm following aSAH: Patients with aSAH are at risk for developing delayed neurologic deterioration, most often caused by vasospasm (i.e., DCI) (Diringer et al., 2011).

a. Patients are at highest risk for DCI onset in the first 6–10 days, with the risk extending to approximately 21 days after hemorrhage.

b. Vasospasm occurs when arteries narrow, resulting in decreased blood flow that causes ischemia or infarction. The pathophysiology of vasospasm is poorly understood and is thought to be related to vessel inflammation that results from breakdown of the subarachnoid blood.

c. Patients with aSAH generally are monitored closely in the neurocritical care unit for neurologic deterioration that may signal vasospasm (Diringer et al., 2011).

(1) Detection of a new neurologic deficit in an aSAH patient is a clinical emergency and should be reported to the interdisciplinary team immediately.

d. In addition to neurological clinical assessment, aSAH patients may be monitored with ongoing transcrianial Doppler studies and serial CT angiography studies to identify vasospasm before permanent infarction occurs. However, the timing and frequency of monitoring varies across centers, and there is no established best practice (Diringer et al., 2011).

e. Nimodipine is a calcium channel blocker shown to improve outcomes in patients with aSAH. Nimpodipine should be administered to patients orally, 60 mg every 4 hours for 21 days (Diringer et al., 2011).

(1) If nimodipine decreases the patient's blood pressure significantly, dosing may be changed to 30 mg every 2 hours to minimize hypotension.

f. After the aneurysm is secured, blood pressure parameters are generally liberalized to allow permissive hypertension, and fluids are administered to maintain euvolemia.

g. If the patient develops neurologic deterioration that is suggestive of vasospasm or clinical testing indicates vasospasm, several interventions may be instituted to reverse ischemia (Diringer et al., 2011).

(1) Hypervolemia used to be the standard treatment for patients in vasospasm. However, current practice is to maintain euvolemia and consider fluid boluses to augment cerebral blood flow.

(2) Hypertension: A trial of induced hypertension should be offered using vasopressor therapy. Target blood pressure goals should be tailored to the individual patient with the minimum elevation necessary to achieve symptom improvement.

(3) If the patient is in suspected or confirmed vasospasm and nimodipine continues to cause hypotension despite dosing adjustments, the medication may be discontinued.

(4) Endovascular therapy may be considered for the treatment of large vessel vasospam. Endovascular options include intra-arterial administration of vasodilators and angioplasty of narrowed vessels.

4. Additional medical management
   a. Patients with aSAH are at risk for aspiration, VTE, and other stroke complications outlined in the care of ischemic and ICH patients. Prophylaxis and prevention strategies as discussed for the care of ischemic stroke and ICH should be implemented for patient with SAH (Connolly et al., 2012).

E. AVMs represent a number of abnormal vessel conditions characterized by abnormal arteriovenous shunting. Unlike normal vasculature, in which a capillary and tissue bed lies between arterial and venous vessels, AVMs are abnormal connections of arteries and veins with no tissue bed or capillaries between them. Abnormal vessel connections and pressures within the vessels make the malformations prone to hemorrhage (Ogilvy et al., 2001).
   1. Cerebral AVM: Cerebral AVM is a venous malformation that occurs in the cerebral tissue. When AVMs rupture, they result in hemorrhage into the cerebral tissue or the subarachnoid space. Supportive medical management generally follows care outlined for ICH. Surgical management of the AVM includes microsurgical resection, radiosurgery, and endovascular embolization. Some AVMs require multiple treatment modalities for full resection.

F. Dural AV fistula (DAVF): DAVF is a direct connection between the meningeal artery and the meningeal vein or dural venous sinus. Patients may experience a variety of symptoms, including headache, tinnitus, bruit, and cranial nerve deficits according to DAVF size and location (Miller, 2012).

G. Cavernous angioma: *Cavernous angioma* is a hemangioma or series of abnormal adjacent capillaries with slow blood flow that may occur anywhere in the central nervous system. Cavernous angiomas are congenitally acquired, and most are benign and never hemorrhage. When symptomatic, patients generally present with headache, seizure, or cerebral hemorrhage. Cavernous angiomas may be treated with radiosurgery or medical management (Batra, Rigamonti, & Rigamonti, 2012).

H. Intraventricular hemorrhage (IVH): IVH may occur as an extension of an ICH or SAH, or, in rare cases, may be spontaneous. Primary or spontaneous IVH without ICH or SAH is rare and is generally caused by hypertension or vascular malformation (Morgenstern et al., 2010).
   1. Intraventricular thrombolysis: Hemorrhage into the ventricular space often results in hydrocephalus and elevated ICP. Placement of an external ventricular drain (EVD) may be adequate to drain cerebrospinal fluid (CSF) and the blood clot. However, studies are currently underway to evaluate the role of administering a small amount of tPA into the ventricular space to expedite clot breakdown and drainage. This use of tPA is currently off label because trials are ongoing. However, many centers have adopted this practice when an EVD becomes clogged due to a thick clot or when a patient has a significant amount of ventricular blood (Staykov & Schwab, 2013).

I. CSF diversion: CSF diversion may be necessary with a number of stroke types, including cerebellar ischemic stroke, ICH, and SAH. Indications for acute CSF diversion in the form of an EVD include significant blood in the ventricular space, obstructive hydrocephalus, and elevated ICP (Morgenstern et al., 2010).
   1. EVD: A drainage catheter is placed through a small burr hole into the ventricular space. ICP may be transduced, and the drain is either closed, left open continuously at

a particular level, or closed and opened to drain periodically. The nursing management of EVD in a stroke patient should follow AANN guidelines for ventricular drain management (American Association of Neuroscience Nurses, 2011).

2. Ventriculoperitoneal shunt (VPS): Attempts to discontinue ventricular drains that were placed acutely after stroke are generally made prior to placement of a permanent VPS. EVD weaning techniques vary across centers, with little science to guide patient management during EVD weaning. If the EVD is unable to be successfully weaned and discontinued, a VPS becomes necessary for the patient to continue to progress in rehabilitation and leave the acute stroke setting.

J. Management of elevated ICP: Elevated ICP is most likely to occur in ICH and SAH, and may be an issue in large vessel ischemic stroke as previously outlined. Multiple tools are available for management of elevated ICP and are listed below from least to most invasive. Most patients require a multimodal approach to ICP management, and each intervention has varying levels of evidence to support the approach, depending on the underlying cause of intracranial hypertension (Wijdicks et al., 2014).
   1. Elevate head of bed to facilitate venous drainage.
   2. Keep head and neck in neutral alignment to facilitate venous drainage.
   3. Osmotherapy
      a. Mannitol therapy
      b. Hypertonic saline
   4. CSF diversion
   5. Targeted temperature management including mild hypothermia
   6. Mechanical ventilation and management of oxygenation and carbon dioxide
   7. Barbiturate coma
   8. Surgical exision of hemorrhage
   9. Craniectomy

Additional Stroke Disorders

A. TIA: TIA is an episode of focal cerebral ischemia and subsequent neurologic dysfunction that does not result in permanent cerebral infarction. TIAs are a warning sign that the patient is at high risk for a significant stroke event (Easton et al., 2009).
   1. The TIA diagnostic criteria is evolving. Traditionally, a TIA was diagnosed according to time to symptom resolution. Any patient with focal ischemia symptoms that resolved within 24 hours was diagnosed as having a TIA. Currently, clinicians should combine the clinical picture, including symptom resolution, with neuroimaging such as MRI to determine TIA versus ischemic stroke diagnosis (Easton et al., 2009).
   2. Patients with TIA are at high risk for having an ischemic stroke. The $ABCD^2$ score stratifies risk of stroke in the days, weeks, and months following ischemic stroke and is discussed earlier in this chapter.
   3. Patients with TIA are generally admitted to the hospital for an expedited workup to assess their risk for recurrent stroke and institute prevention measures immediately. Some programs utilize a rapid hospital workup process with immediate clinical follow up to provide prevention measures (Easton et al., 2009).

B. Cerebral venous thrombosis (CVT): *CVT* is a rare type of stroke during which a clot forms in the dural sinuses or the cerebral veins. CVT often occurs in younger individuals; risk factors include thrombophylias, inflammatory bowel disease, use of oral contraceptives, substance abuse, and head trauma (Saposnik et al., 2011).

1. Patients with CVT generally present with symptoms associated with elevated ICP, venous infarct, or hemorrhage. They often report headache, either of acute onset or insidious, and cranial nerve dysfunction according to venous infarct or hemorrhage location. Patients may also present with seizure.
2. Initial management includes supportive care similar to ICH management. Diagnostic imaging may include venous imaging to identify thrombosis.
3. In addition to supportive treatment for ICH and elevated ICP, patients with CVT may be considered for acute anticoagulation to stop the ongoing thrombotic process that is continuing to cause elevated ICP.
   a. Acute anticoagulation generally begins with heparin infusion and is continued with oral anticoagulation for several months. Patients must be monitored for continued cerebral hemorrhage through close neurologic examination and serial neuroimaging until deemed stable (Saposnik et al., 2011).

C. Cervicocerebral arterial dissection is a rare cause of ischemic stroke and should be considered in any patient who has experienced trauma or is young or middle aged. Cervicocerebral arterial dissection occurs in the carotid or vertebral arteries after an intimal vessel tear allows an intramural hematoma to form (Mohr et al., 2011).
   1. Causes: Dissection is generally either spontaneous or due to severe trauma. Connective tissue disorders should be considered in patients with spontaneous dissection. Some patients report a precipitating event such as sneezing, coughing, vomiting, or exercising.
   2. Carotid artery dissection: Patients report pain in the ipsilateral face, head, or neck with focal ischemic changes that may include Horner's syndrome.
   3. Vertebral artery dissection: Patients generally report an ipsilateral and occipital throbbing or a pressure-like headache. Patients may have focal ischemic changes depending on the location and extent of ischemia.
   4. Intracranial dissection: Dissection of intracranial vessels is possible, although rare, and is often associated with blood in the subarachnoid space.
   5. Treatment of dissection is controversial, and few studies exist to guide management. Patients are generally started on antiplatelet medication, and acute oral anticoagulation may be considered in some cases. Intra-arterial management of the dissection may be considered, including intra-arterial administration of thrombolysis, angioplasty, and stenting.

D. Moyamoya disease: Moyamoya is a chronic, vaso-occlusive disease that was initially recognized in young Asian women. However, the disease is now recognized to affect other nationalities. The full etiology of the vessel disease is unknown and likely has genetic as well as environmental factors that contribute to disease development (Smith & Scott, 2010).
   1. Moyamoya is characterized by progressive narrowing and eventual occlusion of the internal carotid arteries and major branching vessels. Patients with Moyamoya develop an abnormal vessel network in an attempt to support cerebral perfusion. The small collateral vessels result in the characteristic "puff-of-smoke" picture on diagnostic imaging.
   2. Patients with Moyamoya are at risk for ischemic stroke, ICH, SAH, and seizure.
   3. Moyamoya is a progressive disease, and treatment is generally supportive, including primary and secondary prevention of all types of strokes.

E. Hypercoaguable states: A number of thrombophilias place individuals at increased risk for ischemic stroke. Thrombophilias generally are categorized as acquired or inherited. Overall, hypercoaguable state as the cause of stroke is rare (Bushnell & Goldstein, 2003).

1. The most commonly acquired thrombophilia associated with stroke is antiphospholipid antibody syndrome.
2. The most commonly inherited conditions associated with stroke include activated protein C resistance; factor V Leiden mutation; prothrombin gene mutation; or deficiencies of protein C, protein S, or antithrombin III.
3. Other conditions such as elevated homocystine and lipoprotein may place patients at higher risk for atherosclerosis and clot formation.
4. Several temporary or situational factors including pregnancy, severe infection, neoplasm, and trauma may cause patients to be more prone to developing ischemic and hemorrhagic stroke.
5. Hypercoaguable state is generally considered as a cause of stroke in patients without clear mechanisms for stroke, such as clear risk factors or an age profile that is common for stroke.
6. When suspected, laboratory tests are sent to evaluate for the presence of hypercoaguable states. Patient management is then tailored according to the results.

F. Vasculitis: Vasculitis as a cause for stroke represents a number of poorly understood inflammatory diseases that cause inflammation and cell wall death. Vasculitis is a rare cause of stroke. However, vasculitis usually is treatable and should be considered as a causative factor for stroke when no clear etiology is determined. Vasculitides are generally categorized according to the size of the vessel affected and granulomatous status (Berlit, 2010).
   1. Large vessel granulomatous vasculitides include giant cell arteritis, cranial arteritis, and Takayasu arteritis. Medium cell nongranulomatous vasculitides include polyarteritis nodosa and Kawasaki disease. Small vessel antineutrophil cytoplasmic antibodies positive granulomatous disorders include Wegener granulomatosis and Churg-Strauss syndrome. Small vessel nongranulomatous vasculidities include Behcet syndrome and cryoglobulinemic vasculitis (Berlit, 2010).
   2. Diagnosis for vasculitides disorders includes clinical picture, laboratory markers for inflammation including erythrocyte sedimentation rate and c-reactive protein, neuroimaging, and biopsy of the vessel wall for pathologic investigation.
   3. Treatment is disease dependent and often includes a prolonged course of high-dose steroid treatment.

References

Agency for Healthcare Research and Quality. (2013). Fall response and management program. Retrieved from www.ahrq.gov/professionals/systems/long-term-care/resources/injuries/fallspx/fallspxman2.html

Agency for Healthcare Research and Quality. (2014). Preventing pressure ulcers in hospitals: A toolkit for improving quality of care. Retrieved from www.ahrq.gov/professionals/systems/long-term-care/resources/pressure-ulcers/pressureulcertoolkit/putoolkit.pdf

American Association of Neuroscience Nurses. (2011). *Care of the patient undergoing intracranial pressure monitoring/external ventricular drainage or lumbar drainage.* Glenview, IL: American Association of Neuroscience Nurses.

Arbique, D., Cheek, D., Welliver, M., & Vongpatanasin, W. (2014). Management of neurogenic orthostatic hypotension. *Journal of the American Medical Directors Association, 15*(4), 234–239. doi: 10.1016/j.jamda.2013.10.014

Badjatia, N. (2009a). Fever control in the neuro-ICU: Why, who, and when? *Current Opinion in Critical Care, 15*(2), 79–82. doi: 10.1097/MCC.0b013e32832922e9

Badjatia, N. (2009b). Hyperthermia and fever control in brain injury. *Critical Care Medicine, 37*(7 Suppl), S250–257. doi: 10.1097/CCM.0b013e3181aa5e8d

Batra, S., Rigamonti, K., & Rigamonti, D. (2012). Management of hemorrhage from cavernous malformations. *Current Atherosclerosis Reports, 14*(4), 360–365. doi: 10.1007/s11883-012-0261-0

Bayer-Karpinska, A., Schwarz, F., Wollenweber, F. A., Poppert, H., Boeckh-Behrens, T., Becker, A., … Saam, T. (2013). The carotid plaque imaging in acute stroke (CAPIAS) study: Protocol and initial baseline data. *BMC Neurology, 13*, 201. doi: 10.1186/1471-2377-13-201

Berlit, P. (2010). Diagnosis and treatment of cerebral vasculitis. *Therapeutic Advances in Neurological Disorders, 3*(1), 29–42. doi: 10.1177/1756285609347123

Bouri, S., Thapar, A., Shalhoub, J., Jayasooriya, G., Fernando, A., Franklin, I. J., & Davies, A. H. (2011). Hypertension and the post-carotid endarterectomy cerebral hyperperfusion syndrome. *European Journal of Vascular and Endovascular Surgery, 41*(2), 229–237. doi: 10.1016/j.ejvs.2010.10.016

Brott, T. G., Hobson, R. W., 2nd, Howard, G., Roubin, G. S., Clark, W. M., Brooks, W., … Meschia, J. F. (2010). Stenting versus endarterectomy for treatment of carotid-artery stenosis. *New England Journal of Medicine, 363*(1), 11–23. doi: 10.1056/NEJMoa0912321

Bushnell, C., & Goldstein, L. B. (2003). Screening for hypercoagulable syndromes following stroke. *Current Atherosclerosis Reports, 5*(4), 291–298.

Cavanagh, S. J., Hogan, K., Gordon, V., & Fairfax, J. (2000). Stroke-specific FIM models in an urban population. *Journal of Neuroscience Nursing, 32*(1), 17–21.

Chen, B., Grothe, C., & Schaller, K. (2013). Validation of a new neurological score (FOUR Score) in the assessment of neurosurgical patients with severely impaired consciousness. *Acta Neurochirurgica, 155*(11), 2133–2139. doi: 10.1007/s00701-013-1854-2

Collin, C., Wade, D. T., Davies, S., & Horne, V. (1988). The Barthel ADL Index: A reliability study. *International Disability Studies, 10*(2), 61–63.

Connolly, E. S., Jr., Rabinstein, A. A., Carhuapoma, J. R., Derdeyn, C. P., Dion, J., Higashida, R. T., … Council on Clinical Cardiology. (2012). Guidelines for the management of aneurysmal subarachnoid hemorrhage: a guideline for healthcare professionals from the American Heart Association/American Stroke Association. *Stroke, 43*(6), 1711–1737. doi: 10.1161/STR.0b013e3182587839

Cox, N. (2008). Managing the femoral artery in coronary angiography. *Heart, Lung, and Circulation,* 17 Suppl 4, S65–69. doi: 10.1016/j.hlc.2008.08.007

Diringer, M. N., Bleck, T. P., Claude Hemphill, J., 3rd, Menon, D., Shutter, L., Vespa, P., … Neurocritical Care Society. (2011). Critical care management of patients following aneurysmal subarachnoid hemorrhage: Recommendations from the Neurocritical Care Society's Multidisciplinary Consensus Conference. *Neurocritical Care, 15*(2), 211–240. doi: 10.1007/s12028-011-9605-9

Donovan, N. J., Daniels, S. K., Edmiaston, J., Weinhardt, J., Summers, D., Mitchell, P. H., … American Heart Association on Cardiovascular Nursing and Stroke Council. (2013). Dysphagia screening: State of the art: Invitational conference proceeding from the State-of-the-Art Nursing Symposium, International Stroke Conference 2012. *Stroke, 44*(4), e24–e31. doi: 10.1161/STR.0b013e3182877f57

Easton, J. D., Saver, J. L., Albers, G. W., Alberts, M. J., Chaturvedi, S., Feldmann, E., … Interdisciplinary Council on Peripheral Vascular Disease. (2009). Definition and evaluation of transient ischemic attack: A scientific statement for healthcare professionals from the American Heart Association/American Stroke Association Stroke Council; Council on Cardiovascular Surgery and Anesthesia; Council on Cardiovascular Radiology and Intervention; Council on Cardiovascular Nursing; and the Interdisciplinary Council on Peripheral Vascular Disease. The American Academy of Neurology affirms the value of this statement as an educational tool for neurologists. *Stroke, 40*(6), 2276–2293. doi: 10.1161/STROKEAHA.108.192218

Eisenstadt, S. E. (2010). Dysphagia and aspiration pneumonia in older adults. *Journal of the American Academy of Nurse Practitioners, 22*(1), 17–22. doi: 10.1111/j.1745-7599.2009.00470.x

Field, T. S., & Hill, M. D. (2012). Prevention of deep vein thrombosis and pulmonary embolism in patients with stroke. *Clinical and Applied Thrombosis/Hemostasis, 18*(1), 5–19. doi: 10.1177/1076029611412362

Frontera, J. A., Fernandez, A., Claassen, J., Schmidt, M., Schumacher, H. C., Wartenberg, K., ... Mayer, S. A. (2006). Hyperglycemia after SAH: Predictors, associated complications, and impact on outcome. *Stroke, 37*(1), 199–203. doi: 10.1161/01.STR.0000194960.73883.0f

Godoy, D. A., Di Napoli, M., & Rabinstein, A. A. (2010). Treating hyperglycemia in neurocritical patients: Benefits and perils. *Neurocritical Care, 13*(3), 425–438. doi: 10.1007/s12028-010-9404-8

Gur, A. Y., Lampl, Y., Gross, B., Royter, V., Shopin, L., & Bornstein, N. M. (2007). A new scale for assessing patients with vertebrobasilar stroke-the Israeli Vertebrobasilar Stroke Scale (IVBSS): Inter-rater reliability and concurrent validity. *Clinical Neurology and Neurosurgery, 109*(4), 317–322. doi: 10.1016/j.clineuro.2006.12.008

Guyatt, G. H., Akl, E. A., Crowther, M., Gutterman, D. D., Schuunemann, H. J., American College of Chest Physicians Antithrombotic, Therapy, & Prevention of Thrombosis Panel. (2012). Executive summary: Antithrombotic Therapy and Prevention of Thrombosis, 9th ed: American College of Chest Physicians Evidence-Based Clinical Practice Guidelines. *Chest, 141*(2 Suppl), 7S–47S. doi: 10.1378/chest.1412S3

Hannawi, Y., Hannawi, B., Rao, C. P., Suarez, J. I., & Bershad, E. M. (2013). Stroke-associated pneumonia: Major advances and obstacles. *Cerebrovascular Diseases, 35*(5), 430–443. doi: 10.1159/000350199

Hemphill, J. C., 3rd, Bonovich, D. C., Besmertis, L., Manley, G. T., & Johnston, S. C. (2001). The ICH score: A simple, reliable grading scale for intracerebral hemorrhage. *Stroke, 32*(4), 891–897.

Honeybul, S., & Ho, K. M. (2013). The current role of decompressive craniectomy in the management of neurological emergencies. *Brain Injury, 27*(9), 979–991. doi: 10.3109/02699052.2013.794974

Jauch, E. C., Saver, J. L., Adams, H. P., Jr., Bruno, A., Connors, J. J., Demaerschalk, B. M., ... Council on Clinical, Cardiology. (2013). Guidelines for the early management of patients with acute ischemic stroke: A guideline for healthcare professionals from the American Heart Association/American Stroke Association. *Stroke, 44*(3), 870–947. doi: 10.1161/STR.0b013e318284056a

Johnston, S. C., Rothwell, P. M., Nguyen-Huynh, M. N., Giles, M. F., Elkins, J. S., Bernstein, A. L., & Sidney, S. (2007). Validation and refinement of scores to predict very early stroke risk after transient ischaemic attack. *Lancet, 369*(9558), 283–292. doi: 10.1016/S0140-6736(07)60150-0

Kasner, S. E. (2006). Clinical interpretation and use of stroke scales. *Lancet Neurology, 5*(7), 603–612. doi: 10.1016/S1474-4422(06)70495-1

Kong, K. H., & Chuo, A. M. (2003). Incidence and outcome of orthostatic hypotension in stroke patients undergoing rehabilitation. *Archives of Physical Medicine and Rehabilitation, 84*(4), 559–562. doi: 10.1053/apmr.2003.50040

Kornbluth, J., & Bhardwaj, A. (2011). Evaluation of coma: A critical appraisal of popular scoring systems. *Neurocritical Care, 14*(1), 134–143. doi: 10.1007/s12028-010-9409-3

Kutty, S., Sengupta, P. P., & Khandheria, B. K. (2012). Patent foramen ovale: The known and the to be known. *Journal of the American College of Cardiology, 59*(19), 1665–1671. doi: 10.1016/j.jacc.2011.09.085

Li, H., Pan, R., Wang, H., Rong, X., Yin, Z., Milgrom, D. P., ... Peng, Y. (2013). Clipping versus coiling for ruptured intracranial aneurysms: A systematic review and meta-analysis. *Stroke, 44*(1), 29–37. doi: 10.1161/STROKEAHA.112.663559

Lin, C. H., Chen, K. H., Chang, C. H., Chen, C. M., Huang, Y. C., Hsu, H. C., & Hong, C. Z. (2013). Muscle pain intensity and pressure pain threshold changes in different periods of stroke patients. *American Journal of Physical Medicine and Rehabilitation, 93*(4), 299–309. doi: 10.1097/PHM.0000000000000003

Linares, G., & Mayer, S. A. (2009). Hypothermia for the treatment of ischemic and hemorrhagic stroke. *Critical Care Medicine, 37*(7 Suppl), S243–249. doi: 10.1097/CCM.0b013e3181aa5de1

Luitse, M. J., Biessels, G. J., Rutten, G. E., & Kappelle, L. J. (2012). Diabetes, hyperglycaemia, and acute ischaemic stroke. *Lancet Neurology, 11*(3), 261–271. doi: 10.1016/S1474-4422(12)70005-4

Marmagkiolis, K., Nikolaidis, I. G., Politis, T., & Goldstein, L. (2008). Approach to and management of the acute stroke patient with atrial fibrillation: A literature review. *Journal of Hospital Medicine, 3*(4), 326–332. doi: 10.1002/jhm.343

McNett, M., Amato, S., Gianakis, A., Grimm, D., Philippbar, S. A., Belle, J., & Moran, C. (2014). The FOUR Score and GCS as predictors of outcome after traumatic brain injury. *Neurocritical Care*. [epub ahead of print] doi: 10.1007/s12028-013-9947-6

Meyer, B. C., & Lyden, P. D. (2009). The modified National Institutes of Health Stroke Scale: Its time has come. *International Journal of Stroke, 4*(4), 267–273. doi: 10.1111/j.1747-4949.2009.00294.x

Miller, N. R. (2012). Dural carotid-cavernous fistulas: Epidemiology, clinical presentation, and management. *Neurosurgery Clinics of North America, 23*(1), 179–192. doi: 10.1016/j.nec.2011.09.008

Mohr, J. P., Grotta, J. C., Wolf, P. A., Moskowitz, M. A., Mayberg, M. R., & Von Kummer, R. (2011). *Stroke: Pathophysiology, diagnosis, and management* (5th ed.). Philadelphia: Saunders.

Morgenstern, L. B., Hemphill, J. C., 3rd, Anderson, C., Becker, K., Broderick, J. P., Connolly, E. S., Jr., ... Council on Cardiovascular Nursing. (2010). Guidelines for the management of spontaneous intracerebral hemorrhage: A guideline for healthcare professionals from the American Heart Association/American Stroke Association. *Stroke, 41*(9), 2108–2129. doi: 10.1161/STR.0b013e3181ec611b

Ogilvy, C. S., Stieg, P. E., Awad, I., Brown, R. D., Jr., Kondziolka, D., Rosenwasser, R., ... Stroke Council, American Stroke Association. (2001). Recommendations for the management of intracranial arteriovenous malformations: A statement for healthcare professionals from a special writing group of the Stroke Council, American Stroke Association. *Circulation, 103*(21), 2644–2657.

Poisson, S. N., Johnston, S. C., & Josephson, S. A. (2010). Urinary tract infections complicating stroke: Mechanisms, consequences, and possible solutions. *Stroke, 41*(4), e180–184. doi: 10.1161/STROKEAHA.109.576413

Purkayastha, S., & Sorond, F. (2012). Transcranial doppler ultrasound: Technique and application. *Seminars in Neurology, 32*(4), 411–420. doi: 10.1055/s-0032-1331812

Radermecker, R. P., & Scheen, A. J. (2010). Management of blood glucose in patients with stroke. *Diabetes and Metabolism, 36*(Suppl 3), S94–S99. doi: 10.1016/S1262-3636(10)70474-2

Rosen, D. S., & Macdonald, R. L. (2005). Subarachnoid hemorrhage grading scales: A systematic review. *Neurocritical Care, 2*(2), 110–118. doi: 10.1385/NCC:2:2:110

Rowe, S. A., Goodwin, H., Brophy, G. M., Bushwitz, J., Castle, A., Deen, D., ... for the Neurocritical Care Society Pharmacy, Section. (2013). Seizure prophylaxis in neurocritical care: A review of evidence-based support. *Pharmacotherapy, 34*(4), 396-409. doi: 10.1002/phar.1374

Saposnik, G., Barinagarrementeria, F., Brown, R. D., Jr., Bushnell, C. D., Cucchiara, B., Cushman, M., ... American Heart Association Stroke Council and the Council on Epidemiology and Prevention. (2011). Diagnosis and management of cerebral venous thrombosis: A statement for healthcare professionals from the American Heart Association/American Stroke Association. *Stroke, 42*(4), 1158–1192. doi: 10.1161/STR.0b013e31820a8364

Siddiqui, F. M., Bekker, S. V., & Qureshi, A. I. (2011). Neuroimaging of hemorrhage and vascular defects. *Neurotherapeutics, 8*(1), 28–38. doi: 10.1007/s13311-010-0009-x

Smith, E. R., & Scott, R. M. (2010). Moyamoya: Epidemiology, presentation, and diagnosis. *Neurosurgery Clinics of North America, 21*(3), 543–551. doi: 10.1016/j.nec.2010.03.007

Staykov, D., & Schwab, S. (2013). Clearing bloody cerebrospinal fluid: Clot lysis, neuroendoscopy and lumbar drainage. *Current Opinion in Critical Care, 19*(2), 92–100. doi: 10.1097/MCC.0b013e32835cae5e

Summers, D., Leonard, A., Wentworth, D., Saver, J. L., Simpson, J., Spilker, J. A., ... the American Heart Association Stroke Council on Cardiovascular Nursing and the Stroke Council. (2009). Comprehensive overview of nursing and interdisciplinary care of the acute ischemic stroke patient: A scientific statement from the American Heart Association. *Stroke, 40*(8), 2911–2944. doi: 10.1161/STROKEAHA.109.192362

The National Institute of Neurological Disorders and Stroke rt-PA Stroke Study Group. (1995). Tissue plasminogen activator for acute ischemic stroke. *New England Journal of Medicine, 333*(24), 1581–1587. doi: 10.1056/NEJM199512143332401

Titler, M. G., Shever, L. L., Kanak, M. F., Picone, D. M., & Qin, R. (2011). Factors associated with falls during hospitalization in an older adult population. *Research and Theory for Nursing Practice, 25*(2), 127–148.

Tong, E., Hou, Q., Fiebach, J. B., & Wintermark, M. (2014). The role of imaging in acute ischemic stroke. *Neurosurgical Focus, 36*(1), E3. doi: 10.3171/2013.10.FOCUS13396

Wiegand, D. L. (2011). *AACN procedure manual for critical care* (6th ed.). Philadelphia: Saunders.

Wijdicks, E. F., Sheth, K. N., Carter, B. S., Greer, D. M., Kasner, S. E., Kimberly, W. T., … American Heart Association Stroke Council. (2014). Recommendations for the management of cerebral and cerebellar infarction with swelling: A statement for healthcare professionals from the American Heart Association/ American Stroke Association. *Stroke, 45*(4), 1222–1238. doi: 10.1161/01.str.0000441965.15164.d6

Wilson, J. T., Hareendran, A., Grant, M., Baird, T., Schulz, U. G., Muir, K. W., & Bone, I. (2002). Improving the assessment of outcomes in stroke: Use of a structured interview to assign grades on the modified Rankin Scale. *Stroke, 33*(9), 2243–2246.

Wu, T. C., Kasam, M., Harun, N., Hallevi, H., Bektas, H., Acosta, I., … Savitz, S. I. (2011). Pharmacological deep vein thrombosis prophylaxis does not lead to hematoma expansion in intracerebral hemorrhage with intraventricular extension. *Stroke, 42*(3), 705–709. doi: 10.1161/STROKEAHA.110.600593

Chapter

6

Medications

Gretchen Brophy, PharmD BCPS FCCP FCCM; Amber Castle, PharmD BCPS; Ron Neyens, PharmD BCPS; Christina M. Szabo, PhD RN CCRN CNRN

Knowledge and the ability to apply information regarding stroke pharmacology are extremely important for the expert stroke nurse. The expert stroke nurse should understand the application of pharmacology in patient care including recognizing the indication, dosage, and administration; evaluating and monitoring therapeutic effect; and minimizing adverse effects and interactions. The expert stroke nurse also must be able to effectively educate patients and families about the medication name, dose and schedule, route and technique of administration, expected therapeutic response, symptoms of major adverse effects, significant drug-drug and food-drug interactions, and who to contact if there is a therapeutic failure or adverse drug event. This chapter will focus on the pharmacology of pertinent medications used in stroke patients.

Objectives

1. Identify commonly used classes of medications for patients with neurological injury.
   - Antiplatelets
   - Anticoagulants
   - Thrombolytics
   - Antihypertensives and diuretics
   - Vasopressors and inotropes
   - Lipid-lowering agents
   - Nimodipine
   - Osmotic agents
   - Anticonvulsants
   - Glycemic control
   - Antispasmodics
   - Antidepressants
   - Neurostimulants
   - Atypical neuroleptics
   - Analgesics
   - Sedatives
   - Antipyretics

2. Compare and contrast the indications for use of these medications for various disease states.
3. Describe the mechanisms of action, drug interactions, and adverse effects associated with these medications.
4. Discuss the timing and duration of therapy for selected medications for patients with neurological injury.
5. Discuss the dosage of specific medications based on their therapeutic indications.

Antiplatelets

A. Indication
 1. Primary prevention of ischemic stroke
  a. Indications—risk to benefit assessment (Goldstein et al., 2011)
   (1) Ten-year risk for cardiovascular disease 6% or higher
   (2) High-risk women, with greatest benefit if 65 years of age or older
  b. Aspirin 81 mg is preferred to minimize bleeding complications (Goldstein et al., 2011)
   (1) No other antiplatelet agents have indications for primary prevention.
 2. Secondary prevention of ischemic stroke
  a. All antiplatelet agents are reasonable options, with agent selection being patient specific and dependent on factors such as effectiveness, safety, tolerability, and cost
  b. Long-term combination antiplatelet therapy for stroke prevention generally is not recommended because of an increased risk of bleeding (Furie et al., 2011).
  c. Short-term combination antiplatelet therapy may be indicated in specific scenarios (Furie et al., 2011).
   (1) New ischemic stroke and recent coronary stent
    (a) Duration dependent on stent type and date of placement
   (2) Cerebral circulation stent
   (3) Minor stroke and transient ischemic attack (Wang et al., 2013)

B. Mechanism (**Table 6-1** and **Figure 6-1**)
 1. Antiplatelet medications decrease platelet aggregation via various mechanisms (Siller-Matula, Krumphuber, & Jilma, 2010).
  a. Cyclooxygenase (COX) inhibition to decrease production of thromboxane A_2
  b. Antagonizes P2Y12 component of adenosine diphosphate (ADP) receptor
  c. Phosphodiesterase (PDE) inhibition to decrease breakdown of cyclic adenosine monophosphate
  d. Antagonizes glycoprotein IIb/IIIa (GPIIb/IIIa) receptor

C. Dose (Table 6-1)

D. Adverse drug reactions (Lexi-Comp, 2013)
 1. Consistent with its mechanism; the most common adverse reaction is bleeding.

E. Contraindications (Lexi-Comp, 2013)
 1. Severe hypersensitivity or active pathological bleeding

F. Interactions (Table 6-1; Lexi-Comp, 2013)
 1. Increased bleeding risk if taken in combination with specific medications
  a. Anticoagulants
  b. Nonsteroidal antiinflammatory drugs (NSAIDs)
  c. Herbals
   (1) Examples include ginkgo, garlic, ginger, ginseng

G. Monitoring (Lexi-Comp, 2013)
 1. Bleeding

Table 6-1. Antiplatelet Medications (Furie et al., 2011; Serebruany et al., 2005; Levine et al., 2011; Lexi-Comp, 2013)

Indication	Medication	Dose	Interactions	Clinical Pearls
Primary prevention	*Cyclooxygenase inhibitor*			
	Aspirin	81–325 mg daily	Aspirin may ↑ methotrexate levels (aspirin dose dependent) ↓ aspirin effects: Nonselective nonsteroidal antiinflammatory drug (avoid if possible)	Irreversible—inhibits for life of platelet (5–7 days) GI bleed is most common complication: – Dose-dependent risk: ≤ 325 mg/day = ~0.4%/yr – 81 mg vs 325 mg—higher dose may ↑ risk 2x – Risk is not decreased with buffered or enteric-coated dosage formulations.
Secondary prevention	**Aspirin**	see above	see above	see above
	PDE inhibitor			
	Dipyridamole/ Aspirin (Aggrenox®)	200 mg/25 mg BID	No significant	Irreversible—inhibits for life of platelet (5–7 days) Headache in up to 40% of patients – Tolerance often develops within 1–2 weeks
	Adenosine diphosphate inhibitors			
	Clopidogrel (Plavix®)	75 mg daily	↓ clopidogrel effects: Proton pump inhibitors	Pro-drug—CYP conversion to active metabolite – Impacted by genetic polymorphisms (CYP2C19) Irreversible—inhibits for life of platelet (5–7 days) Hypersensitivity (usually rash) in 4%–6% – Cross reactivity to ticlopidine in up to 27% ADR: TTP is rare (ticlopidine > clopidogrel)
	Ticlopidine (Ticlid®)	250 mg BID	No significant	Pro-drug—CYP conversion to active metabolite Irreversible—inhibits for life of platelet (5–7 days) Replaced by clopidogrel—delayed onset and ↑ ADRs ADRs: GI intolerance, neutropenia, aplastic anemia, and TTP

ADR indicates adverse drug reaction; BID, twice daily; CYP, cytochrome P450; GI, gastrointestinal; PDE, phosphodiesterase; TTP, thrombotic thrombocytopenic purpura.

Figure 6-1. Antiplatelet Mechanism

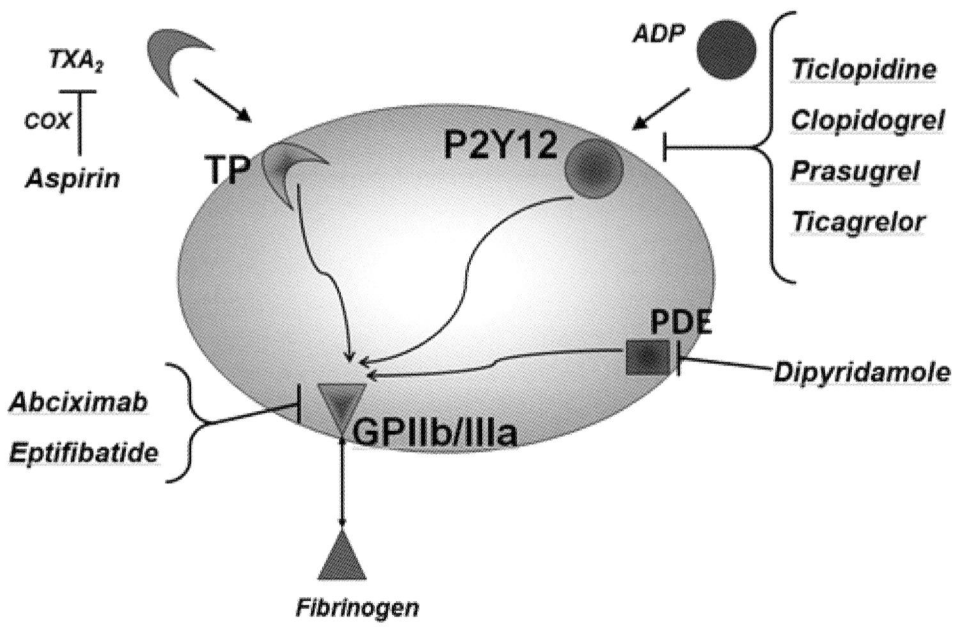

Antiplatelet medications and their respective receptor or enzyme target.

ADP indicates adenosine diphosphate; COX, cyclooxygenase; GPIIb/IIIa, glycoprotein IIb/IIIa; PDE, phosphodiesterase; TP, thromboxane prostanoid; TXA_2, thromboxane A_2.

Reprinted from "Pharmacokinetic, Pharmacodynamic and Clinical Profile of Novel Antiplatelet Drugs Targeting Vascular Diseases," by J. M. Siller-Matula, J. Krumphuber, and B. Jilma, 2010, British Journal of Pharmacology, 159*(3), pp. 502–517. © 2010 by the British Pharmacological Society. Reprinted with permission.*

2. Platelet resistance (or inadequate antiplatelet response; Eikelboom, Hirsh, Spencer, Baglin, & Weitz, 2012)
   a. Incidence varies based on the test used, medical comorbidities, ethnicity of the patient, medication compliance, drug interactions, and genetic polymorphisms
      (1) Incidence is higher for clopidogrel in comparison with aspirin.
   b. The role of testing and any reactant therapeutic strategy remains undefined.
   c. Accumetrics (VerifyNow®) is the most common test used.
      (1) Reported as aspirin reaction units or P2Y12 reaction units

H. Drug-specific information
1. Aspirin
   a. The NSAID interaction is not definite; however, it is best to avoid the combination if feasible (Medwatch, 2010).
2. Clopidogrel
   a. Genetic polymorphisms, specifically cytochrome P450 (CYP2C19), may impair or enhance conversion to active metabolite (Eikelboom et al., 2012).
      (1) The role of genetic testing remains undefined.
   b. Clopidogrel plus proton pump inhibitors (PPIs) may impair the conversion to active metabolite (Levine et al., 2011).
      (1) A meaningful difference in clinical outcome does not exist.
      (2) Clinical relevance may exist in CYP2C19 poor metabolizers.
      (3) Remains reasonable to utilize a PPI in those at risk for gastrointestinal bleeding.

(a) If clinical concern exists, pantoprazole (Protonix®) or rabeprazole (Aciphex®) may be a safer alternative.

3. Dipyridamole/aspirin
   a. It is more effective than aspirin alone in secondary prevention of ischemic stroke; however, it may be poorly tolerated (Verro, Gorelick, & Nguyen, 2008).
   b. For patients with intolerable headache, a once-daily regimen can be used until tolerance develops before increasing to the usual twice-daily schedule (Lexi-Comp, 2013).
4. Abciximab (Reopro®) and eptifibatide (Integrilin®)
   a. GPIIb/IIIa inhibitors used during endovascular procedures for stroke
5. Others
   a. Prasugrel (Effient®) and ticagrelor (Brilinta®) are more potent P2Y12/ADP inhibitors but only have indications for acute coronary syndromes (ACS; Eikelboom et al., 2012).
      (1) Contraindications exist for utilization in stroke.

Anticoagulants

A. Indication (**Table 6-2**; Furie et al., 2012)
   1. Warfarin
      a. Indicated as anticoagulant in all forms of cardioembolic stroke
   2. Novel oral anticoagulants
      a. Indicated as anticoagulant for nonvalvular atrial fibrillation
         1) Dabigatran has an increased risk of embolic events if used as an anticoagulant for patients with valvular disease (Van de Werf et al., 2012).

B. Mechanism (Table 6-2 and **Figure 6-2**; Furie et al., 2012; Ageno et al., 2012)
   1. Anticoagulant medications decrease clot formation via various mechanisms.
      a. Vitamin K epoxide reductase complex 1 inhibition to decrease activation of vitamin K-dependent clotting factors (II, VII, IX, and X)
      b. Direct inhibition of free and fibrin-bound thrombin
      c. Direct inhibition of free and clot-bound factor Xa

C. Initiation of anticoagulation is typically deferred for several days after acute ischemic stroke because of the risk of hemorrhagic transformation (Furie et al., 2011)

D. Dose (Table 6-2; Lexi-Comp, 2013)
   1. Warfarin dosing is highly variable and dependent on indication, drug-drug interactions, dietary vitamin K intake, and genetic polymorphisms.
   2. Novel oral anticoagulant dosing may vary based on age, renal function, drug-drug interactions, and bleeding risk factors (Eikelboom et al., 2011; Furie et al., 2012).
      a. Limited data for use in the elderly older than 75 years of age
         1) Bleed risk varies based on dose, age, end-organ function, drug-drug interactions, and concomitant risk factors that may increase bleeding.
      b. Risk stratification, dosing strategy, and place in therapy may vary depending on referenced guideline (Heidbuchel et al., 2013).

E. Adverse drug reactions (Lexi-Comp, 2013)
   1. Consistent with its mechanism, the most common adverse reaction is bleeding.

F. Contraindications (Table 6-2; Lexi-Comp, 2013)
   1. Severe hypersensitivity or active pathological bleeding
   2. Recommend avoiding use with severe organ impairment
      a. Warfarin
         (1) Caution and close monitoring with severe hepatic impairment
      b. Dabigatran
         (1) Avoid use with severe renal impairment

Table 6-2. Anticoagulant Medications (Ageno et al., 2012; Furie et al., 2012; Lexi-Comp, 2013)

	Warfarin (Coumadin®)	Dabigatran (Pradaxa®)	Rivaroxaban (Xarelto®)	Apixaban (Eliquis®)
Mechanism	Vitamin K antagonist	Direct thrombin inhibitor	Direct Xa inhibitor	Direct Xa inhibitor
Indication	Cardioembolic stroke	Nonvalvular afib VTE treatment	Nonvalvular afib VTE treatment VTE prophylaxis (ortho)	Nonvalvular afib VTE prophylaxis (ortho)
Dose	Variable; titrate to INR 2–3 (goal 2.5–3.5 in some indications)	75–150 mg BID†	15–20 mg daily† (afib) Other indications: dose varies	2.5–5 mg BID†
Onset	48–120+ hr	1–2 hr	2–4 hr	3–4 hr
Half-Life	20–60 hr (variable)	12–17 hr‡	5–13 hr‡	8–15 hr‡
Drug Interactions	↑ warfarin effects: Herbals Amiodarone/ Dronedarone Antibiotics Antifungals HIV medications Phenytoin Acute ethanol ingestion ↓ warfarin effects: Phenobarbital Carbamazepine Rifampin Vitamin K (food as well) Chronic ethanol ingestion	↑ dabigatran effects: Dronedarone Ketoconazole ↓ dabigatran effects: Rifampin	↑ rivaroxaban effects: Clarithromycin/ Erythromycin Ketoconazole/ Fluconazole Ritonavir ↓ rivaroxaban effects: Phenytoin Phenobarbital Carbamazepine Rifampin	↑ apixaban effects: Clarithromycin/ Erythromycin Ketoconazole/ Fluconazole Ritonavir ↓ apixiban effects: Phenytoin Phenobarbital Carbamazepine Rifampin
Contraindications	Child-Pugh C (caution)	CrCl ≤15 ml/min	CrCl ≤15 ml/min Child-Pugh C	CrCl ≤15-25 ml/min Child-Pugh C
Reversal Agent	Vitamin K + FFP or PCC (life threatening) Not dialyzable	No antidote PCC or rFVIIa (life threating) Dialyzable	No antidote PCC or rFVIIa (life threating) Not dialyzable	No antidote PCC or rFVIIa (life threating) Not dialyzable
Peri-Procedural Discontinuation	1–7 days (surgery risk dependent)	1–7 days (renal function and surgery risk dependent)	1–5 days (renal function and surgery risk dependent)	1–5 days (renal function and surgery risk dependent)
Clinical Pearls	Numerous drug-drug-food interactions	Prodrug—hydrolysis to active form Do not open/ crush (~75% ↑ in exposure)	Can crush and administer via feeding tube (as long as not given post-pyloric)	No data for feeding tube administration

afib indicates atrial fibrillation; BID, twice daily; CrCl, creatinine clearance; FFP, fresh frozen plasma; INR, international normalized ratio; PCC, prothrombin complex concentrate; ortho, orthopedic; rFVIIa, activated recombinant factor VII.

†Dose depends on age, renal function, and drug-drug interactions

‡Half-life can be prolonged with end-organ dysfunction: dabigatran (renal), rivaroxaban, and apixaban (renal/hepatic)

Figure 6-2. Anticoagulant Mechanism

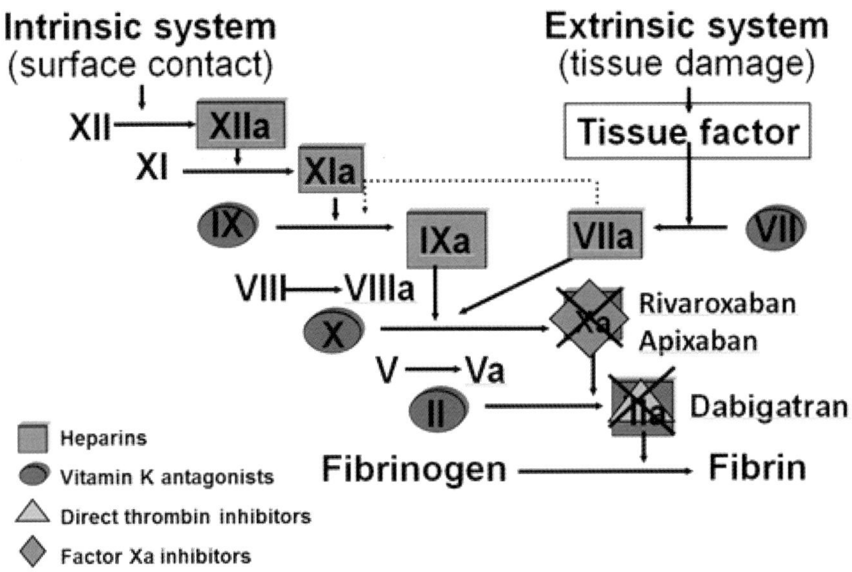

Anticoagulant medications used in the management of stroke and their respective receptor target.

Reprinted from "Oral Anticoagulant Therapies: Balancing the Risks," by E. A. Nutescu, 2013, American Journal of Health System Pharmacy, *70(10 Suppl 1), pp. S3–S11. © 2013 by the American Society of Health-System Pharmacists. Reprinted with permission.*

c. Rivaroxaban and apixaban
(1) Avoid use with severe renal or hepatic impairment

G. Interactions (Table 6-2; Lexi-Comp, 2013)
1. Increased bleeding risk if taken with medications that decrease the ability to clot
a. Antiplatelets
b. NSAIDs
c. Herbals
(1) Examples include ginkgo, garlic, ginger, and ginseng
2. Warfarin has numerous drug-drug and drug-food interactions.
a. An interaction check should be conducted with the addition or removal of any medication.
b. Consistent dietary vitamin K intake is necessary.
c. Binge alcohol use and chronic alcohol abuse must be avoided.
3. Novel oral anticoagulants have fewer drug-drug and drug-food interactions than warfarin, but limited documentation currently exists (Heidbuchel et al., 2013).

H. Monitoring (Lexi-Comp, 2013)
1. Bleeding
2. Coagulation assays (Douxfils, Mullier, Robert, et al., 2012; Douxfils, Mullier, Loosen, et al., 2012; Douxfils, Chatelain, Chatelain, Dogne, & Mullier, 2013)
a. Warfarin and international normalized ratio (INR) monitoring are well validated.
(1) Target INR range for stroke prevention in nonvalvular atrial fibrillation patients is 2–3.
(2) Percentage of time in target INR range is approximately 60% in clinical practice (Furie et al., 2012).
b. Novel oral anticoagulants do not have clinically validated monitoring assays.

(1) Routine monitoring not recommended but may be beneficial in specific scenarios
    (a) Emergent bleeding
    (b) Drug compliance assessment
    (c) Drug accumulation assessment in presence of uncertain end-organ function
(2) Dabigatran
    (a) Activated partial thromboplastin time—reagent variability, does not correlate with therapeutic serum concentrations at high concentrations
    (b) Thrombin time—highly sensitive, does not quantify serum concentrations, but may be useful to determine presence of dabigatran
    (c) Hemoclot thrombin inhibitor assay—good correlation to therapeutic serum concentrations but not routinely available
(3) Rivaroxaban
    (a) Prothrombin time (PT)—reagent variability, may be elevated, but does not correlate to therapeutic serum concentrations and clinical effect
    (b) Agent specific anti-Xa assay—good correlation to therapeutic serum concentrations but not routinely available
(4) Apixaban
    (a) PT—reagent variability, not sensitive enough to prolong with therapeutic serum concentrations
    (b) Agent-specific anti-Xa assay—good correlation to therapeutic serum concentrations but not routinely available

Thrombolytics

A. Alteplase (Activase®; also known as tissue plasminogen activator [tPA]) is the only thrombolytic approved for the treatment of stroke.

B. Indication
  1. Acute ischemic stroke, must be given within 4.5 hours of symptom onset (Jauch et al., 2013)

C. Mechanism (Lansberg et al., 2012; Lexi-Comp, 2013)
  1. Promotes fibrinolysis of a fibrin clot via activation of plasminogen to plasmin
  2. Highly specific for clot-bound fibrin, which minimizes systemic fibrinolysis

D. Dose (Lexi-Comp, 2013)
  1. 0.9 mg/kg, 10% as an intravenous bolus over 1 minute, with remainder infused over 60 minutes
  2. Maximum dose is 90 mg for patients weighing more than 100 kg.
  3. Specific guidelines exist for reconstitution. The vial should not be shaken; otherwise, the medication may be ineffective as a result of protein destruction.
  4. Line should be flushed after alteplase administration to ensure delivery of the total dose.
  5. Within 10 minutes after infusion is complete, 80% of the drug is cleared from the body.

E. Adverse drug reactions (Jauch et al., 2013; Lexi-Comp, 2013)
  1. Consistent with its mechanism, the most common adverse reaction is bleeding.
     a. Intracranial hemorrhage occurs in up to 6% of patients but can be minimized with appropriate patient selection, dosing, monitoring, and post-infusion supportive care.
  2. Orolingual angioedema
     a. Occurs in up to 5%
        (1) Often unilateral and contralateral to ischemic hemisphere
        (2) Risk factors—angiotensin-converting enzyme inhibitor (ACEI) use, strokes involving the insular and frontal cortex
  3. Anaphylaxis
     a. Rare, occurs in <0.5%

F. Contraindications (Jauch et al., 2013; Lexi-Comp, 2013)
  1. Severe hypersensitivity or active pathological bleeding
  2. An extensive list of relative and absolute contraindications exist (a few are listed in **Table 6-3**; however, refer to the package insert or another reliable reference for more complete information).

G. Interactions (Lexi-Comp, 2013)
  1. No significant interactions exist

H. Monitoring (Jauch et al., 2013; Lexi-Comp, 2013)
  1. Frequent neurological assessments—every 15 minutes during infusion, then every 30 minutes for the next 6 hours, then hourly until 24 hours after treatment
     a. A significant neurological change, severe headache, acute hypertension, or new onset nausea and vomiting require interruption of the thrombolytic infusion (if applicable) and emergent assessment for possible hemorrhagic conversion.
  2. Blood pressure—every 15 minutes for initial 2 hours, then every 30 minutes for the next 6 hours, then hourly until 24 hours after treatment
     a. Goal—systolic blood pressure ≤180 mmHg and diastolic blood pressure ≤105 mmHg

I. Clinical pearls (Jauch et al., 2013)
  1. Thrombolytic success rate depends on several factors, including clot composition and clot burden
     a. Larger clots, typically located in more proximal arteries (e.g., internal carotid, proximal middle cerebral artery), are more resistant to successful intravenous (IV) thrombolytic therapy.
  2. Following thrombolytic therapy, antiplatelet agents and deep vein thrombosis (DVT) prophylaxis are usually withheld for the initial 24 hours until the patient is deemed clinically stable without hemorrhagic transformation.

Table 6-3. Alteplase Relative and Absolute Contraindications

Inclusion	Contraindications
Onset within 3 hr	Active internal bleeding
	Evidence or history of intracranial hemorrhage
	Suspicion of subarachnoid hemorrhage
	Intracranial or intraspinal surgery, serious head trauma, or previous stroke within the past 3 months
	Uncontrolled hypertension, SBP >185 mmHg or DBP >110 mmHg
	Intracranial neoplasm or vascular malformation
	Recent warfarin use with an INR >1.7 or use of heparin or novel oral anticoagulation in the past 2 days with abnormal coagulation assays
	Platelet count <100,000/m^3
Onset within 3–4.5 hr	Above contraindications plus any of the following:
	Age >80 years
	History of prior stroke and diabetes
	Anticoagulant use prior to admission, regardless of coagulation assays
	NIHSS ≥25

DBP indicates diastolic blood pressure; INR, international normalized ratio; NIHSS, National Institutes of Health stroke scale; SBP, systolic blood pressure.

Antihypertensives and Diuretics

A. Indication (Lexi-Comp, 2013)

1. Blood pressure or rate control depending on agent selected
   a. Agent selection is dependent on patient and disease-specific factors
   b. Blood pressure
      (1) Beta blockers with alpha antagonism, dihydropyridine calcium channel blockers, ACEIs, angiotensin II receptor blockers, renin antagonist, thiazide diuretics, potassium-sparing diuretics, direct vasodilators, alpha-1 antagonists, nitrates, and central alpha-2 agonists
   c. Rate control
      (1) Beta blockers and nondihydropyridine calcium channel blockers (e.g., verapamil and diltiazem)

B. Mechanism (Dasta et al., 2010; Lexi-Comp, 2013)

1. Blood pressure = cardiac output (CO) x systemic vascular resistance (SVR)
2. Blood pressure medications decrease blood pressure via various mechanisms—See **Table 6-4** for IV blood pressure medications. (Oral agents are excluded because of the numerous options, yet mechanisms of specific classes are summarized below.)
   a. $Beta_1$ antagonist to decrease heart rate and CO
      (1) Beta blockers (generic name ends with -lol)
   b. $Alpha_1$ antagonist to decrease systemic vascular resistance
      (1) Beta blockers with $alpha_1$ antagonism (e.g., carvedilol, labetalol)
      (2) $Alpha_1$ selective (generic name ends with -zosin)
   c. $Alpha_2$ agonist to decrease catecholamine outflow
      (1) Central acting (e.g., clonidine, guanfacine, guanabenz, methyldopa)
   d. Calcium channel antagonist to decrease heart rate (nondihydropyridine) or systemic vascular resistance (dihydropyridine)
      (1) Nondihydropyridine (e.g., verapamil, diltiazem)
      (2) Dihydropyridine (generic name ends with -dipine)
   e. Renin-angiotensin system modulation to decrease systemic vascular resistance and/or to reduce sodium and water retention
      (1) ACEI (generic name ends with -pril)
      (2) Angiotensin-II blockers (generic name ends with -artan)
      (3) Renin inhibitor (e.g., aliskiren)
      (4) Aldosterone antagonist (e.g., spironolactone, eplerenone)
   f. Direct vasodilation to reduce systemic vascular resistance
      (1) Vasodilators (e.g., hydralazine, minoxidil)
   g. Nitric oxide and cyclic guanosine monophosphate modulation to decrease systemic vascular resistance
      (1) Nitrates (e.g., nitroglycerin in various dosage formulations)
   h. Diuretics to decrease sodium and water retention (e.g., thiazide and loop, and potassium-sparing diuretics) and systemic vascular resistance via antagonism of vascular sodium channels (e.g., thiazide diuretics)
      (1) Thiazide (e.g., hydrochlorothiazide, chlorthalidone, indapamide)
      (2) Loop (e.g., furosemide, bumetanide, torsemide, ethacrynic acid)
         (a) Estimated dose conversion ratio is furosemide:torsemide:bumetanide (40:20:1)
         (b) Ethacrynic acid used if severe sulfa allergy; however, it has a greater degree of ototoxicity.

Table 6-4. Intravenous Antihypertensives (Dasta et al., 2010; Lexi-Comp, 2013)

Medication	Pharmacokinetics	Dosing	Cautions/CI	Clinical Pearls
Beta Blockers				
Labetalol (Trandate®)	O: 2–5 min D: 2–18 hr	Bolus: 10–20 mg Infusion: 1–3 mg/min Max: ~ 300 mg/day	Caution: heart failure, aortic stenosis, bradycardia CI: 2nd-/3rd-degree heart block	Nonselective ($alpha_1$/$beta_{1,2}$) Blood pressure control Short-term use—oral transition Respiratory distress (COPD patients)
Metoprolol (Lopressor®)	O: 2–5 min D: 5–8 hr	Bolus: 1.25–5 mg q6h Max: 15 mg q3h		B_1 selective Heart rate control
Esmolol (Brevibloc®)	O: 2–10 min D: 10–20 min	Bolus: 500 mcg/kg Infusion: 50–300 mcg/kg/min		B_1 selective Heart rate control Thrombophlebitis risk
Calcium Channel Blockers				
Nicardipine (Cardene®)	O: 10 min D: ≤8 hr	Infusion: 5–15 mg/hr	Caution: heart failure, aortic stenosis	PIV = risk for volume overload CIV = concentration > 0.2 mg/mL
Clevidipine (Cleviprex®)	O: 2–4 min D: 5–15 min	Infusion: 1–32 mg/hr (usually controlled on <10 mg/hr)		20% lipid—caution for soy or egg allergy Short-term use—oral transition
ACE Inhibitors				
Enalaprilat (Vasotec®)	O: 15 min D: 6 hr	Bolus: 1.25 mg q6h Max: 5 mg q6h	Caution: hyperkalemia, aortic stenosis, renal artery stenosis, renal insufficiency CI: allergy, angioedema	Not first line—unpredictable effects Drug cough (ACEI cough) Angioedema
Vasodilators				
Hydralazine	O: 5–20 min D: 1–4 hr	Bolus: 10–20 mg q4-6h Max: 40 mg q4-6h	Caution: coronary disease, rheumatic heart disease	Not first line—unpredictable effects Tachycardia, angina (CAD patients)
Nitroglycerin	O: 1–2 min D: 3–5 min	Infusion: 5–200 mcg/min	CI: restrictive cardiomyopathy, constrictive pericarditis	Coronary selectivity Tachyphylaxis (nitrate tolerance)
Nitroprusside (Nitropress®)	O: 1–2 min D: 1–10 min	Infusion: 0.3–10 mcg/kg/min	Caution: heart failure, renal or hepatic insufficiency	Venous and arterial dilator Cyanide or thiocyanate toxicity May ↑ ICP with large dose titrations

ACEI indicates angiotensin converting enzyme inhibitor; CAD, coronary artery disease; CI, contraindication; CIV, central intravenous line; COPD, chronic obstructive pulmonary disease; D, duration; ICP, intracranial pressure; mcg, micrograms; mg, milligrams; O, onset; PIV, peripheral intravenous line; q, every.

Adapted from "Intravenous to Oral Conversion of Antihypertensives: A Toolkit for Guideline Development [Review]," by J. F. Dasta, B. A. Boucher, G. M. Brophy, H. Cohen, E. Hassan, R. Maclaren, … A. L. Seybert, 2010, The Annals of Pharmacotherapy, *44(9), pp. 1430–1447. © 2010 by SAGE Publications. Adapted with permission.*

(3) Potassium-sparing (e.g., amiloride, spironolactone, eplerenone, triamterene)
(4) Carbonic anhydrase inhibitors (e.g., acetazolamide)
(a) Weak diuretic, primarily used for chloride-unresponsive metabolic alkalosis to decrease tubular reabsorption of bicarbonate

C. Dose (intravenous antihypertensives) (Table 6-4)

D. Adverse drug reactions (Lexi-Comp, 2013)

1. Adverse drug reactions are agent (or class) specific, with the most common listed below
2. Beta blockers
   a. Nonselective (B_1 and B_2) blockers may cause bronchospasm, with the highest risk of occurrence being in those patients with hyperactive airway disease
   b. Bradycardia
3. $Alpha_1$ antagonist
   a. Orthostasis and syncope
4. $Alpha_2$ agonist
   a. Drowsiness, fatigue, and depression
   b. Rebound hypertension upon abrupt discontinuation
5. ACEI and angiotensin-II blockers
   a. ACEI—dry, nonproductive cough ("ACEI cough") and angioedema; patients experiencing adverse effects with ACEI often will tolerate angiotensin-II blockers.
   b. Hyperkalemia
6. Nitrates
   a. Headache
7. Diuretics
   a. Thiazide and loop—hyponatremia and hypokalemia
   b. Thiazide—hypercalcemia and hyperuricemia
   c. Loop—ototoxicity, which is dose and administration rate dependent
   d. Potassium-sparing—hyperkalemia
   e. Carbonic anhydrase inhibitors—paresthesia and metabolic acidosis

E. Contraindications (Lexi-Comp, 2013)

1. Severe hypersensitivity
2. Agent specific
   a. Beta blockers
      (1) Second- or third-degree heart block
   b. Nondihydropyridine calcium channel blockers
      (1) Second- or third-degree heart block
      (2) Supraventricular arrhythmia with an accessory bypass tract (e.g., Wolff-Parkinson-White)
   c. ACEI and angiotensin-II blockers
      (1) Acute kidney injury
      (2) Bilateral renal artery stenosis
      (3) Pregnancy—may harm developing fetus
      (4) Concomitant use with aliskiren (renin inhibitor) in diabetic patients
   d. Nitrates
      (1) Concomitant use with PDE-5 inhibitors (sildenafil, tadalafil, or vardenafil) can cause severe hypotension.

Vasopressors and Inotropes

A. Indication
   1. Blood pressure or cardiac contractility augmentation depending on agent selected
      a. Agent selection is dependent on patient and disease-specific factors as well as type of shock
B. Mechanism (**Table 6-5**; Lexi-Comp, 2013; Hollenberg, 2011)
   1. Vasoactive medications increase blood pressure and cardiac output via various mechanisms
   2. Increase in SVR
      a. Agonism of $alpha_1$ or $vasopressin_1$ receptors
   3. Increase in cardiac contractility
      a. Agonism of $beta_1$ receptors or inhibition of PDE
C. Dose (Table 6-5)
   1. Agents should be initiated at a low dose and titrated slowly to achieve hemodynamic goals.
   2. Agents should be infused via a central line.
   3. Vital signs should be continuously monitored.
   4. Vasopressors may be less effective in acidemic patients; however, effects of vasopressin may be spared.
D. Adverse drug reactions (Hollenberg, 2011; Kellum & Pinsky, 2002)
   1. Agents can cause similar adverse reactions (e.g., tachyarrhythmias, tissue and end-organ ischemia, extravasation); however, some agents have a higher propensity than others.
   2. Tachyarrhythmias
      a. Dopamine, dobutamine, and epinephrine have a higher rate than norepinephrine.
      b. Phenylephrine may result in a reflexive bradycardia.
   3. Extravasation
      a. Treatment—phentolamine 5–10 mg diluted in 10 mL 0.9% NaCl, infiltrated as soon as possible

Table 6-5. Vasopressor and Inotropes (Hollenberg, 2011; Kellum & Pinsky, 2002)

Drug	Dose	Receptors						Cardiac Effects		Peripheral Vasculature Effects	
		α_1	β_1	β_2	D_1	PDE	V_1	HR	CO	Vasoconstriction	Vasodilation
Dobutamine	2–20 mcg/kg/min	+	+++	+	0	0	0	++	++++	+	++
Dopamine	1–3 mcg/kg/min	+/-	++	+/-	++++	0	0	+	+	0	+
	4–10 mcg/kg/min	++	+++	+	++	0	0	++	+++	+	0
	11–20 mcg/kg/min	++++	+++	0	+	0	0	++	+/-	+++	0
Epinephrine (Adrenalin®)	1–20 mcg/min	+++	+++	++	0	0	0	++++	++++	++++	+++
Milrinone (Primacor®)	0.375–0.75 mcg/kg/min	0	0	0	0	++++	0	+	+++	0	++
Norepinephrine (Levophed®)	2–30 mcg/min	++++	+++	0	0	0	0	+	++	++++	0
Phenylephrine (Neo-Synephrine®)	40–200 mcg/min	++++	0	0	0	0	0	0	0	+++	0
Vasopressin (Pitressin®)	0.01–0.03 units/min	0	0	0	0	0	++++	0	0	++++	0

α_1 *indicates alpha*$_1$*;* β_1*, beta*$_1$*;* β_2*, beta*$_2$*; CO, cardiac output;* D_1*, dopamine*$_1$ *HR, heart rate; PDE, phosphodiesterase;* V_1*, vasopressin*$_1$*.*

Adapted from "Vasoactive Drugs in Circulatory Shock," by S. M. Hollenberg, 2011, American Journal of Respiratory and Critical Care Medicine, 183*(7), pp. 847–855.*

Lipid-Lowering Agents

A. Indication (Furie et al., 2011; Goldstein et al., 2011; McKenney, 2003)
   1. Various pharmacologic agents exist. Each affect the low-density lipoprotein (LDL), high-density lipoprotein (HDL), and triglycerides to differing amounts, with the statin class of medications having the best clinical literature for primary and secondary risk reduction.
   2. The treatment goal is to improve the cholesterol profile by targeting LDL and non-HDL levels defined by risk-assessment strategies.
      a. In the adult treatment panel (ATP) III guidelines that were published in 2003, if a stroke is caused by atherosclerosis, high-intensity statin therapy with atorvastatin, rosuvastatin, or simvastatin was recommended to target LDL levels <100 mg/dL (ideally <70 mg/dL; McKenney, 2003).
      b. The 2013 ATP IV (American College of Cardiology/American Heart Association) guidelines do not recommend specific treatment goals, but they do recommend high-intensity therapy (i.e., atorvastatin or rosuvastatin doses that lower LDL cholesterol [LDL-C] by 50% or more) for adults 75 years of age or younger and moderate intensity statin therapy (i.e., statin doses that lower LDL-C by 30% to less than 50%) for those older than 75 years of age or those who cannot tolerate intensive therapy for secondary stroke prevention (Stone et al., 2013).

B. Mechanism (**Table 6-6**; Lexi-Comp, 2013)
   1. Statins
      a. 3-hydroxyl-3-methylglutaryl coenzyme A reductase inhibition to decrease cholesterol synthesis
   2. Fibric acid derivatives
      a. Peroxisome proliferator-activated receptor agonist that modifies lipoprotein expression, resulting in increased catabolism and fatty acid oxidation
   3. Nicotinic acid
      a. Enzymatic cofactor that enhances physiologic cholesterol metabolism
   4. Cholesterol-absorption inhibitors
      a. Inhibit transport proteins within the small intestine to decrease absorption of cholesterol
   5. Bile acid sequestrants
      a. Binds bile acid within the small intestine and increases bile acid elimination via the feces, which results in increased hepatic cholesterol oxidation to resynthesize bile acids
   6. Omega-3 fatty acids
      a. Enhances hepatic cholesterol oxidation and reduces synthesis of triglycerides

C. Dose (Table 6-6)

D. Adverse drug reactions (Lexi-Comp, 2013)
   1. Statins
      a. Transaminitis (increases in aspartate aminotransferase and alanine aminotransferase), myositis, and rhabdomyolysis
         (1) Risk is agent specific and appears to be highest with simvastatin
   2. Fibric acid derivatives
      a. Transaminitis, myositis, and rhabdomyolysis
      b. Dyspepsia and abdominal pain
   3. Nicotinic acid
      a. Transaminitis, myositis, and rhabdomyolysis

b. Flushing
    (1) More severe with immediate-release dosage forms but can be prevented by pretreatment with aspirin
c. Hyperpigmentation
d. Hyperglycemia and hyperuricemia

4. Cholesterol-absorption inhibitors
    a. Transaminitis
5. Bile acid sequestrants
    a. Transaminitis
    b. Bloating and abdominal cramping
6. Omega-3 fatty acids
    a. Transaminitis
    b. Dyspepsia

E. Contraindications (Lexi-Comp, 2013)
1. Severe hypersensitivity
2. Agent specific
    a. Statins and cholesterol-absorption inhibitors
        (1) Pregnancy—may harm developing fetus

F. Interactions (Lexi-Comp, 2013)
1. Combination therapy with statins and fibric acid derivatives, nicotinic acid derivatives, or ezetimibe may increase the risk of transaminitis, myositis, or rhabdomyolysis.
2. Numerous interactions exist with statins (inhibitors of metabolism), which are agent specific with various degrees of clinical relevance. It is best to consult a drug reference or pharmacist.
    a. Examples—warfarin, immunosuppressants, erythromycin, protease inhibitors, amiodarone, diltiazem, verapamil, grape fruit.
    b. Pravastatin, rosuvastatin, and pitavastatin have the fewest drug-drug interactions.
3. Bile acid sequestrants may decrease the absorption of fat-soluble medications. It is best to consult a drug reference or pharmacist.
    a. Examples—warfarin, digoxin, thyroxine, antiepileptics

G. Monitoring (Lexi-Comp, 2013)
1. Fasting lipid panel, liver function test, and muscle weakness or pain

Table 6-6. Lipid-Lowering Medications (Lexi-Comp, 2013; Wiviott & Cannon, 2006)

Medication	Dose	Cholesterol Lowering Effect		
		LDL	HDL	Triglycerides
Statins				
Lovastatin (Mevacor®)	20–80 mg daily	↓ 20%–45%	↑ 5%–10%	↓ 10%–30%
Pravastatin (Pravachol®)	10–80 mg daily	↓ 20%–45%		
Simvastatin (Zocor®)	5–40 mg daily	↓ 20%–45%		
Fluvastatin (Lescol®)	20–80 mg daily	↓ 20%–30%		
Atorvastatin (Lipitor®)	10–80 mg daily	↓ 30%–60%		
Rosuvastatin (Crestor®)	5–40 mg daily	↓ 30%–65%		
Pitavastatin (Livalo®)	1–4 mg daily	↓ 30%–45%		
Fibric Acid Derivatives				
Gemfibrozil (Lopid®)	600 mg BID	↓ 5%–20%	↑ 5%–20%	↓ 35%–50%
Fenofibrate (Tricor®)	Dosage-form dependent			
Nicotinic Acid				
Niacin	Dosage-form dependent	↓ 10%–25%	↑ 15%–35%	↓ 25%–30%
Cholesterol Absorption Inhibitor				
Ezetimibe (Zetia®)	10 mg daily	↓ 15%	----	↓ 7%–8%
Bile Acid Sequestrants				
Cholestyramine (Questran®)	4–12 gm BID	↓ 15%–30%	----	----
Colesevelam (Welchol®)	Dosage-form dependent			
Colestipol (Colestid®)	Dosage-form dependent			
Omega-3 Fatty Acids				
Omega-3 Ethyl Esters (Lovaza®)	2 gm BID 4 gm daily	↑ 5%–45%	↑ 5%–10%	↓ 25%–45%
Icosapent Ethyl (Vascepa®)	2 gm BID			

BID indicates twice daily; HDL, high density lipoprotein; LDL, low density lipoprotein.

Nimodipine

A. Indication (Chen, Fuh, & Wang, 2010; Diringer et al., 2011)
   1. Aneurysmal subarachnoid hemorrhage
      a. Nimodipine has not been shown to decrease the incidence of cerebral vasospasm, but it does decrease delayed ischemic deficits and improves functional outcome (assessed by Modified Rankin Scale).
   2. Reversible cerebrovascular vasoconstriction syndrome

B. Mechanism (Diringer et al., 2011; Lexi-Comp, 2013)
   1. Dihydropyridine calcium channel blocker with increased lipid solubility and greater blood brain barrier (BBB) penetration than alternative dihydropyridines

C. Dose (Lexi-Comp, 2013)
   1. Product availability—30 mg capsule or 60 mg/20 mL oral solution
      a. Caution: if removing capsule liquid contents, it is only to be given enterally (NOT intravenously).
   2. Standard—60 mg by mouth (PO) every 4 hours for 21 days
   3. If hypotensive, may consider 30 mg PO every 2 hours
   4. High cost prohibits continued outpatient therapy for many patients

D. Adverse drug reactions (Lexi-Comp, 2013)
   1. Hypotension, otherwise well tolerated

E. Contraindications (Lexi-Comp, 2013)
   1. Severe hypersensitivity

F. Interactions (Lexi-Comp, 2013)
   1. Few interactions, with varying degrees of clinical relevance, exist with nimodipine. It is best to consult a drug reference or pharmacist.
      a. Examples include conivaptan, phenytoin, immunosuppressants, grapefruit

Osmotic Agents

A. Indication (Forsyth, Liu-DeRyke, Parker, & Rhoney, 2008; Rangel-Castilla, Gopinath, & Robertson, 2008)
   1. Cerebral edema
   2. Intracranial hypertension

B. Mechanism (Forsyth et al., 2008; Rangel-Castilla et al., 2008)
   1. Biphasic
      a. First—reduction in blood viscosity and optimization of cerebral blood flow with a resultant reflexive vasoconstriction and reduction in cerebral blood volume and intracranial pressure (ICP)
         (1) Occurs within 3–5 minutes but is dependent on intact pressure autoregulation
      b. Second—osmotic gradient and cellular dehydration with a resultant reduction in brain water content and cerebral edema
         (1) Delayed 15–30 minutes but is dependent on intact BBB

C. Dose (**Table 6-7**)
   1. Mannitol
      a. Renal elimination, scheduled dosing, or repetitive high doses should be avoided if significant renal impairment exists.

Table 6-7. Pharmacological Agents Used for Intracranial Pressure Control (Forsyth et al., 2008; Papangelou, Lewin, Mirski, & Stevens, 2009)			
Agent	**Dosing**	**Concerns**	**Clinical Pearls**
Mannitol	0.5–1 gm/kg over 5–15 min Can be redosed every 4–6 hr	• Rebound ICP elevation • Acute kidney injury • Dehydration • Hypotension	• Dose response curve unknown • Requires in-line filter (precipitates-crystal formation) but may require warming to dissolve crystals before administration • May be given via peripheral access • Monitor serum osmolality (<320 mOsm/kg) and osmolar gap (<55 mOsm/Kg). An osmolar gap of <20 mOsm/L is commonly used in clinical practice for redosing in neurocritical care patients.
Hypertonic Saline	*Crisis* 3%: 250–500 mL over 20 min (2.5–5 mL/kg) 7.5%: 100–200 mL over 20 min (1.5–2.5 mL/kg) 23.4%: 30 mL over 20 min *Maintenance* 2%–3% continuous at 0.5–2 mL/kg/hr	• Rebound ICP elevation • Myelinolysis • Pulmonary edema • Heart failure • Acute kidney injury • Coagulopathy • Hypernatremia • Metabolic acidosis	• Central access if >2% (particularly if continuous infusion) • Rapid availability via ADC may be limited • Monitor serum sodium every 4–6 hr, avoid prolonged hypernatremia >160 meq/L • Decrease chloride and increase acetate content if patient develops metabolic acidosis

ADC indicates automatic dispensing cabinet; ICP, intracranial pressure.

Anticonvulsants

A. Anticonvulsant agents commonly used in neurological injury patients are summarized in **Table 6-8**.

B. Mechanism of action
   1. These agents work by inhibiting neuronal excitability and the propagation of seizures via multiple mechanisms, with a majority of medications inhibiting sodium channels or stimulating gamma-aminobutyric acid receptors.

C. Indications
   1. Prophylaxis
      a. Unclear if seizure prevention improves outcomes
      b. Ischemic stroke
         (1) Not indicated (Jauch et al., 2013)
      c. Intracerebral hemorrhage
         (1) Not indicated (Morgenstern et al., 2010)
      d. Aneurysmal subarachnoid hemorrhage (aSAH)
         (1) May be considered in the immediate posthemorrhagic period
         (2) Short course, such as 3–7 days, is recommended in place of long-term use for most patients.

(3) Longer duration of prophylactic anticonvulsants may be appropriate for patients with risk factors for developing a seizure disorder such as prior seizure, middle cerebral artery aneurysm, infarction, or parenchymal clot.
(4) The use of prophylactic anticonvulsants following aSAH, most commonly phenytoin, has been associated with worse neurologic outcomes (Connolly et al., 2012; Diringer et al., 2011).

2. Treatment
   a. Recurrent seizures after stroke should be treated with anticonvulsants (Jauch et al., 2013).
   b. No single agent has been shown to be superior, therefore patient-specific factors should guide the selection of an appropriate anticonvulsant agent (Jauch et al., 2013).
   c. Commonly used anticonvulsants for the treatment of seizures in patients with recurrent post-stroke seizures are summarized below.
      (1) Emergent treatment
         (a) Benzodiazepines are utilized to terminate ongoing seizure activity.
         (b) Lorazepam (Ativan®) is first-line; however other agents may be used for administration by alternate routes as outlined in Table 6-8.
      (2) Maintenance
         (a) Phenytoin (Dilantin®)
         (b) Fosphenytoin (Cerebyx®)
            1) Prodrug of phenytoin, dosed in milligrams of phenytoin equivalents
            2) Unlike phenytoin, can administer intramuscularly
         (c) Levetiracetam (Keppra®)
         (d) Lacosamide (Vimpat®)
         (e) Valproic acid (Depakote®)
      (3) Refractory
         (a) Pentobarbital (Nembutal®)
            1) Pentobarbital, a potent inducer of CYP3A4 and CYP2A6, is associated with numerous drug interactions.
            2) Frequent neurologic assessments may be confounded due to long duration of action.

Table 6-8. Anticonvulsant Agents Commonly Used in Neurological Injury Patients (Brophy et al., 2012; Lexi-Comp, 2013)

Generic (Brand) Formulations	Dose	Adverse Drug Reactions	Drug Interactions	Monitoring	Comments
Lorazepam (Ativan®) injection, oral liquid, tablet	0.1 mg/kg IV up to 4 mg per dose, may repeat in 5–10 min IV: maximum administration rate 2 mg/min	Hypotension, respiratory depression	↑ lorazepam concentration: valproate, probenecid	Blood pressure, respiratory status	Pregnancy category D Propylene glycol contained in injectable formulation can accumulate with prolonged infusions and cause a metabolic acidosis
Midazolam (Versed®) injection, oral syrup	0.2 mg/kg IM up to maximum of 10 mg 0.2 mg/kg intranasal 0.5 mg/kg buccal	Hypotension, respiratory depression	↑ midazolam concentration: cimetidine, erythromycin, diltiazem, verapamil, ketoconazole, itraconazole	Blood pressure, respiratory status	Pregnancy category D
Diazepam (Valium®) injection, tablet, oral solution, rectal gel	0.15 mg/kg IV up to 10 mg per dose, may repeat in 5 min 0.2 mg/kg PR	Hypotension, respiratory depression	↑ diazepam concentration: cimetidine, ketoconazole, fluvoxamine, fluoxetine, omeprazole	Blood pressure, respiratory status	Pregnancy category D Propylene glycol contained in injectable formulation can accumulate with prolonged infusions and cause a metabolic acidosis
Phenytoin (Dilantin®) and **Fosphenytoin** (Cerebryx®) Phenytoin: injection, chewable tablet, extended-release capsule, oral suspension Fosphenytoin: injection	*Loading dose*: 10–20 mg/kg (phenytoin) or mg PE/kg (fosphenytoin) *Maintenance dose:* 3–7 mg/kg/day or mg PE/kg/day (ideal body weight) in 2–3 divided doses *IV:* maximum administration rate 50 mg/min phenytoin, 150 mg PE/min fosphenytoin	Hypotension during infusion and cardiovascular depression following intravascular administration; phlebitis; hypersensitivity reactions; rash; nystagmus; blood dyscrasias; hepatotoxicity; at high serum levels delirium, psychosis, encephalopathy	↑ phenytoin level: amiodarone, diazepam, fluoxetine, fluvoxamine, omeprazole, methylphenidate, sertraline, sulfonamides, trazodone ↓ phenytoin level: carbamazepine, sucralfate, calcium, enteral feeds, dexamethasone Variable effect on phenytoin level: alcohol intake, phenobarbital, valproate sodium Phenytoin may reduce efficacy: azole antifungals, corticosteroids, furosemide, paroxetine, warfarin, sertraline, vitamin D	Therapeutic serum phenytoin level: total 10–20 mcg/ml, free 1–2 mcg/ml Blood pressure, heart rate, CBC, LFTs, albumin	Pregnancy category D Injectable formulation of phenytoin is not stable in dextrose-containing solutions.

continued

Table 6-8. Anticonvulsant Agents Commonly Used in Neurological Injury Patients (Brophy et al., 2012; Lexi-Comp, 2013) continued

Generic (Brand) Formulations	Dose	Adverse Drug Reactions	Drug Interactions	Monitoring	Comments
Levetiracetam (Keppra®) injection, oral solution, immediate-release tablet, extended-release tablet	1000–3000 mg/day in 2 divided doses *IV*: administer over 15 min	Somnolence; asthenia; fatigue; infection; dizziness; coordination difficulties; behavior disturbances including psychotic symptoms, depression, nervousness, anxiety, emotional lability	No significant	Drug level monitoring not routinely recommended	Pregnancy category C Reduce dose in renal impairment
Lacosamide (Vimpat®) injection, oral solution, immediate-release tablet	50–400 mg/day in 2 divided doses *IV*: administer over 30–60 min	Diplopia, headache, dizziness, syncope, ataxia, nausea, hypersensitivity reactions, PR interval prolongation	No significant	Drug level monitoring not routinely recommended EKG	Pregnancy category C Use caution in patients with known cardiac conduction problems or severe cardiac disease Reduce dose in severe renal or hepatic impairment Schedule V narcotic
Valproic Acid (Depakote®) immediate-release capsule, delayed-release tablet, extended-release tablet, oral-solution, injection	*Loading dose*: 15–30 mg/kg *Maintenance dose*: 15 mg/kg/day in 2–4 divided doses, then titrate to therapeutic level *IV*: maximum administration rate 1.5–6 mg/kg/min	Headache, somnolence, dizziness, alopecia, nausea, vomiting, anorexia, insomnia, nervousness, weight gain, menstrual changes, diarrhea, thrombocytopenia, tremor, weakness, diplopia, infection, hepatotoxicity, hyperammonemia, hypersensitivity reaction, pancreatitis	↓ valproic acid concentration: carbapenems, rifampin ↑ valproic acid concentration: clarithromycin, erythromycin, felbamate valproic acid ↑ concentration: lamotrigine, lorazepam, rufinamide	Therapeutic valproate level: 50–100 mcg/ml; higher goal may be appropriate in selected patients Ammonia, LFTs, CBC	Pregnancy category D Contraindicated in severe hepatic impairment, patients with mitochondrial polymerase gamma gene mutation disorder.

continued

Table 6-8. Anticonvulsant Agents Commonly Used in Neurological Injury Patients (Brophy et al., 2012; Lexi-Comp, 2013) continued

Generic (Brand) Formulations	Dose	Adverse Drug Reactions	Drug Interactions	Monitoring	Comments
Pentobarbital (Nembutal®) C-II injection	*Loading dose*: 10–15 mg/kg *Maintenance infusion*: 1–4 mg/kg/hr *IV*: Maximum administration rate 50 mg/min	Hypotension, respiratory depression, syncope, bradycardia, confusion, fever, depression, dizziness, hallucinations, headache, nightmares, psychiatric disturbances, angioedema, rash, constipation, anemia, hepatotoxicity, bowel edema	Pentobarbital ↓ concentration: alfuzosin, amiodarone, amlodipine, apixaban, atorvastatin, aripiprazole, azole antifungals, benzodiazepines, bisoprolol, buspirone, citalopram, clarithromycin, cyclosporine, dantrolene, dapsone, dexamethasone, diltiazem, doxazosin, efavirenz, erythromycin, escitalopram, estrogen, ethosuximide, felbamate, guanfacine, haloperidol, isosorbide, lansoprazole, lidocaine, losartan, lovastatin, maraviroc, methadone, mirtazapine, modafinil, montelukast, nefazodone, nicardipine, nimodipine, ondansetron, oxycodone, protease inhibitors, quetiapine, quinidine, ranolazine, sildenafil, simvastatin, sirolimus, tacrolimus, tamoxifen, tamsulosin, tetracycline, theophylline, ticlopidine, tramadol, trazodone, venlafaxine, verapamil Pentobarbital is contraindicated: apixiban, axitinib, clozapine, dronedarone, itraconazole, lapatinib, lurasidone, nifedipine, nisoldipine, ranolazine, rivaroxaban, ticagrelor, tolvaptan	Continuous EEG monitoring EKG, blood pressure, respiratory status	Reserved for patients with refractory ICP elevation or refractory status epilepticus Also has sedative properties Propylene glycol contained in IV pentobarbital can accumulate with prolonged infusions and cause metabolic acidosis. Reduce dose in renal or hepatic dysfunction. Accumulates during prolonged infusions, which may delay awakening

CBC indicates complete blood count; EEG, Electroencephalography; EKG, electrocardiogram; ICP, intracranial pressure; IM, intramuscular; IV, intravenous; LFTs, liver function tests; PE, phenytoin equivalent; PR, rectal administration.

Glycemic Control

A. Agents commonly used to prevent and treat hyperglycemia are summarized in **Tables 6-9–6-11**.

Table 6-9. Insulin Products (Inzucchi, 2012; Lexi-Comp, 2013)

Medication	Route	Onset	Peak (hr)	Duration (hr)	Clinical Pearls
Insulin Lispro (Humalog®)	SC	10–15 min	1–2	3–5	Rapid-acting insulins are best for sliding scale doses for patients who can eat because they can be administered with meals and adjusted for variable oral intake.
Insulin Aspart (Novolog®)	SC	10–15 min	1–2	3–5	
Insulin Glulisine (Apidra®)	SC	10–15 min	1–2	3–5	Monitor glucose every 4 hr in unstable patients.
Insulin Regular	SC, IV	0.5–1hr	2–4	4–8	Short-acting regular insulin is ideal for sliding scale doses in patients who are NPO or on continuous tube feeds. Monitor glucose every 6 hr in unstable patients. Only regular insulin can be administered as an IV infusion.
Insulin NPH	SC	1–3	4–10	10–18	
Insulin Detemir (Levemir®)	SC	1	none	Up to 24	Long-acting insulin doses are intended to meet basal insulin needs and generally do not account for mealtime insulin needs.
Insulin Glargine (Lantus®)	SC	2–3	none	24	Holding doses of long-acting insulins, even when patients are NPO, may result in severe hyperglycemia; when necessary, a dose reduction is generally preferred.

IV indicates intravenous; NPH, neutral protamine Hagedorn; NPO, nothing by mouth; SC, subcutaneous.

B. Therapeutics
   1. Hypoglycemia can cause neurologic symptoms that can mimic a stroke; rapid correction of hypoglycemia can reverse these symptoms.
   2. Hyperglycemia is common and compared to patients with normoglycemia has been associated with worse clinical outcomes, especially in patients with neurologic injury.
   3. The ideal blood glucose level is unknown; however, both hypoglycemia and hyperglycemia are associated with harm and should be avoided (Connolly et al., 2012; Jauch et al., 2013; Morgenstern et al., 2010).

C. Monitoring
   1. Glucose monitoring is recommended for patients with acute ischemic and hemorrhagic strokes, as well as any acutely ill critical care patient.
   2. Patients should be monitored every 4–6 hours when receiving subcutaneous insulin injections or oral hypoglycemic agents until they are stabilized.
   3. Patients on continuous insulin infusions should be monitored every 1–2 hours until glucose levels and insulin dose stabilize. Less frequent monitoring may be considered

once the patient is stable, however most patients will continue to require frequent blood glucose checks because of changes in overall clinical status and delivery of nutrition.

4. It may be reasonable to adjust serum glucose to avoid low cerebral glucose in aSAH patients who are monitored with microdialysis (Diringer et al., 2011).

D. Treatment goals

1. In the absence of evidence to support a goal glucose range specifically for patients with acute stroke, normoglycemia is recommended (Connolly et al., 2012; Jauch et al., 2013; Morgenstern et al., 2010).
2. The American Diabetes Association recommendation of a blood glucose range of 140–180 mg/dl for hospitalized patients is a reasonable goal (Jauch et al., 2013).
3. Hypoglycemia (<60 mg/dl) should be corrected immediately to prevent secondary brain injury (Jauch et al., 2013). A more conservative treatment threshold (<80 mg/dl) has been suggested for patients with aSAH (Diringer et al., 2011). The Society of Critical Care Medicine guidelines have the most conservative definition of hypoglycemia (<100 mg/dl) for neurocritically ill patients.

E. Management

1. Hypoglycemia
   a. Discontinue the offending hypoglycemic agent until the patient is stabilized or the cause (e.g., feedings held, nausea or vomiting, supratherapeutic dose) is corrected.
   b. A single dose of dextrose 50% 25 mL slow IV push is preferred.
   c. Alternatively, oral glucose-containing solutions can be administered. These are limited by their slow onset and difficult administration in the presence of dysphagia (Jauch et al., 2013).
2. Hyperglycemia
   a. Insulin products are preferred in the acute setting because they can be rapidly titrated, whereas oral agents are typically held until the patient is stable.
   b. Agents associated with hypoglycemia (e.g. sulfonylureas, meglinitides) should be avoided in the acute setting.
   c. Metformin (Glucophage®) should be held for at least 48 hours after administration of iodinated contrast and can be restarted when there is evidence of normal kidney function.

Table 6-10. Oral Agents (Inzucchi, 2012; Lexi-Comp, 2013)

Class/Mechanism of Action	Medication and Usual Dose (mg/day)	Peak Effect (hr)	Duration (hr)	Adverse Drug Reactions	Drug Interactions	Clinical Pearls
Sulfonylureas Stimulate insulin release through beta cells	**Glyburide** (Micronase®) 1.25–20	4	12–24	Hypoglycemia, weight gain	↑ glyburide concentration: fluconazole, ranitidine, voriconazole Beta blockers and GLP-1 agonists may enhance hypoglycemic effect.	Avoid use in the elderly and in patients with renal impairment due to potential accumulation of active metabolite. Avoid in patients with sulfa allergy or G6PD deficiency.
	Glipizide (Glucotrol®) 2.5–40 Also available in extended-release formulation	1–3	12–24	Hypoglycemia, weight gain	↑ glipizide concentration: fluconazole, ranitidine, voriconazole Beta blockers and GLP-1 agonists may enhance hypoglycemic effect.	Avoid in patients with sulfa allergy or G6PD deficiency.
	Glimepiride (Amaryl®) 1–8	2–3	24	Hypoglycemia, weight gain	↑ glimepiride concentration: fluconazole, ranitidine, voriconazole Beta-blockers and GLP-1 agonists may enhance hypoglycemic effect	Avoid in patients with sulfa allergy or G6PD deficiency.

continued

Table 6-10. Oral Agents (Inzucchi, 2012; Lexi-Comp, 2013) continued

Class/Mechanism of Action	Medication and Usual Dose (mg/day)	Peak Effect (hr)	Duration (hr)	Adverse Drug Reactions	Drug Interactions	Clinical Pearls
Thiazolidinediones Increase peripheral insulin sensitivity through activation of peroxisome proliferator-activated receptor-gamma	**Pioglitazone** (Actos®) 15–45	n/a	Days to weeks	Heart failure, edema, weight gain, bone fractures	↓ pioglitazone absorption: bile acid squestrants ↑ pioglitazone concentration: gemfibrozil Pioglitazone ↓ concentration: aripiprazole	Not associated with hypoglycemia Avoid in patients with congestive heart failure, hepatic impairment, or osteoporosis.
Biguanides Decrease hepatic gluconeogenesis, increase insulin sensitivity	**Metformin** (Glucophage®) 1,000–2,550 Also available in extended-release formulation	2–3	12–18	Lactic acidosis, nausea, diarrhea, abdominal pain	↑ metformin concentration: cephalexin, lamotrigine, trimethoprim Metformin ↓ absorption: folic acid, vitamin B12	Contraindicated when SCr ≥ 1.4 mg/dl in women, ≥ 1.5 mg/dl in men Avoid use in patients with dehydration, or congestive heart failure.

continued

Table 6-10. Oral Agents (Inzucchi, 2012; Lexi-Comp, 2013) continued

Class/Mechanism of Action	Medication and Usual Dose (mg/day)	Peak Effect (hr)	Duration (hr)	Adverse Drug Reactions	Drug Interactions	Clinical Pearls
Dipeptidyl peptidase-4 inhibitors Increase glucose-dependent insulin release, supress glucagon secretion	**Sitaglipitin** (Januvia®) 100	1–4	24	Urticaria, hypersensitivity reaction angioedema, pancreatitis	Sitagliptin ↑ concentration: Digoxin	Not associated with hypoglycemia Reduce dose in patients with renal impairment.
	Saxagliptin (Onglyza®) 5	2	24	Urticaria	↓ saxagliptin concentration: clarithromycin, nefazodone, protease inhibitors	Not associated with hypoglycemia Reduce dose in patients with renal impairment.
	Linagliptin (Trandjenta®) 5	1.5	24	Urticaria	↓ linagliptin concentration: clarithromycin, nefazodone, protease inhibitors	No dose adjustment required for renal or hepatic failure

continued

Table 6-10. Oral Agents (Inzucchi, 2012; Lexi-Comp, 2013) continued

Class/Mechanism of Action	Medication and Usual Dose (mg/day)	Peak Effect (hr)	Duration (hr)	Adverse Drug Reactions	Drug Interactions	Clinical Pearls
Meglinitides Stimulate insulin release through beta cells	**Repaglinide** (Prandin®) 1.5–16	1	4–6	Hypoglycemia, weight gain	↓ repaglinide concentration: clarithromycin, nefazodone, protease inhibitors ↑ repaglinide concentration: gemfibrozil,	Administer with meals; hold while NPO Patients with adrenal, hepatic, or renal insufficiency may experience enhanced hypoglycemic effects. Avoid coadministration with NPH insulin.
	Nateglinide (Starlix®) 180–360	0.3	4	Hypoglycemia, weight gain	↓ nateglinide concentration: clarithromycin, nefazodone, protease inhibitors	Administer with meals; hold while NPO. Patients with adrenal, hepatic, or renal insufficiency may experience enhanced hypoglycemic effects. Avoid coadministration with sulfonylureas because of lack of benefit.

continued

Table 6-10. Oral Agents (Inzucchi, 2012; Lexi-Comp, 2013) continued

Class/Mechanism of Action	Medication and Usual Dose (mg/day)	Peak Effect (hr)	Duration (hr)	Adverse Drug Reactions	Drug Interactions	Clinical Pearls
α-glucosidase inhibitors Slows carbohydrate absorption from the gut by inhibiting α-glucosidases	**Acarbose** (Precose®) 150–300	n/a	2–3	Gas, abdominal pain, diarrhea	Acarbose ↓ serum concentration: digoxin	Administer with meals; hold while NPO. Not associated with hypoglycemia Avoid in patients with significant renal or hepatic impairment or inflammatory bowel disease.
	Miglitol (Glyset®) 150–300	n/a	2–3	Gas, abdominal pain, diarrhea		Administer with meals; hold while NPO. Not associated with hypoglycemia Avoid in patients with significant renal impairment or inflammatory bowel disease.

GLP-1 indicates glucagon-like polypeptide-1; NPO, nothing by mouth; SCr, serum creatinine.

Table 6-11. Noninsulin Injectable Agents (Inzucchi, 2012; Lexi-Comp, 2013)

Class/Mechanism of Action	Medication and Usual dose/day	Peak Effect (hr)	Duration (hr)	Adverse Drug Reactions	Drug Interactions	Clinical Pearls
Glucagon-like polypeptide-1 mimetics Stimulates insulin release in presence of glucose, suppresses glucagons release, slows gastric emptying, and produces early satiety	**Exenatide** (Byetta®) Immediate-release: 10–20 mcg divided twice daily Extended-release: 2 mg weekly Available in extended-release formulation	2–3	5	Nausea, weight loss, necrotizing pancreatitis, thyroid tumors	↓ absorption of oral agents Exenatide ↓ ↑ concentration: estrogens, progestins Exenatide ↑ concentration: warfarin	Not associated with hypoglycemia unless used in combination with sulfonylureas Should not be used in combination with insulin except insulin glargine Avoid use in patients with gastroparesis, severe gastrointestinal disease, or renal impairment.
	Liraglutide (Victoza®) 1.2–1.8 mcg	8–12	5	Nausea, weight loss, necrotizing pancreatitis, thyroid tumors	↓ absorption of oral agents	Not associated with hypoglycemia unless used in combination with sulfonylureas Avoid use in patients with gastroparesis or renal impairment. Contraindicated if personal or family history of medullary cancer or multiple endocrine neoplasm type 2 present
Amylinomimetic Amylin receptor agonist that suppresses glucagon release, slows gastric emptying, produces early satiety	**Pramlintide** (Symlin®) 45–360 mcg	0.3	3	Hypoglycemia, weight loss, nausea, anorexia	Pramlintide may potentiate gastrointestinal anticholinergic effects of anticholinergic drugs	Administer prior to meals. Avoid use in patients with gastroparesis.

Antispasmodics

A. Spasticity
   1. Spasticity is common after stroke and is associated with significant functional disability and pain (Miller et al., 2010).
   2. Exercise and stretching can increase range of motion and prevent permanent shortening of muscle tissue. Medications can be used in combination with physical therapy for the symptomatic management of muscle spasticity (Miller et al., 2010).

B. Medical management
   1. Injectable medications administered locally may prevent systemic adverse effects associated with oral agents.
   2. Geriatric patients are particularly susceptible to the effects of some antispasmodics anticholinergic effects that can worsen dementia and lead to falls (Fick & Semla, 2012).
   3. Oral medications
      a. Benzodiazepines should be avoided when possible because of sedation and potentially detrimental effects on neurologic recovery (Duncan et al., 2005; Department of Veteran Affairs & Department of Defense, 2010).
      b. Tizanidine (Zanaflex®)
         (1) Tizanidine is a centrally acting muscle relaxant and beta$_2$ noradrenergic agonist.
         (2) Tizanidine is usually initiated at 4 mg per day then slowly titrated up to a maintenance dose of 8 mg every 6–8 hours up to a maximum of 36 mg per day.
         (3) Adverse effects of tizanidine include xerostomia, lethargy, hypotension, asthenia, dizziness, and weakness; it is rarely associated with hepatotoxicity and hallucinations.
         (4) The following medications may increase tizanidine concentrations: acyclovir, amiodarone, cimetidine, ciprofloxacin, famotidine, fluvoxamine, mexiletine, propafenone, verapamil, and oral contraceptives.
         (5) A dose reduction may be required for patients with renal impairment, and tizanidine should be avoided in patients with significant hepatic impairment.
         (6) Patients who have received high doses for an extended period of time may experience withdrawal symptoms (e.g., hypertension, tachycardia, hypertonia, tremor, anxiety) with abrupt discontinuation, therefore tapering is recommended.
      c. Baclofen (oral)
         (1) Baclofen is believed to reduce muscle spasticity through inhibition of monosynaptic and polysynaptic reflexes at the spinal cord.
         (2) The usual dose is 5–10 mg three or four times per day up to a maximum of 80 mg per day.
         (3) Baclofen may cause excessive sedation and be less effective for spasticity due to stroke (Pedersen, Arlien-Soborg, & Mai, 1974).
         (4) Adverse effects of baclofen include lethargy, constipation, dizziness, insomnia, ataxia, hypotonia, and weakness.
         (5) Central nervous system (CNS) adverse effects may be enhanced when baclofen is used in combination with other CNS depressants.
      d. Dantrolene (Dantrium®)
         (1) Dantrolene reduces muscle contraction through the modulation of calcium release from sarcoplasmic reticulum of skeletal muscle.
         (2) The starting dose of dantrolene is 25 mg per day, which is slowly titrated up to a maximum of 100 mg four times per day.

(3) The most common adverse effects are nausea, headache, dizziness, weakness, and diarrhea, which are dose related and often transient; however, significant muscle weakness and severe diarrhea may require discontinuation in some cases. Reportedly, dantrolene has no cognitive adverse effects (Ketel & Kolb, 1984).

(4) Hepatic function should be monitored at baseline and periodically throughout the treatment course. Dantrolene should be discontinued if benefit is not observed after 45 days of therapy due to the risk of hepatotoxicity. Baseline liver enzyme abnormalities and concurrent use of estrogen in women older than 35 years of age have been identified as possible risk factors.

(5) Similar to baclofen, CNS adverse effects may be enhanced when dantrolene is used in combination with other CNS depressants.

(6) Cardiovascular collapse has rarely been associated with concurrent intravenous dantrolene and verapamil. Although this has not been reported with the oral formulation, concomitant use of calcium channel blockers should be avoided.

4. Injectable medications

a. Botulinum toxin A (Botox®)

(1) Botulinum toxin is often used in conjunction with oral agents. It exerts its therapeutic effect through inhibition of acetylcholine release at the neuromuscular junction.

(2) The dose of botulinum toxin varies by the formulation and intended site of administration. Different botulinum toxin preparations are not interchangeable, and there are no recommendations for dose conversion between agents. Please consult the individual prescribing information for dosing information for a specific product.

(3) Adverse effects vary by injection site. Common adverse effects include infection, pain, and headache.

(4) Distant spread of toxin effects is a rare complication of botulinum toxin. Symptoms, including life-threatening swallowing and breathing problems, may occur hours to weeks following an injection.

(5) Concurrent administration of aminoglycosides, muscle relaxants, or neuromuscular blockers may potentiate the effects of botulinum toxin.

(6) Doses should not exceed the maximum recommended dose or be administered more than once every 3 months to prevent the formation of antibodies and resistance.

b. Baclofen (intrathecal; Lioresal®)

(1) Intrathecal baclofen is administered via an implantable intrathecal pump that requires intermittent refills.

(2) Patients with chronic lower extremity spasticity who fail or are intolerant of oral antispasmodic therapy may be candidates for intrathecal baclofen. A test dose in a medically supervised setting with resuscitative equipment available is required prior to initiation to evaluate tolerability and response.

(3) After a positive response to a test dose of 25–100 mcg, the initial rate is typically 1–2 times the test dose administered over 24 hours. The dose is then titrated to effect, with most patients requiring 100–800 mcg per day.

(4) Adverse effects of intrathecal baclofen are similar to oral baclofen; however, lower doses are required when baclofen is administered directly into the intrathecal space and dose-related effects such as constipation and lethargy are reduced.

(5) If the intrathecal pump malfunctions or is programmed incorrectly, a potentially life-threatening overdose or withdrawal syndrome can occur.
  (a) Baclofen overdose may cause CNS depression, seizure, cardiovascular collapse, and respiratory failure.
  (b) Baclofen withdrawal syndrome is characterized by fever, rash, seizure, and cardiovascular instability.

Antidepressants

A. Depression
  1. Depression is present in more than 25% of ischemic stroke patients, can negatively affect cognitive and motor recovery, and has been associated with increased mortality (Miller et al., 2010; Paolucci, Gandolfo, Provinciali, Torta, & Toso, 2006).
  2. American Heart Association guidelines recommend screening for depression for 6 months following a stroke and, if present, use of antidepressants. Antidepressants improve outcomes in stroke survivors with, and possibly in those without, depression (Mead et al., 2012; Mikami et al., 2011; Teasell et al., 2009).

B. Medical management
  1. A summary of agents used for the treatment of poststroke depression are outlined in **Table 6-12**.
  2. It may take 4–6 weeks for patients to feel the full effects of antidepressant treatment.
  3. Significant drug interactions
    a. Concomitant administration of drugs with serotonergic properties may increase the risk for serotonin syndrome.
    b. Additive QTc interval prolongation may occur with coadministration of drugs that also prolong the QTc interval.
    c. Alcohol should be avoided during therapy because it may increase the toxicity of selective serotonin reuptake inhibitors (SSRIs).
    d. Concomitant use of anticoagulant or antiplatelet agents with SSRIs may increase the risk of bleeding.
  4. Abrupt discontinuation should be avoided because patients can experience withdrawal effects, such as flu-like symptoms, nausea and vomiting, and abdominal pain.
  5. There are several proposed mechanisms for the effectiveness of antidepressants post stroke (Burns & Greenberg, 2010).
    a. Antidepressants may protect against acute ischemic neuronal injury.
    b. Antidepressants may enhance ischemia-induced neurogenesis.
  6. Treatment of depression
    a. Antidepressants are effective in producing remission and improving depressive symptoms, although their use is also associated with an increased incidence of adverse effects (Hackett, Anderson, House, & Xia, 2008; Teasell et al., 2009).
    b. SSRIs are often selected as first-line therapy because of their favorable adverse effect profile, particularly for patients with stroke and heart disease. Based on observational studies, there may be a small absolute risk of hemorrhagic stroke with SSRI use (Hackam & Mrkobrada, 2012).
    c. Tricyclic antidepressants appear to be equally effective; however, their use is limited by a high rate of anticholinergic adverse effects.
    d. There is insufficient evidence to support the use of the serotonin/norepinephrine reuptake inhibitor venlafaxine (Effexor®) for post-stroke depression.

e. Although methylphenidate (Ritalin®) is primarily used after stroke as a neurostimulant, there is some evidence that it may improve depressive symptoms and functional recovery. The onset of action is more rapid than traditional antidepressants; however, it is associated with adverse cardiac effects (Teasell et al., 2009).

7. Treatment of anxiety
   a. Paroxetine (Paxil®) or buspirone (Buspar®) may be effective options for patients with comorbid depression and anxiety (Teasell et al., 2009).
8. Prevention of depression
   a. A 2008 Cochrane review was unable to conclude that antidepressants are effective for the prevention of depression; however, more recent data suggest that there may be some benefit (Chollet et al., 2011; Hackett, Anderson, House, & Halteh, 2008).
   b. There is no clear advantage of using one SSRI over another for the prevention of depression; however, there are differences in adverse effects that may guide drug selection (Hackett et al., 2008).
9. Improved recovery
   a. SSRIs may improve recovery after stroke, even in patients who are not depressed.
   b. There is no clear advantage of using one SSRI over another to improve recovery after stroke (Mead et al., 2012).

Table 6-12. Agents Used for the Treatment or Prevention of Post-Stroke Depression (Lexi-Comp, 2013)

Generic Name (Brand Name) and Dose	Class	Adverse Drug Reactions	Drug Interactions	Clinical Pearls
Fluoxetine (Prozac®) Usual dose: Immediate-release 20–80 mg daily Controlled-release 90 mg per week	SSRI	Sleep disturbances, nausea, headache, somnolence, anxiety, anorexia, xerostomia, decreased libido, weakness, tremor, prolonged QTc, rare serotonin syndrome, suicidal ideation, bleeding, SIADH, may lower seizure threshold	Fluoxetine ↑ concentration: aripiprazole, atomoxetine, captopril, carbamazepine, carvedilol, chlorpromazine, dextromethorphan, doxepin, doxorubicin, haloperidol, imipramine, methamphetamine, metoprolol, nefazodone, nortriptyline, perphenazine, promethazine, propafenone, propranolol, risperidone ↑ fluoxetine concentration: capecitabine, cimetidine, fluconazole, fluorouracil, gemfibrozil, ketoconazole, nicardipine, sulfadiazine ↓ fluoxetine concentration: carbamazepine, phenobarbital, phenytoin, primidone, rifampin MAOIs, linezolid, and tamoxifen are contraindicated with fluoxetine.	Monitor for SIADH because low serum sodium levels can induce seizures (all SSRIs). Lacks anticholinergic adverse effects Use caution in patients with renal or hepatic insufficiency. Withdrawal symptoms less severe than other SSRIs because of long half-life Available in once-weekly and oral solution formulations

continued

Table 6-12. Agents Used for the Treatment or Prevention of Post-Stroke Depression (Lexi-Comp, 2013) continued

Generic Name (Brand Name) and Dose	Class	Adverse Drug Reactions	Drug Interactions	Clinical Pearls
Paroxetine (Paxil®) Usual dose: Immediate-release 20–50 mg daily Controlled release 25–62.5 mg daily	SSRI	Similar to fluoxetine	Paroxetine ↑ concentration: aripiprazole, atomoxetine, captopril, carbamazepine, carvedilol, chlorpromazine, dextromethorphan, doxepin, doxorubicin, haloperidol, imipramine, methamphetamine, metoprolol, nefazodone, nortriptyline, perphenazine, promethazine, propafenone, propranolol, risperidone ↑ paroxetine concentration: cimetidine MAOIs and linezolid are contraindicated with paroxetine.	More anticholinergic effects than other SSRIs; fewer anticholinergic effects than TCAs Use caution in patients with renal or hepatic insufficiency. Available as controlled-release tablet and oral suspension
Sertraline (Zoloft®) Usual dose: 50–200 mg daily	SSRI	Similar to fluoxetine	Similar to paroxetine	Lacks anticholinergic adverse effects Use caution in patients with renal or hepatic insufficiency or with uric acid nephropathy. Available as an oral solution
Citalopram (Celexa®) Usual dose: 20–40 mg daily 40 mg dose not recommended in patients >60 years, who are poor CYP2C19 metabolizers, or who are on drugs that significantly inhibit CYP2C19	SSRI	Similar to fluoxetine, risk of torsades de pointe	↑ citalopram concentration: azole antifungals, chloramphenicol, cimetidine, clarithromycin, conivaptan, gemfibrozil, isoniazid, modafinil, nefazodone, nicardipine, protease inhibitors, ticlopidine ↓ citalopram concentration: carbamazepine, dexamethasone, efavirenz, nafcillin, oxcarbazepine, pentobarbital, phenobarbital, primidone, phenytoin, rifampin MAOIs and linezolid are contraindicated with citalopram.	Dose reductions or avoidance may be necessary in some patients (the elderly, hepatic insufficient, others) because of its propensity to prolong the QTc interval. Available as an oral solution

continued

Table 6-12. Agents Used for the Treatment or Prevention of Post-Stroke Depression (Lexi-Comp, 2013) continued

Generic Name (Brand Name) and Dose	Class	Adverse Drug Reactions	Drug Interactions	Clinical Pearls
Escitalopram (Lexapro®) Usual dose: 10–20 mg daily	SSRI	Similar to citalopram	Similar to citalopram	Escitalopram is the more active enantiomer of citalopram. Available as an oral solution
Nortriptyline (Pamelor®) Usual dose: 75–150 mg daily, may be given in divided doses	TCA	Constipation, xerostomia, urinary retention, blurred vision, confusion, orthostatic hypotension, hypertension, sleep disturbances, sedation, rare hyperpyrexia, bone marrow suppression, conduction abnormalities, serotonin syndrome, suicidal ideation, bleeding, SIADH, may lower seizure threshold	May enhance sympathomimetic effects of alpha and beta agonists Additive effects when used in combination with drugs that have anticholinergic properties MAOIs and linezolid are contraindicated with nortriptyline.	Use caution in patients with hyperthyroidism, cardiovascular disease, and renal or hepatic insufficiency. Potentially fatal in overdose Available as an oral solution
Amitriptyline (Elavil®) Usual dose: 50–300 mg daily at bedtime, may be given in divided doses	TCA	Similar to nortriptyline; however, there is a higher incidence of adverse effects including anticholinergic effects.	Similar to nortriptyline	Use caution in patients with hyperthyroidism, cardiovascular disease, and renal or hepatic insufficiency. Potentially fatal in overdose
Trazodone (Desyrel®) Usual dose: 50–200 mg three times daily	SARI	Sedation, headache, dizziness, xerostomia, nausea, blurred vision, gastrointestinal disturbances, orthostatic hypotension, edema, rare priapism, QTc prolongation, serotonin syndrome, SIADH, suicidal ideation	↑ trazodone concentration: carbamazepine, dexamethasone, oxcarbazepine, phenobarbital, phenytoin, primidone, rifampin ↓ trazodone concentration: azole antifungals, clarithromycin, nefazodone, nicardipine, protease inhibitors MAOIs and linezolid are contraindicated with trazodone.	Use caution in patients with hyperthyroidism, cardiovascular disease, and renal or hepatic insufficiency.

CYP indicates cytochrome P450; MAOI, monoamine oxidase inhibitor; SARI, serotonin antagonist/reuptake inhibitor; SIADH, syndrome of inappropriate antidiuretic hormone; SSRI, selective serotonin reuptake inhibitors; TCA, tricyclic antidepressants.

Neurostimulants

A. Mood, behavior, and cognitive symptoms are common after stroke.

B. Neurostimulants are sometimes employed to accelerate and improve motor and cognitive recovery, although the data supporting their use in this setting are limited (Zorowitz, Smout, Gassaway, & Horn, 2005).

C. Pharmacologic management

1. Medications used as neurostimulants post-stroke are summarized in **Table 6-13**.
2. Methylphenidate with or without levodopa may improve motor recovery when used in combination with physical therapy (Grade, Redford, Chrostowski, Toussaint, & Blackwell, 1998; Lokk, Salman Roghani, & Delbari, 2011).
3. Levodopa alone may be effective in the treatment of motor deficits following stroke, though results have been mixed (Scheidtmann, Fries, Muller, & Koenig, 2001; Sonde & Lokk, 2007).
4. Levodopa may also improve aphasia in combination with speech and language therapy (Seniow, Litwin, Litwin, Lesniak, & Czlonkowska, 2009).
5. SSRIs may enhance motor recovery. These agents are summarized in the antidepressant section (Mead et al., 2012).
6. A small, open-label study associated donepezil with some improvement in language function (Berthier, Hinojosa, Martín Mdel, & Fernandez, 2003).
7. Currently, there is insufficient evidence to recommend the use of dextroamphetamine to improve motor rehabilitation after stroke (Martinsson, Hardemark, & Eksborg, 2007).
8. There is insufficient evidence to recommend the use of bromocriptine to improve verbal function after stroke (Ashtary, Janghorbani, Chitsaz, Reisi, & Bahrami, 2006; Gupta, Mlcoch, Scolaro, & Moritz, 1995).

Table 6-13. Neurostimulants (Lexi-Comp, 2013)

Generic (Brand) and Formulations	Mechanism of Action	Usual Oral Dose (mg/day)	Adverse Drug Reactions	Drug Interactions	Contraindications	Clinical Pearls
Methylphenidate (Ritalin®, Concerta®, Daytrana®) Tablet, chewable tablet, extended-release tablet, extended-release capsule, oral solution, transdermal patch	Inhibits reuptake of norepinephrine and dopamine	5–60	Anorexia, tic, headache, insomnia, anxiety, aggression, tremor, blurred vision, psychosis, hypertension, tachycardia, may lower seizure threshold, rare cardiac events	Methylphenidate may have additive sympathomimetic effects when used with other sympathomimetics.	Alcohol, MAOIs, and linezolid are contraindicated with methylphenidate.	Avoid use in patients with significant cardiovascular disease, tics, severe anxiety or agitation, psychosis, or bipolar disorder. Immediate-release dosage forms should be divided BID and given at 8 am and noon. Controlled substance (C-II), avoid in patients with a history of substance abuse.
Dextroamphetamine (Dexedrine®) Tablet, extended-release capsule, oral solution	Enhances synaptic release of norepinephrine and dopamine	10–60	Similar to methylphenidate	Alkalinizing agents such as sodium bicarbonate ↓ excretion of amphetamines. Dextroamphetamine may have additive sympathomimetic effects when used with other sympathomimetics.	MAOIs and linezolid are contraindicated with dextroamphetamine.	Similar to methylphenidate Avoid in patients with hyperthyroidism and glaucoma. Controlled substance (C-II), avoid in patients with a history of substance abuse.

continued

Table 6-13. Neurostimulants (Lexi-Comp, 2013) continued

Generic (Brand) and Formulations	Mechanism of Action	Usual Oral Dose (mg/day)	Adverse Drug Reactions	Drug Interactions	Contraindications	Clinical Pearls
Amantadine (Symmetrel®) Capsule, tablet, oral solution	NMDA receptor antagonist; inhibits dopamine reuptake	200–400	Orthostatic hypotension, peripheral edema, agitation, confusion, delirium, fatigue, headache, insomnia, anorexia, constipation, xerostomia, nausea, livedo reticularis, prolonged QTc interval, may lower seizure threshold	Antipsychotics ↓ effectiveness of amantadine Amantadine may cause additive QTc prolongation with other agents that prolong the QTc interval.	None	Reduce dose in patients with renal impairment. Avoid in patients with untreated angle closure glaucoma and uncontrolled psychosis. May exacerbate impulse control disorder Abrupt withdrawal or dose reduction may cause agitation, delirium, delusions, depression, hallucinations, slurred speech, stupor, or neuroleptic malignant syndrome.

continued

Table 6-13. Neurostimulants (Lexi-Comp, 2013) continued

Generic (Brand) and Formulations	Mechanism of Action	Usual Oral Dose (mg/day)	Adverse Drug Reactions	Drug Interactions	Contraindications	Clinical Pearls
Carbidopa-levodopa (Sinemet®, Parcopa®) Tablet, orally disintegrating tablet, extended-release tablet	Levodopa is converted to dopamine in the CNS; carbidopa inhibits the peripheral metabolism of levodopa.	75/300–200/2000	Orthostatic hypotension, arrhythmia, syncope, somnolence, agitation, alopecia, confusion, delusions, dementia, falling, hallucinations, insomnia, nightmares, psychosis, hyperglycemia, hypokalemia, hypersexuality, nausea, constipation, diarrhea, duodenal ulcer, dyspepsia, sialorrhea, taste alterations, discoloration of urine, sweat and saliva, priapism, proteinuria, urinary retention, constipation, blood dyscrasias, paresthesia, diplopia, may exacerbate dyskinesias, rare hypersensitivity reactions, myocardial infarction	Antipsychotics and pyridoxine ↓ effectiveness of levodopa. High protein diets ↓ levodopa absorption.	Carbidopa-levodopa is contraindicated with MAOIs. Carbidopa-levodopa should not be used in patients with narrow-angle glaucoma.	Levodopa is only commercially available as a combination product due to improved tolerability with carbidopa. Use with caution in patients with cardiovascular disease, respiratory disease, peptic ulcer disease, seizures, glaucoma, or renal or hepatic impairment. May exacerbate impulse control disorder Levodopa should be taken with food to reduce nausea and at least 2 hours apart from iron salts to maximize absorption. Abrupt discontinuation may result in syndrome similar to neuroleptic malignant syndrome.

continued

Table 6-13. Neurostimulants (Lexi-Comp, 2013) continued

Generic (Brand) and Formulations	Mechanism of Action	Usual Oral Dose (mg/day)	Adverse Drug Reactions	Drug Interactions	Contraindications	Clinical Pearls
Donepezil (Aricept®) Tablet, orally disintegrating tablet	Reversible, noncompetitive inhibition of centrally-active acetylcholinesterase	5–23	Weight loss, anorexia, nausea, vomiting, diarrhea, insomnia, infection, bradycardia, hypertension, headache, pain, dizziness, bruising, muscle cramps	Duration of effect of donepezil ↑ succinylcholine		Use caution in patients with cardiac conduction abnormalities, peptic ulcer disease, respiratory disease, or seizure disorder.
Bromocriptine (Parlodel®) Capsule, tablet	Dopamine receptor agonist	2.5–100	Dizziness, fatigue, headache, constipation, nausea, weakness, rhinitis, hypotension, syncope, drowsiness, somnolence, hypoglycemia, anorexia, diarrhea, dyspepsia, vomiting, xerostomia, gastrointestinal bleeding, rare cardiac valvular fibrosis, seizures, myocardial infarction, stroke, pleural/retroperitoneal fibrosis	Antipsychotics ↓ effectiveness of bromocriptine. Beta blockers ↑ vasoconstricting effects of bromocriptine. Clarithromycin and erythromycin may enhance the adverse effects of bromocriptine. ↑ bromocriptine level: Azole antifungals, chloramphenicol, nefazodone, nicardipine, and protease inhibitors Concomitant use of other serotonergic agents ↑ the risk of serotonin syndrome.	Bromocriptine is contraindicated in patients with uncontrolled hypertension or psychosis. Bromocriptine is contraindicated with ephedrine, epinephrine, nitroglycerin, norepinephrine, protease inhibitors, pseudoephedrine, midodrine, phenylephrine, and triptans.	Use with caution in patients with cardiovascular disease, dementia, hepatic or renal impairment, or peptic ulcer disease. May exacerbate impulse control disorder Abrupt discontinuation may result in syndrome similar to neuroleptic malignant syndrome.

BID indicates twice a day; CNS, central nervous system; MAOI, monoamine oxidase inhibitor; NMDA, N-methyl-D-aspartate.

Atypical Neuroleptics

A. Delirium is common in critically ill patients and has been associated with poor outcomes, including increased mortality (Barr et al., 2013).

B. Patients in the intensive care unit (ICU) should be routinely evaluated for the presence of delirium and, if present, treated (Barr et al., 2013).

C. Standardized tools such as the Confusion Assessment Method for the Intensive Care Unit (CAM-ICU) and the Intensive Care Delirium Screening Checklist (ICDSC) are effective in the detection of delirium in general ICU populations; however, their use has not yet been validated in patients with neurologic injury (Barr et al., 2013).

D. Medications

1. Neuroleptics commonly used post stroke are summarized in **Table 6-14**, **Table 6-15**, and **Figure 6-3**.
2. Prevention
   a. Benzodiazepines, narcotics, and anticholinergic agents may exacerbate delirium, therefore these agents should be avoided when possible (Makii, Mirski, & Lewin, 2010).
3. Prophylaxis
   a. Prophylactic treatment with neuroleptics to prevent delirium is not recommended.
4. Treatment
   a. Neuroleptics are generally employed to treat acute agitation or aggression that is associated with delirium and psychoses.
   b. Although haloperidol (Haldol®) is commonly used in the treatment of ICU delirium, only atypical antipsychotics have been shown to reduce its duration.
   c. In patients with delirium that is not due to alcohol or benzodiazepine withdrawal, substituting dexmedetomidine (Precedex®) or propofol (Diprivan®) for a benzodiazepine infusion may reduce the delerium's duration (Barr et al., 2013; Fraser et al., 2013).
   d. Neuroleptics have several important drug interactions:
      (1) All antipsychotics may prolong the QTc interval to varying degrees, increasing the risk of ventricular arrhythmias such as torsades de pointe. Hypokalemia and hypomagnesemia should be avoided.
      (2) Neuroleptics may diminish the effectiveness of stimulants and dopamine agonists.
      (3) Neuroleptics with anticholinergic properties will have additive effects when administered with other anticholinergic agents.
   e. Adverse effects
      (1) The U.S. Food and Drug Administration (FDA) issued black box warnings describing the risk of cerebrovascular adverse events, including stroke, when atypical antipsychotics are used in elderly individuals with dementia-related psychosis. Even brief exposure to antipsychotics is associated with an increased risk of stroke (Wang et al., 2012).
      (2) Neuroleptics have the potential to lower the seizure threshold.

Table 6-14. Adverse Effects of Selected Neuroleptics (The Medical Letter, 2013)

Generic (Brand)	**EPS**	**Sedation**	**Weight Gain/ Diabetes Mellitus**	**Dyslipidemia**	**Anticholinergic**	**Orthostatic Hypotension**	**QTc Prolongation**	**Hyperprolactinemia**
Haloperidol (Haldol®)	+++	++	+	+	0	0	+	+++
Aripiprazole (Abilify®)	+	+	0	0	0	0	0	0
Quetiapine (Seroquel®)	0	++	++	+++	+	++	++	0
Risperidone (Risperdal®)	++	+	++	+	0	++	+	+++
Ziprasidone (Geodon)	+	+	0	0	0	+	++	+
Olanzapine (Zyprexa®)	+	++	+++	+++	++	+	+	0

EPS indicates extrapyramidal symptoms.

Table 6-15. Pharmacologic Properties of Selected Neuroleptics (Lexi-Comp, 2013)

Generic (Brand) and Formulations	Usual Oral Dose (mg/day)	Drug Interactions	Contraindications	Clinical Pearls
Haloperidol (Haldol®) Tablet, oral solution, immediate-acting and long-acting injection	Oral: 5–10 IV: 0.5–10 mg per dose	↓ haloperidol concentration: carbamazepine, dexamethasone, efavirenz, fosphenytoin, glycopyrrolate, oxcarbazepine, pentobarbital, phenobarbital, phenytoin, primidone, rifampin ↑ haloperidol concentration: azole antifungals, bupropion, chloramphenicol, clarithromycin, cinacalcet, fluoxetine, nefazodone, nicardipine, paroxetine, protease inhibitors, quinidine, thioridazine Haloperidol ↑ concentration: colchicine, eplerenone, fentanyl, metoprolol, thioridazine	Haloperidol is contraindicated with ipratropium, metoclopramide, and tiotropium.	
Aripiprazole (Abilify®) Tablet, ODT, oral solution, immediate-acting and long-acting injection	10–30	↓ aripiprazole concentration: carbamazepine, dexamethasone, efavirenz, fosphenytoin, oxcarbazepine, pentobarbital, phenobarbital, phenytoin, primidone, rifampin ↑ aripiprazole concentration: bupropion, chloramphenicol, clarithromycin, cinacalcet, fluoxetine, itraconazole, ketoconazole, nefazodone, nicardipine, paroxetine, posaconazole, protease inhibitors, quinidine, thioridazine, voriconazole	Aripiprazole is contraindicated with metoclopramide.	Delayed onset of action Partial DA agonist

continued

Table 6-15. Pharmacologic Properties of Selected Neuroleptics (Lexi-Comp, 2013) continued

Generic (Brand) and Formulations	Usual Oral Dose (mg/day)	Drug Interactions	Contraindications	Clinical Pearls
Quetiapine (Seroquel®) Tablet, extended-release tablet	300–800	↓ quetiapine concentration: carbamazepine, dexamethasone, efavirenz, fosphenytoin, oxcarbazepine, pentobarbital, phenobarbital, phenytoin, primidone, rifampin, St John's wort ↑ quetiapine concentration: chloramphenicol, clarithromycin, nefazodone, nicardipine, protease inhibitors, azole antifungals	Quetiapine is contraindicated with ipratropium, metoclopramide, and tiotropium.	
Risperidone (Risperdal®) Tablet, ODT, oral solution, long-acting injection	4–8	↑ risperidone concentration: bupropion, cinacalcet, fluoxetine, paroxetine, quinidine, ritonavir, thioridazine Loop diuretics ↑ toxicity associated with risperidone	Risperidone is contraindicated with ipratropium, metoclopramide, and tiotropium.	At high doses adverse effects similar to typical antipsychotics
Ziprasidone (Geodon) Capsule, oral solution, immediate-acting injection	120–160	↓ ziprasidone concentration: carbamazepine ↑ ziprasidone concentration: ketoconazole	Ziprasidone is contraindicated with fluoxetine and metoclopramide.	Ziprasidone should be taken with food to maximize absorption.
Olanzapine (Zyprexa®) Tablet, ODT, immediate-acting and long-acting injection	10–20	↓ olanzapine concentration: carbamazepine, phenobarbital, primidone, rifampin, tobacco use ↑ olanzapine concentration: ciprofloxacin, fluvoxamine, ketoconazole, mexilitene, ofloxacin, primaquine	Olanzapine is contraindicated with ipratropium, metoclopramide, and tiotropium. IM olanzapine is contraindicated with parenteral benzodiazepines.	

DA indicates dopamine; IM, intramuscular; IV, intravenous; ODT, orally disintegrating tablet.

Figure 6-3. Atypical Antipsychotic Receptor Characteristics*

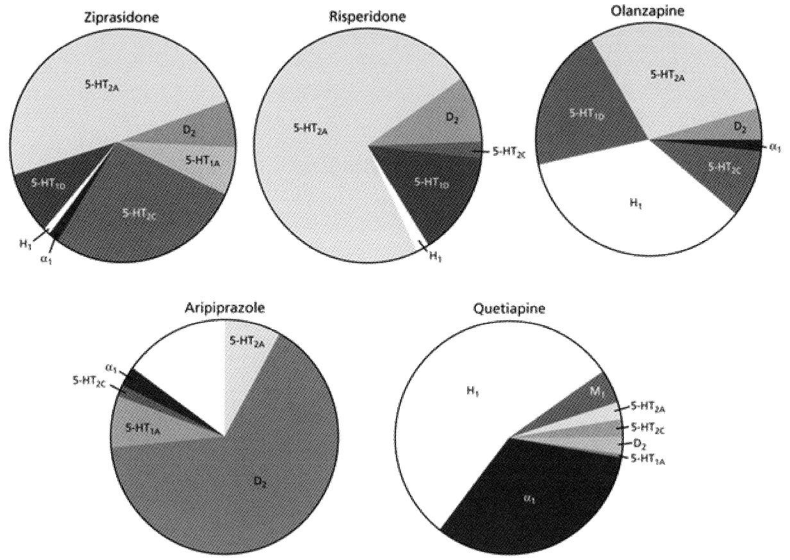

**5-HT indicates serotonin; D, dopamine; H, histamine; M, Muscarine.*

Reprinted from "The Science of Antipsychotics: Mechanistic Insight," by C. A. Tamminga, 2003, CNS Spectrums, *8(11 Suppl 2), pp. 5–9. © 2003 by Cambridge. Reprinted with permission.*

Analgesics

A. Pain is common in the ICU, and untreated pain has been associated with long-lasting psychological consequences, deleterious effects on health-related quality of life, and chronic pain (Barr et al., 2013).

B. Pain should be routinely assessed in all critically ill patients (Barr et al., 2013).

C. Pain can be systematically assessed in neurocritically ill patients by self-report, or when self-report is not possible, by standardized tools such as the Behavioral Pain Scale (BPS) and BPS-nonintubated (BPS-NI) for intubated and nonintubated patients, respectively (Yu et al., 2013).

D. Medications commonly employed in the treatment of pain in neurocritically ill patients are summarized in **Table 6-16**.

1. IV opiates are considered first-line for non-neuropathic pain in critically ill patients.
    a. Along with the analgesic effects of opiate agonists, opiates also possess sedative properties.
    b. Opiates have the potential to increase ICP, generally through hypercarbia.
    c. Elderly patients tend to be more sensitive to opiates and more likely to experience toxicity associated with these agents. Lower doses may be required for this population.
    d. Partial opiate agonists, such as buprenorphine, butorphanol, and nalbuphine, may diminish the analgesic effect of other opiates.
    e. Opiates may produce tolerance and dependence. Opiate-tolerant patients may require higher than usual doses. Patients should be monitored for withdrawal symptoms when abruptly discontinuing after prolonged use.

f. Opiates are contraindicated in patients with paralytic ileus. Alvimopan should not be initiated in patients receiving long-term (at least 1 week) opiates.

2. Acetaminophen and NSAIDs are effective for less severe pain and notably are unlikely to affect the neurologic exam. They also are effective antipyretics. Please see the antipyretic section for more information about these agents.

E. Analgesia should not be interrupted during neuromuscular blockade.

Table 6-16. Analgesics (Lexi-Comp, 2013)

Drug Class Generic (Brand), Schedule, and Formulations	Usual Dose	Adverse Drug Reactions	Drug Interactions	Contraindications	Clinical Pearls
Fentanyl (Duragesic®) C-II Buccal "lollipop," transdermal patch, lozenge, sublingual spray, nasal spray, sublingual tablet, injection	Bolus 12.5–100 mcg or 1–2 mcg/kg IVP Maintenance IV infusion 0.7–10 mcg/kg/hr or 25–700 mcg/hr	Bradycardia, chest wall rigidity, confusion, constipation, dependency, diaphoresis, edema, headache, miosis, mood changes, myoclonus, nausea, respiratory depression, sedation, vomiting, xerostomia	↑ fentanyl concentration: amiodarone, azole antifungals, cimetidine, clarithromycin, cyclosporine, desipramine, diltiazem, dronedarone, erythromycin, grapefruit juice, haloperidol, metronidazole, nefazodone, nicardipine, protease inhibitors, sertraline, verapamil	Fentanyl is contraindicated with MAOIs.	Use caution in patients with renal or hepatic impairment. The fentanyl patch cannot be rapidly titrated because it has a delayed onset (6–24 hr, longest with first dose) and prolonged duration of action even if the patch is removed; the transdermal route should be avoided in patients with significant edema or who are undergoing therapeutic hypothermia due to erratic absorption. Fentanyl patch should be changed every 72 hours. Transmucosal, immediate-release fentanyl products are approved for use in opiate-tolerant patients and are only available through a restricted access program. Fentanyl is not administered via the oral route because of significant first-pass metabolism. Accumulation in lipid tissues is possible with prolonged infusions or repeated bolus doses.

continued

Table 6-16. Analgesics (Lexi-Comp, 2013) continued

Drug Class Generic (Brand), Schedule, and Formulations	Usual Dose	Adverse Drug Reactions	Drug Interactions	Contraindications	Clinical Pearls
Hydrocodone/ Acetaminophen (Vicodin®, Lortab®) C-III Tablet, oral solution	5–10 mg of hydrocodone component every 4–6 hr, not to exceed 4 g of acetaminophen in 24 hr	Bradycardia, dependency, diaphoresis, dyspepsia, hepatotoxicity (due to acetaminophen component), hypersensitivity reactions, hypotension, mood changes, rare myelosuppression,respiratory depression, sedation	See text, p. 191, D.1.d	Contraindicated with paralytic ileus	Not available as hydrocodone alone; acetaminophen content varies. Use caution in patients with G6PD deficiency or renal or hepatic impairment. Hydromorphone is an active metabolite of hydrocodone.
Hydromorphone (Dilaudid®) C-II Tablet, extended-release tablet, oral-solution, injection, rectal suppository	Oral: 2–4 mg every 4–6 hr IV: 0.2–1 mg every 4–6 hr	Bradycardia, confusion, constipation, dependency, diaphoresis, edema, headache, miosis, mood changes, myoclonus, nausea, respiratory depression, sedation, vomiting, xerostomia	See text, p. 191, D.1.d	Hydromorphone is contraindicated with MAOIs and paralytic ileus.	Use caution in patients with inflammatory or obstructive bowel disorder, cardiovascular disease, or renal or hepatic impairment.
Morphine (Duramorph®, MS Contin®) C-II Tablet, extended-release tablet, oral-solution, injection	Bolus 2–10 mg IVP Intermittent dose 2–8 mg every 3–4 hr Maintenance infusion 0.8–30 mg/hr	Antidiuretic hormone release, constipation, dependency, dizziness, fever, headache, hypotension, itching, may elevate ICP due to hypercarbia, mood changes, myoclonus, nausea, pain at injection site, pruritis, respiratory depression, sedation, urinary retention, vomiting, xerostomia	See text, p. 191, D.1.d	Contraindicated with paralytic ileus	Active metabolites may accumulate in renal dysfunction; reduced dose recommended. Can induce a histamine release that causes itching

continued

Table 6-16. Analgesics (Lexi-Comp, 2013) continued

Drug Class Generic (Brand), Schedule, and Formulations	Usual Dose	Adverse Drug Reactions	Drug Interactions	Contraindications	Clinical Pearls
Oxycodone (Roxicodone®, Oxycontin®) C-II Oral tablet, extended-release tablet, oral solution	Usual immediate-release oral dose 5–20 mg every 4–6 hr	Confusion, constipation, dependency, diaphoresis, dizziness, headache, mood changes, myoclonus, nausea, orthostatic hypotension, respiratory depression, somnolence, vomiting, xerostomia	↓ oxycodone concentration: carbamazepine, dexamethasone, efavirenz, fosphenytoin, oxcarbazepine, pentobarbital, phenobarbital, phenytoin, primidone, rifampin ↑ oxycodone concentration: azole antifungals, chloramphenicol, clarithromycin, protease inhibitors, nefazodone, nicardipine	Contraindicated with paralytic ileus, gastrointestinal obstruction	Active metabolites may accumulate in patients with renal dysfunction. Often coformulated with acetaminophen

ICP indicates intracranial pressure; IVP, intravenous push; MAOI, monoamine oxidase inhibitor.

Sedatives

A. Sedatives are often required in the ICU to facilitate necessary care and relieve emotional and physical stress; however, their use must be minimized so that they do not compromise the ability to obtain frequent, high-quality neurologic examinations.

B. Pain should always be assessed and, if present, treated before initiating sedatives.

C. Sedation can and should be routinely and systematically assessed in neurocritically ill patients using standardized tools such as the Richmond Agitation-Sedation Scale (RASS) (Barr et al., 2013; Yu et al., 2013).

D. Medications used for sedation in patients with neurologic injury are summarized in **Table 6-17**.

1. Sedation should be employed for the shortest duration and at the lowest dose tolerated. This correlates to a goal RASS -1 to +1 or Riker Sedation-Agitation Scale 3 to 4 (Barr et al., 2013). Deeper levels of sedation may be required for selected patients with difficult to control elevated ICP.
2. Goals of sedation in neurocritically ill patients:
   a. Reduce ICP
   b. Suppress central hyperventilation
   c. Calm agitated or combative patients
   d. Adjunct treatment of refractory status epilepticus
   e. Treat intoxication or drug withdrawal (Keegan, 2008)
3. Benzodiazepines and propofol also possess anticonvulsant effects.
4. As in the general ICU population, propofol (Diprivan®) and dexmedetomidine (Precedex®) generally are preferred in place of benzodiazepines because they have been associated with a shorter ICU length of stay and duration of mechanical ventilation, and possibly less delirium. Nonetheless, benzodiazepines may be particularly beneficial in the treatment seizures or alcohol withdrawal (Barr et al., 2013).
5. Avoiding benzodiazepine use or substituting an agent such as dexmedetomidine (Precedex®) or propofol (Diprivan®) may reduce the risk of developing delirium (Barr et al., 2013; Fraser et al., 2013).
6. Sedatives have several important adverse effects that may be particularly problematic in patients with neurologic injury.
   a. There is the potential to confound the neurologic exam, thus obscuring subtle signs of neurologic deterioration.
   b. Many sedative agents are associated with hypotension, which can compromise cerebral perfusion.
   c. Elderly patients are particularly susceptible to toxicity associated with sedatives because of reduced clearance and increased sensitivity. Therefore, low initial doses and slow titration of sedatives generally are recommended.
   d. Tachyphylaxis and withdrawal are possible with prolonged infusions of benzodiazepines or dexmedetomidine.

E. Although some benefit has been observed with the daily interruption of sedation in a mixed medical intensive-care population, more evidence is needed before its use can be routinely recommended for neurocritically ill patients (Barr et al., 2013).

1. Daily interruption of sedation should be implemented cautiously in patients with a significant history of alcohol use or uncontrolled elevated ICP.
2. Sedation should not be interrupted during neuromuscular blockade.

Table 6-17. Sedatives (Lexi-Comp, 2013)

Drug Class, Generic (Brand), and Schedule	Mechanism of Action	Usual Intravenous Dose for Sedation	Adverse Drug Reactions	Drug Interactions	Contraindications	Clinical Pearls
Propofol (Diprivan®)	Propofol produces sedation through agonism of GABAa receptors	5–100 mcg/kg/min	Apnea, hypertriglyceridemia, hypotension, movement, pain at the injection site, pancreatitis, PRIS (hyperkalemia, dysrhythmia, lipemia, metabolic acidosis, heart failure, +/- rhabdomyolysis)	Rifampin may enhance hypotensive effects.	Allergy to soy or egg	Use with caution in patients with cardiovascular disease. Rapid onset and offset that can facilitate frequent neurologic exams Lipid vehicle is particularly susceptible to bacterial contamination; IV tubing and bottle should be changed every 12 hr. The risk of PRIS is increased when propofol is administered at high doses (>50 mcg/kg/min) for a prolonged duration (>48 hr). Blue-green discoloration of urine may occur. Propofol delivers 1.1 kcal/ml.

continued

Table 6-17. Sedatives (Lexi-Comp, 2013) continued

Drug Class, Generic (Brand), and Schedule	Mechanism of Action	Usual Intravenous Dose for Sedation	Adverse Drug Reactions	Drug Interactions	Contraindications	Clinical Pearls
Dexmedetomidine (Precedex®)	Alpha-2 agonist producing anesthesia and sedation	Optional loading dose 1 mcg/ kg over 10 min; the loading dose generally is not recommended in critically ill patients because of the risk of severe bradycardia, hypotension, and sinus arrest. Maintenance infusion 0.2–0.7 mcg/ kg/hr, some literature supports doses up to 1.4 mcg/ kg/hr	Bradycardia, dry mouth, hypotension, transient hypertension during loading dose	Dexmedetomidine may enhance bet blocker-induced AV blockade; beta blockers may enhance rebound hypertensive effects. ↑ dexmedetomidine concentration: letrozole	None	Also has analgesic properties Patients are arousable with stimulation, even during infusion, and then return to sedated state without stimulation. Manufacturer recommends 24-hr infusion; however postmarketing trials support infusions of longer duration. Does not require mechanical ventilation Use with caution in patients with diabetes mellitus, severe hepatic dysfunction, cardiovascular disease, chronic hypertension, or hypovolemia.

continued

Table 6-17. Sedatives (Lexi-Comp, 2013) continued

Drug Class, Generic (Brand), and Schedule	Mechanism of Action	Usual Intravenous Dose for Sedation	Adverse Drug Reactions	Drug Interactions	Contraindications	Clinical Pearls
Lorazepam (Ativan®) C-IV	Enhances the inhibitory effects of GABA	Loading dose 0.02–0.04 mg/kg Intermittent dose 0.02–0.06 mg/kg q 2–6 hr Maintenance infusion 0.01–0.1 mg/kg/hr	akathisia, amnesia, confusion, dependency, drowsiness, hypotension, nausea, pain at injection site, rash, respiratory depression, visual disturbances, vomiting	Benzodiazepines may ↑ toxicity of clozapine. ↑ lorazepam concentration: theophylline, valproic acid	Benzodiazepines are contraindicated with intramuscular olanzapine. Acute narrow-angle glaucoma	Propylene glycol contained in IV lorazepam can accumulate with prolonged infusions and cause a metabolic acidosis. Precipitation is possible; an in-line filter is recommended.
Midazolam (Versed®) C-IV	Enhances the inhibitory effects of GABA	Loading dose 0.01–0.05 mg/kg Maintenance infusion 0.01–0.1 mg/kg/hr	Similar to lorazepam	Benzodiazepines ↑ toxicity of clozapine ↑ midazolam concentration: grapefruit juice, azole antifungals, chloramphenicol, clarithromycin, diltiazem, erythromycin, nefazodone, nicardipine, verapamil ↓ midazolam concentration: carbamazepine, dexamethasone, fosphenytoin, oxcarbazepine, pentobarbital, phenobarbital, phenytoin, primidone, rifampin, theophylline	Benzodiazepines are contraindicated with intramuscular olanzapine. Midazolam is contraindicated with conivaptan, efavirenz, ketoconazole, itraconazole, and protease inhibitors.	Also has anticonvulsant properties Midazolam has a rapid onset and short duration, however prolonged infusions may result in altered pharmacokinetics as midazolam accumulates in lipid tissues. Midazolam has active metabolites that may accumulate in patients with renal dysfunction.

AV indicates atrioventricular; GABA gamma-aminobutyric acid; IV, intravenous; PRIS, propofol-related infusion syndrome.

Antipyretics

A. Temperature goal
  1. Normothermia is a reasonable goal for patients with acute ischemic or hemorrhagic stroke.
  2. The potential role of hypothermia in stroke is actively under investigation. Currently, there is insufficient evidence to support its routine use in this setting (Connolly et al., 2012; Diringer et al., 2011; Jauch et al., 2013; Morgenstern et al., 2010).
  3. Fever is common and has been associated with poor outcomes in patients with neurologic injury (Connolly et al., 2012; Diringer et al., 2011; Jauch et al., 2013).

B. Fever
  1. Patients with stroke should be monitored for fever and, if present, treated. However, evidence of improved outcomes with successful fever management is lacking (Diringer et al., 2011; Morgenstern et al., 2010).
  2. For patients with aSAH, cooling devices may be effective when pharmacologic interventions fail; however, its use is limited by adverse effects such as shivering (Diringer et al., 2011).

C. Medications used to prevent or treat fever in patients with neurologic injury.
  1. Acetaminophen (Tylenol®)
     a. Acetaminophen is available in oral, rectal, and intravenous formulations. Rectal formulations are not very well absorbed and achieve lower serum concentrations at comparative doses. Liquid formulations may contain sorbitol and can cause diarrhea.
     b. Acetaminophen exerts its antipyretic effects through inhibition of the hypothalamic thermoregulatory center.
     c. The usual dose is 650–1,000 mg every 4–6 hours up to a maximum 4,000 mg per day.
     d. A new dose limit of 325 mg per prescription product has been recommended by the FDA due to the risk of hepatotoxity with combination products.
     e. Adverse effects include nausea, vomiting, headache, insomnia, rash (can be severe), and electrolyte disturbances; overdose can result in nephrotoxicity and hepatotoxicity.
     f. Acetaminophen may cause increased hepatotoxicity when used in combination with other drugs that are associated with liver injury.
     g. Avoid use in patients with severe liver disease; use with caution in patients with significant renal impairment or G6PD deficiency.
     h. Importantly, acetaminophen is devoid of antiplatelet effects.
  2. Aspirin
     a. Aspirin is available in oral and rectal formulations.
     b. Aspirin decreases prostaglandin formation through irreversible inhibition of COX-1 and COX-2.
     c. The usual dose for fever is 325–650 mg orally or 300–600 mg rectally every 4–6 hours up to 4,000 mg daily.
     d. Please refer to the antiplatelet section for additional information about aspirin.
  3. Ibuprofen (Motrin®)
     a. Ibuprofen is available in oral and intravenous formulations.
     b. Ibuprofen decreases prostaglandin formation through reversible inhibition of COX-1 and COX-2.
     c. The usual dose is 200–400 mg every 4–6 hours up to a maximum of 3,200 mg per day.

d. Adverse effects include nausea, gastric and duodenal ulcer, edema, hypertension, dizziness, bleeding, hyperkalemia, rash, asthma exacerbation, tinnitus, blood dyscrasias, nephrotoxicity, and hepatotoxicity.
e. Ibuprofen may increase the bleeding risk associated with antiplatelet and anticoagulant drugs. A lithium dose reduction may be required upon initiation of ibuprofen, and there is an increased risk of lithium toxicity. Ibuprofen may diminish the effect of loop diuretics and the protective cardiovascular effects of aspirin. Avoid concurrent administration of cyclosporine or methotrexate.
f. Avoid use in patients with aspirin-sensitive asthma, bleeding disorders, kidney injury, or severe hepatic insufficiency.

References

Ageno, W., Gallus, A. S., Wittkowsky, A., Crowther, M., Hylek, E. M., Palareti, G., & American College of Chest Physicians. (2012). Oral anticoagulant therapy: Antithrombotic therapy and prevention of thrombosis, 9th ed: American College of Chest Physicians evidence-based clinical practice guidelines. *Chest, 141*(2 Suppl), e44S–88S. doi: 10.1378/chest.11-2292

Ashtary, F., Janghorbani, M., Chitsaz, A., Reisi, M., & Bahrami, A. (2006). A randomized, double-blind trial of bromocriptine efficacy in nonfluent aphasia after stroke. *Neurology, 66*(6), 914–916. doi: 10.1212/01.wnl.0000203119.91762.0c

Barr, J., Fraser, G. L., Puntillo, K., Ely, E. W., Gelinas, C., Dasta, J. F., . . . Jaeschke, R. (2013). Clinical practice guidelines for the management of pain, agitation, and delirium in adult patients in the intensive care unit. *Critical Care Medicine, 41*(1), 263–306. doi: 10.1097/CCM.0b013e3182783b72

Berthier, M. L., Hinojosa, J., Martín Mdel, C., & Fernandez, I. (2003). Open-label study of donepezil in chronic poststroke aphasia. *Neurology, 60*(7), 1218–1219.

Brophy, G. M., Bell, R., Classen, J., Alldredge, B., Bleck, T. P., Glauser, T., ... Neurocritical Care Society Status Epilepticus Guideline Writing Committee. (2012). Guidelines for the evaluation and management of status epilepticus. *Neurocritical Care, 17*(1), 3–23. doi: 10.1007/s12028-012-9695.z

Burns, M. M., & Greenberg, D. A. (2010). Antidepressants in the treatment of stroke. *Expert Review of Neurotherapeutics, 10*(8), 1237–1241. doi: 10.1586/ern.10.96

Chen, S. P., Fuh, J. L., & Wang, S. J. (2010). Reversible cerebral vasoconstriction syndrome: An underrecognized clinical emergency. *Therapeutic Advances in Neurological Disorders, 3*(3), 161–171. doi: 10.1177/1756285610361795

Chollet, F., Tardy, J., Albucher, J. F., Thalamas, C., Berard, E., Lamy, C., . . . Loubinoux, I. (2011). Fluoxetine for motor recovery after acute ischaemic stroke (FLAME): A randomised placebo-controlled trial. *Lancet Neurology, 10*(2), 123–130. doi: 10.1016/S1474-4422(10)70314-8

Connolly, E. S., Jr., Rabinstein, A. A., Carhuapoma, J. R., Derdeyn, C. P., Dion, J., Higashida, R. T., . . . Vespa, P. (2012). Guidelines for the management of aneurysmal subarachnoid hemorrhage: A guideline for healthcare professionals from the American Heart Association/American Stroke Association. *Stroke, 43*(6), 1711–1737. doi: 10.1161/STR.0b013e3182587839

Dasta, J. F., Boucher, B. A., Brophy, G. M., Cohen, H., Hassan, E., Maclaren, R., . . . Seybert, A. L. (2010). Intravenous to oral conversion of antihypertensives: a toolkit for guideline development. [Review]. *The Annals of Pharmacotherapy, 44*(9), 1430–1447. doi: 10.1345/aph.1P086

Department of Veterans Affairs & Department of Defense. (2010). The management of stroke rehabiliation. Retrieved from www.healthquality.va.gov/stroke/stroke_full_221.pdf

Diringer, M. N., Bleck, T. P., Claude Hemphill, J., 3rd, Menon, D., Shutter, L., Vespa, P., . . . Neurocritical Care Society. (2011). Critical care management of patients following aneurysmal subarachnoid hemorrhage: Recommendations from the Neurocritical Care Society's Multidisciplinary Consensus Conference. *Neurocritical Care, 15*(2), 211–240. doi: 10.1007/s12028-011-9605-9

Douxfils, J., Chatelain, C., Chatelain, B., Dogne, J. M., & Mullier, F. (2013). Impact of apixaban on routine and specific coagulation assays: A practical laboratory guide. *Thrombosis and Haemostasis, 110*(2), 283–294. doi: 10.1160/TH12-12-0898

Douxfils, J., Mullier, F., Loosen, C., Chatelain, C., Chatelain, B., & Dogne, J. M. (2012). Assessment of the impact of rivaroxaban on coagulation assays: Laboratory recommendations for the monitoring of rivaroxaban and review of the literature. *Thrombosis Research, 130*(6), 956–966. doi: 10.1016/j.thromres.2012.09.004

Douxfils, J., Mullier, F., Robert, S., Chatelain, C., Chatelain, B., & Dogne, J. M. (2012). Impact of dabigatran on a large panel of routine or specific coagulation assays. Laboratory recommendations for monitoring of dabigatran etexilate. *Thrombosis and Haemostasis, 107*(5), 985–997. doi: 10.1160/TH11-11-0804

Duncan, P. W., Zorowitz, R., Bates, B., Choi, J. Y., Glasberg, J. J., Graham, G. D., . . . Reker, D. (2005). Management of adult stroke rehabilitation care: A clinical practice guideline. *Stroke, 36*(9), e100–143. doi: 10.1161/01.STR.0000180861.54180.FF

Eikelboom, J. W., Hirsh, J., Spencer, F. A., Baglin, T. P., & Weitz, J. I. (2012). Antiplatelet drugs: Antithrombotic therapy and prevention of thrombosis, 9th ed: American College of Chest Physicians evidence-based clinical practice guidelines. *Chest, 141*(2 Suppl), e89S–119S. doi: 10.1378/chest.11-2293

Eikelboom, J. W., Wallentin, L., Connolly, S. J., Ezekowitz, M., Healey, J. S., Oldgren, J., . . . Yusuf, S. (2011). Risk of bleeding with 2 doses of dabigatran compared with warfarin in older and younger patients with atrial fibrillation: An analysis of the randomized evaluation of long-term anticoagulant therapy (RE-LY) trial. *Circulation, 123*(21), 2363–2372. doi: 10.1161/CIRCULATIONAHA.110.004747

Fick, D. M., & Semla, T. P. (2012). 2012 American Geriatrics Society Beers Criteria: New year, new criteria, new perspective. *Journal of the American Geriatrics Society, 60*(4), 614–615. doi: 10.1111/j.1532-5415.2012.03922.x

Forsyth, L. L., Liu-DeRyke, X., Parker, D., Jr., & Rhoney, D. H. (2008). Role of hypertonic saline for the management of intracranial hypertension after stroke and traumatic brain injury. *Pharmacotherapy, 28*(4), 469–484. doi: 10.1592/phco.28.4.469

Fraser, G. L., Devlin, J. W., Worby, C. P., Alhazzani, W., Barr, J., Dasta, J. F., . . . Spencer, F. A. (2013). Benzodiazepine versus nonbenzodiazepine-based sedation for mechanically ventilated, critically ill adults: A systematic review and meta-analysis of randomized trials. *Critical Care Medicine, 41*(9 Suppl 1), S30–S38. doi: 10.1097/CCM.0b013e3182a16898

Furie, K. L., Goldstein, L. B., Albers, G. W., Khatri, P., Neyens, R., Turakhia, M. P., . . . Council on Peripheral Vascular Disease. (2012). Oral antithrombotic agents for the prevention of stroke in nonvalvular atrial fibrillation: A science advisory for healthcare professionals from the American Heart Association/American Stroke Association. *Stroke, 43*(12), 3442–3453. doi: 10.1161/STR.0b013e318266722a

Furie, K. L., Kasner, S. E., Adams, R. J., Albers, G. W., Bush, R. L., Fagan, S. C., . . . Inter-disciplinary Council on Quality of Care and Outcomes Research. (2011). Guidelines for the prevention of stroke in patients with stroke or transient ischemic attack: A guideline for healthcare professionals from the American Heart Association/American Stroke Association. *Stroke, 42*(1), 227–276. doi: 10.1161/STR.0b013e3181f7d043

Goldstein, L. B., Bushnell, C. D., Adams, R. J., Appel, L. J., Braun, L. T., Chaturvedi, S., . . . Inter-disciplinary Council on Quality of Care and Outcomes Research. (2011). Guidelines for the primary prevention of stroke: A guideline for healthcare professionals from the American Heart Association/American Stroke Association. *Stroke, 42*(2), 517–584. doi: 10.1161/STR.0b013e3181fcb238

Grade, C., Redford, B., Chrostowski, J., Toussaint, L., & Blackwell, B. (1998). Methylphenidate in early poststroke recovery: A double-blind, placebo-controlled study. *Archives of Physical Medicine and Rehabilitation, 79*(9), 1047–1050.

Gupta, S. R., Mlcoch, A. G., Scolaro, C., & Moritz, T. (1995). Bromocriptine treatment of nonfluent aphasia. *Neurology, 45*(12), 2170–2173.

Hackam, D. G., & Mrkobrada, M. (2012). Selective serotonin reuptake inhibitors and brain hemorrhage: A meta-analysis. *Neurology, 79*(18), 1862–1865. doi: 10.1212/WNL.0b013e318271f848

Hackett, M. L., Anderson, C. S., House, A., & Halteh, C. (2008). Interventions for preventing depression after stroke. *The Cochrane Database of Systematic Reviews,* (3), CD003689. doi: 10.1002/14651858.CD003689.pub3

Hackett, M. L., Anderson, C. S., House, A., & Xia, J. (2008). Interventions for treating depression after stroke. *The Cochrane Database of Systematic Reviews,* (4), CD003437. doi: 10.1002/14651858.CD003437.pub3

Heidbuchel, H., Verhamme, P., Alings, M., Antz, M., Hacke, W., Oldgren, J., . . . Kirchhof, P. (2013). EHRA practical guide on the use of new oral anticoagulants in patients with non-valvular atrial fibrillation: Executive summary. *European Heart Journal, 34*(27), 2094–2106. doi: 10.1093/eurheartj/eht134

Hollenberg, S. M. (2011). Vasoactive drugs in circulatory shock. *American Journal of Respiratory and Critical Care Medicine, 183*(7), 847–855. doi: 10.1164/rccm.201006-0972CI

Inzucchi, S. E. (2012). *Diabetes facts and guidelines.* Retrieved from http://endocrinology.yale.edu/patient/diabetescenter.html

Jauch, E. C., Saver, J. L., Adams, H. P., Jr., Bruno, A., Connors, J. J., Demaerschalk, B. M., . . . Council on Clinical Cardiology. (2013). Guidelines for the early management of patients with acute ischemic stroke: A guideline for healthcare professionals from the American Heart Association/American Stroke Association. *Stroke, 44*(3), 870–947. doi: 10.1161/STR.0b013e318284056a

Keegan, M. T. (2008). Sedation in the neurologic intensive care unit. *Current Treatment Options in Neurology, 10*(2), 111–125.

Kellum, J. A., & Pinsky, M. R. (2002). Use of vasopressor agents in critically ill patients. *Current Opinions in Critical Care, 8*(3), 236–241.

Ketel, W. B., & Kolb, M. E. (1984). Long-term treatment with dantrolene sodium of stroke patients with spasticity limiting the return of function. *Current Medical Research and Opinion, 9*(3), 161–169. doi: 10.1185/03007998409109576

Lansberg, M. G., O'Donnell, M. J., Khatri, P., Lang, E. S., Nguyen-Huynh, M. N., Schwartz, N. E., . . . American College of Chest Physicians. (2012). Antithrombotic and thrombolytic therapy for ischemic stroke: Antithrombotic therapy and prevention of thrombosis, 9th ed: American College of Chest Physicians evidence-based clinical practice Guidelines. *Chest, 141*(2 Suppl), e601S–636S. doi: 10.1378/chest.11-2302

Levine, G. N., Bates, E. R., Blankenship, J. C., Bailey, S. R., Bittl, J. A., Cercek, B., . . . Society for Cardiovascular Angiography and Interventions. (2011). 2011 ACCF/AHA/SCAI guideline for percutaneous coronary intervention. A report of the American College of Cardiology Foundation/American Heart Association Task Force on Practice Guidelines and the Society for Cardiovascular Angiography and Interventions. *Journal of the American College of Cardiology, 58*(24), e44–122. doi: 10.1016/j.jacc.2011.08.007

Lexi-Comp, I. L.-D. (2013). Lexi-Drugs. Retrieved from Lexi-Comp, Inc

Lokk, J., Salman Roghani, R., & Delbari, A. (2011). Effect of methylphenidate and/or levodopa coupled with physiotherapy on functional and motor recovery after stroke: A randomized, double-blind, placebo-controlled trial. *Acta Neurologica Scandinavica, 123*(4), 266–273. doi: 10.1111/j.1600-0404.2010.01395.x

Makii, J. M., Mirski, M. A., & Lewin, J. J., 3rd. (2010). Sedation and analgesia in critically ill neurologic patients. *Journal of Pharmacy Practice, 23*(5), 455–469. doi: 10.1177/0897190010372339

Martinsson, L., Hardemark, H., & Eksborg, S. (2007). Amphetamines for improving recovery after stroke. *The Cochrane Database of Systematic Reviews,* (1), CD002090. doi: 10.1002/14651858.CD002090.pub2

McKenney, J. M. (2003). Update on the National Cholesterol Education Program Adult Treatment Panel III guidelines: Getting to goal. *Pharmacotherapy, 23*(9 Pt 2), 26S–33S.

Mead, G. E., Hsieh, C. F., Lee, R., Kutlubaev, M. A., Claxton, A., Hankey, G. J., & Hackett, M. L. (2012). Selective serotonin reuptake inhibitors (SSRIs) for stroke recovery. *The Cochrane Database of Systematic Reviews, 11,* CD009286. doi: 10.1002/14651858.CD009286.pub2

Medwatch. (2010). Information for healthcare professionals: Concomitant use of ibuprofen and aspirin. www.fda.gov/Drugs/DrugSafety/PostmarketDrugSafetyInformationforPatientsandProviders/ucm125222.htm. Retrieved July 10, 2013

Mikami, K., Jorge, R. E., Adams, H. P., Jr., Davis, P. H., Leira, E. C., Jang, M., & Robinson, R. G. (2011). Effect of antidepressants on the course of disability following stroke. *The American Journal of Geriatric Psychiatry, 19*(12), 1007–1015. doi: 10.1097/JGP.0b013e31821181b0

Miller, E. L., Murray, L., Richards, L., Zorowitz, R. D., Bakas, T., Clark, P., & Billinger, S. A. (2010). Comprehensive overview of nursing and interdisciplinary rehabilitation care of the stroke patient: A scientific statement from the American Heart Association. *Stroke, 41*(10), 2402-2448. doi: 10.1161/STR.0b013e3181e7512b

Morgenstern, L. B., Hemphill, J. C., 3rd, Anderson, C., Becker, K., Broderick, J. P., Connolly, E. S., Jr., . . . Tamargo, R. J. (2010). Guidelines for the management of spontaneous intracerebral hemorrhage: A guideline for healthcare professionals from the American Heart Association/American Stroke Association. *Stroke, 41*(9), 2108–2129. doi: 10.1161/STR.0b013e3181ec611b

Nutescu, E. A. (2013). Oral anticoagulant therapies: Balancing the risks. *American Journal of Health System Pharmacy, 70*(10 Suppl 1), S3–S11. doi: 10.2146/ajhp130040

Paolucci, S., Gandolfo, C., Provinciali, L., Torta, R., & Toso, V. (2006). The Italian multicenter observational study on post-stroke depression (DESTRO). *Journal of Neurology, 253*(5), 556–562. doi: 10.1007/s00415-006-0058-6

Papangelou, A., Lewin, J. J., 3rd, Mirski, M. A., & Stevens, R. D. (2009). Pharmacologic management of brain edema. *Current Treatment Options in Neurology, 11*(1), 64–73.

Pedersen, E., Arlien-Soborg, P., & Mai, J. (1974). The mode of action of the gaba derivative baclofen in human spasticity. *Acta Neurologica Scandinavica, 50*(6), 665–680.

Rangel-Castilla, L., Gopinath, S., & Robertson, C. S. (2008). Management of intracranial hypertension. *Neurolgic Clinics, 26*(2), 521–541, x. doi: 10.1016/j.ncl.2008.02.003

Scheidtmann, K., Fries, W., Muller, F., & Koenig, E. (2001). Effect of levodopa in combination with physiotherapy on functional motor recovery after stroke: A prospective, randomised, double-blind study. *Lancet, 358*(9284), 787–790. doi: 10.1016/S0140-6736(01)05966-9

Seniow, J., Litwin, M., Litwin, T., Lesniak, M., & Czlonkowska, A. (2009). New approach to the rehabilitation of post-stroke focal cognitive syndrome: Effect of levodopa combined with speech and language therapy on functional recovery from aphasia. *Journal of the Neurological Sciences, 283*(1–2), 214–218. doi: 10.1016/j.jns.2009.02.336

Serebruany, V. L., Steinhubl, S. R., Berger, P. B., Malinin, A. I., Bhatt, D. L., & Topol, E. J. (2005). Variability in platelet responsiveness to clopidogrel among 544 individuals. *Journal of the American College of Cardiology, 45*(2), 246–251. doi: 10.1016/j.jacc.2004.09.067

Siller-Matula, J. M., Krumphuber, J., & Jilma, B. (2010). Pharmacokinetic, pharmacodynamic and clinical profile of novel antiplatelet drugs targeting vascular diseases. *British Journal of Pharmacology, 159*(3), 502–517. doi: 10.1111/j.1476-5381.2009.00555.x

Sonde, L., & Lokk, J. (2007). Effects of amphetamine and/or L-dopa and physiotherapy after stroke: A blinded randomized study. *Acta Neurologica Scandinavica, 115*(1), 55–59. doi: 10.1111/j.1600-0404.2006.00728.x

Stone, N. J., Robinson, J., Lichtenstein, A. H., Bairey Merz, C. N., Lloyd-Jones, D. M., Blum, C. B., . . . Wilson, P. W. (2013). 2013 ACC/AHA guideline on the treatment of blood cholesterol to reduce atherosclerotic cardiovascular risk in adults: A report of the American College of Cardiology/American Heart Association Task Force on Practice Guidelines. Advance online publication. *Journal of the American College of Cardiology.* doi: 10.1016/j.jacc.2013.11.002

Tamminga, C. A. (2003). The science of antipsychotics: mechanistic insight. *CNS Spectrums, 8*(11 Suppl 2), 5-9.

Teasell, R., Foley, N., Salter, K., Bhogal, S., Jutai, J., & Speechley, M. (2009). Evidence-based review of stroke rehabilitation: Executive summary, 12th edition. *Topics in Stroke Rehabilitation, 16*(6), 463–488. doi: 10.1310/tsr1606-463

The Medical Letter. (2013). Drugs for psychiatric disorders. *Treatment Guidelines, 130*(53), 53–64.

Van de Werf, F., Brueckmann, M., Connolly, S. J., Friedman, J., Granger, C. B., Hartter, S., . . . Eikelboom, J. W. (2012). A comparison of dabigatran etexilate with warfarin in patients with mechanical heart valves: The randomized, phase II study to evaluate the safety and pharmacokinetics of oral dabigatran etexilate in patients after heart valve replacement (RE-ALIGN). *American Heart Journal, 163*(6), 931–937 e931. doi: 10.1016/j.ahj.2012.03.011

Verro, P., Gorelick, P. B., & Nguyen, D. (2008). Aspirin plus dipyridamole versus aspirin for prevention of vascular events after stroke or TIA: A meta-analysis. *Stroke, 39*(4), 1358–1363. doi: 10.1161/STROKEAHA.107.496281

Wang, S., Linkletter, C., Dore, D., Mor, V., Buka, S., & Maclure, M. (2012). Age, antipsychotics, and the risk of ischemic stroke in the Veterans Health Administration. *Stroke, 43*(1), 28–31. doi: 10.1161/STROKEAHA.111.617191

Wang, Y., Wang, Y., Zhao, X., Liu, L., Wang, D., Wang, C., . . . CHANCE Investigators. (2013). Clopidogrel with aspirin in acute minor stroke or transient ischemic attack. [Multicenter Study Randomized Controlled Trial Research Support, Non-U.S. Gov't]. *New England Journal of Medicine, 369*(1), 11–19. doi: 10.1056/NEJMoa1215340

Wiviott, S. D., & Cannon, C. P. (2006). Update on lipid-lowering therapy and LDL-cholesterol targets. *Nature Clinical Practice Cardiovascular Medicine, 3*(8), 424–436. doi: 10.1038/ncpcardio0613

Yu, A., Teitelbaum, J., Scott, J., Gesin, G., Russell, B., Huynh, T., & Skrobik, Y. (2013). Evaluating pain, sedation, and delirium in the neurologically critically ill-feasibility and reliability of standardized tools: A multi-institutional study. *Critical Care Medicine, 41*(8), 2002–2007. doi: 10.1097/CCM.0b013e31828e96c0

Zorowitz, R. D., Smout, R. J., Gassaway, J. A., & Horn, S. D. (2005). Neurostimulant medication usage during stroke rehabilitation: the Post-Stroke Rehabilitation Outcomes Project (PSROP). *Topics in Stroke Rehabilitation, 12*(4), 28–36. doi: 10.1310/2403-B0CY-1UDN-4B6D

Chapter

7

Postacute Care

Patricia Garvin Higgins, MN RN CNS CRRN

Stroke is the leading cause of serious long-term disability in both the United States and in many regions across the globe (National Institute of Neurological Disorders and Stroke [NINDS], n.d.; National Stroke Association [NSA], n.d.; Roger et al., 2012). Although early action in the treatment of stroke is paramount, lifelong rehabilitation and recovery is essential for the achievement of optimal functional outcomes. Many patients who have had a stroke require the services of an interprofessional healthcare team to guide and assist them through the trajectory of care so that prevention and wellness are adopted in an effort toward maintaining an improved quality of life.

Patients who have had a stroke may face myriad lifestyle changes, from very minor issues to significant functional deficits. Rehabilitation and the restoration of function need to be addressed as soon as possible after a patient is admitted to the hospital following a stroke. The rehabilitative philosophy of care should permeate the continuum of care to best prevent secondary complications and improve the patient's quality of life.

The nurse dedicated to the care of the stroke patient must have an adequate understanding of rehabilitation and restorative concepts and the resources that exist to help the patient and his or her family transition to the next level of care, with the utmost goal being the patient's return to his or her home and community as a productive member of society.

Objectives

1. State a working definition of rehabilitation and restorative care concepts.
2. List the typical levels of postacute rehabilitative/restorative care settings that may be available to the person who has had a stroke.
3. Describe the roles of the interprofessional or interdisciplinary rehabilitation care team members.
4. List techniques that rehabilitative and restorative care team members employ to minimize functional deficits.
5. Describe the importance of developing a lifelong plan of care to optimize functional return for the person who has had a stroke.
6. Discuss the latest innovative techniques that are employed in the continued quest for improved stroke care in postacute settings.

Introduction to Rehabilitation and Restorative Care Concepts

A. Definitions and key concepts

1. Rehabilitation is a philosophy of practice and an attitude toward caring for people with disabilities and chronic health conditions. It is practiced across the continuum of patient care (Jacelon, 2011).
2. Rehabilitation comes from the Latin word *habilitas*, meaning to make able or to make fit again.
3. The practice of rehabilitation is designed to achieve the restoration of an individual to the highest practicable functional level that is realistically possible.
4. Emphasis is placed on teaching the person to be self-sufficient and to adopt prevention and wellness as a way of life.
5. The goal of rehabilitation is to restore function and reduce dependency on others. It emphasizes the positive and minimizes the negative. Rehabilitation emphasizes the person's abilities and minimizes any disability.
6. Rehabilitation focuses on specialized skills and retraining patients to help them cope with the effects of an injury or insult (e.g., stroke). It usually involves many members of an interprofessional or interdisciplinary team for the coordination of care.
7. An interprofessional healthcare team involves the continuous collaboration of two or more professionals or disciplines, organized into a common effort, to solve or explore common issues with the best possible participation of the patient and family. It uses patient- and family-centered care (PFCC) concepts and allows for more patient autonomy. The PFCC approach is grounded in mutually beneficial partnerships among healthcare providers, patients, and families. It redefines relationships in health care (Institute for Patient- and Family-Centered Care, n.d.).
8. An interdisciplinary care team is defined as a group of rehabilitation professionals from diverse fields organized to complete a task together toward a common goal for the patient (Treiger & Fink-Samnick, 2013). Ideally, the interdisciplinary team practices within an interprofessional healthcare team model.
9. Interdisciplinary team care focuses on patient needs, ensuring that the health services provided are relevant to the patient and family and based on demographics and community needs.
10. The interdisciplinary team facilitates access to the right service, at the right time, in the right place, and by the right people.
11. The interdisciplinary team works well when individuals respect and learn from one another. Communication and shared decision making are the hallmarks of an effective interdisciplinary team.
12. Although rehabilitative care strives for recovery and restoration to the greatest possible functional level, the concept of restorative care centers on maintaining the patient's optimal level of functioning, achieved through a more intensive rehabilitation program on a longer-term basis. It often is practiced by older adults in long-term care settings and is administered by specially trained restorative nursing assistants under the direction of a licensed nurse.
13. "Rehabilitation nursing practice involves the diagnosis and treatment of human responses of individuals and groups to actual or potential health problems stemming from altered functional ability and altered lifestyle" (Association of Rehabilitation Nurses [ARN], 2008, p. 5).
14. Rehabilitation nursing involves teaching the individual and family that outcomes can be affected—action makes a difference. Self-care is emphasized as much as possible.

15. Rehabilitation nurses work with other members of the interdisciplinary or interprofessional team to improve patients' self-esteem and help them regain their sense of dignity, security, and control over their life.

Levels of Rehabilitative/Restorative Care

A. Acute care setting: Rehabilitation begins soon after the stroke occurs. Patients in this setting need acute medical management; although they are not ready for more intensive rehabilitation therapy, they may be ready to receive therapeutic modalities directed toward increasing endurance and strength. For maximum recovery, these therapies should start within 2 days of the onset of the stroke (NSA, n.d.). The role of the acute care nurse is essential to encouraging patients and families to participate in early rehabilitation care and ensuring they will be ready for a more intensive program, if necessary (Jacelon, 2011).

B. Acute care for elders (ACE) units: This type of unit within a hospital setting provides care to adults who are older than 65 years. These are the patients who may benefit from acute care by a staff specially trained in gerontological rehabilitation care delivery. In these units, daily interdisciplinary rounds often are held, and a holistic approach is fostered with the aim of rapid functional recovery. The role of the ACE unit nurse is to provide gerontological rehabilitation care in a less intense setting than would be offered in an inpatient rehabilitation facility (IRF). An ACE unit is not regulated like a skilled nursing facility (SNF) or IRF but is part of an acute hospital service (Jacelon, 2011).

C. Postacute care settings
   1. Inpatient rehabilitation facility (Jacelon, 2011)
      a. An IRF is the most common type of comprehensive inpatient rehabilitation patient care setting. Approximately 40% of all patients who have had a stroke experience moderate to severe impairments requiring special care. Of these, 10% will require care in a nursing home or other long-term care facility (NSA, 2014).
      b. IRF services may be provided in a general rehabilitation care unit within a hospital through age-specific specialization, by diagnosis (e.g., stroke rehabilitation unit), or in a freestanding rehabilitation center.
      c. Standardized guidelines from the Commission on Accreditation of Rehabilitation Facilities or other models of care are used to treat stroke patients and assist their families.
      d. Patients admitted to an IRF have to meet stringent admission guidelines: The patient must have the tolerance for 3 hours of therapy a day for at least 5 days a week; have a discharge to the community plan in place; and require the services of a specially trained rehabilitation physician and nurse 24 hours a day, 7 days a week. In addition, the patient must require the services of at least two therapeutic modalities (e.g., physical therapy, occupational therapy, speech and language pathology). If a patient only requires one therapy, he or she can receive it in an outpatient setting.
      e. An IRF may be selective regarding which ages and diagnostic categories are considered for admission. The diagnosis of stroke is often the top diagnostic category for admission to an IRF. In addition, most patients admitted to an IRF are older adults; therefore, the nurse working in the IRF setting must be educated in geriatric principles.
      f. Intensive rehabilitation nursing care in an IRF is provided to meet the patient's rehabilitative and functional needs in such areas as bladder and bowel management, medication management, nutritional management, skin management, pain management, pulmonary and cardiovascular management, and safety management.

g. The nurse working on an IRF patient care unit provides care based on the most up-to-date evidence. Texts such as *The Standards and Scope of Rehabilitation Nursing Practice* (ARN, 2008) can be helpful tools for staying abreast of the standards of care.

2. Subacute rehabilitation care facility (Jacelon, 2011)
   a. A lower-cost option for those patients who cannot tolerate the intensity of the therapeutic services offered by a stroke rehabilitation program in an IRF setting, or do not meet the stringent admission guidelines.
   b. A subacute rehabilitation program provides a level of care "needed by a patient who does not require hospital acute care, but who requires more intensive skilled nursing care than is provided to the majority of patients in a skilled nursing facility" (Department of Health Care Services [DHCS], n.d.).
   c. Patients who are admitted to a subacute level of rehabilitation care often are "medically fragile and require special services such as inhalation therapy, tracheotomy care, intravenous tube feeding, and complex wound management care" (DHCS, n.d.).
   d. Patients in a subacute rehabilitation level of care still receive therapies but with less intensity and for a shorter period of time.
3. Skilled nursing facility (Jacelon, 2011)
   a. SNF is another term for a nursing home. Many SNFs also provide rehabilitation services, some as an outpatient service after the patient is discharged to home.
   b. Most patients admitted to an SNF are medically stable but still require the services of a nurse with oversight by a physician and close supervision by at least one registered nurse.
   c. Skilled services that cannot be provided in the home setting (e.g., wound care, intravenous medications, enteral feedings, bladder and bowel management, pulmonary care) may be needed. Some SNFs will provide a higher acuity of care, including ventilator monitoring.
   d. Rehabilitation services from a physical therapist (PT), occupational therapist (OTR), or speech and language pathologist (SLP) still may be needed but often will be provided at a less intense level and typically no more than once a day per modality.
   e. A restorative aide may be assigned in the SNF setting to provide direct restorative care and delegated therapy tasks, including passive and active range of motion exercises, ambulation, special positioning techniques, splint use, assistive feeding device/adaptive equipment use, activities of daily living (ADLs) training, bowel and bladder management, restorative dining, and bladder retraining.
   f. Optimal patient wellness still is the goal in the SNF setting, although research shows higher functional outcomes in an IRF setting.
4. Long-term acute care hospital (Jacelon, 2011)
   a. A *long-term acute care hospital (LTACH)* is defined as an acute care hospital that is focused on those patients who require a stay of more than 25 days. Usually patients requiring this type of care need extended intensive medical and rehabilitative care because they have multiple acute or chronic conditions.
   b. Patients in an LTACH often are too sick to be in a nursing home but not sick enough to be in a traditional hospital setting.
   c. An LTACH also is referred to as a long-term acute care facility.
   d. A stroke patient in an LTACH usually is admitted from a short-term acute care hospital, IRF, or SNF.

   e. An LTACH often is temporary placement until the patient can tolerate a stay in a more traditional nursing home setting or ideally a community setting.
   f. According to the Gerson Lehrman Group, LTACHs started in the 1980s and the number of facilities has grown to nearly 400 nationwide (McDaniel, n.d.).
   g. Medicare usually is the primary payer for LTACH services.
   h. This type of facility often is confused with a subacute rehabilitation facility. An LTACH either may be freestanding or located within another hospital (McDaniel, n.d.). The main difference will be the type and intensity of rehabilitation therapies offered, dependent on what the patient can tolerate. Some LTACHs have separate subacute or rehabilitation rooms or wings.
5. Assisted living center (Assisted Living Federation of America, 2013)
   a. An assisted living center is another postacute care option for a person who has had a stroke and cannot live independently.
   b. A person at an assisted living center is considered a resident and is assigned to their own private room or mini apartment according to availability and the ability to pay. There usually is a tiered system in place, depending on the needs of the resident.
   c. An assisted living center usually is covered by private funds, especially for room and board costs. Some centers accept Medicaid to cover the medical services required by the patient, but each state varies in its coverage of services in this type of setting (Matthews, 2013).
   d. Residents are independent within their rooms but have access to personal care and support services if needed.
   e. Assisted living centers differ from nursing homes in that they don't offer complex medical services.
   f. Most assisted living centers have a nursing staff consisting of one or two registered nurses for the entire facility, along with licensed vocational and practical nurses and nursing assistants.
   g. There are varying levels of nursing care that can be provided to the resident depending on their needs (e.g., medication management; diabetic management; assistance with self-care needs including bathing, grooming, and dressing). A fall alarm also may be used to alert the staff if a patient is at high risk for falls.
   h. Most assisted living centers have a private dining room, television or game room, hair salon, recreation center, and chapel.
   i. Most assisted living centers provide transportation to medical appointments.
   j. Families of residents in an assisted living center usually express relief that their loved one receives a degree of supervision the family might not be able to provide on a consistent basis.
6. Board and care (Hawes et al., 1995)
   a. The most common form of residential setting with services for people with disabilities is a board and care home.
   b. "The term board and care refers to nonmedical community-based residential settings that house two or more unrelated adults and provide some services such as meals, medication supervision or reminders, organized activities, transportation, or help with bathing, dressing, and other ADLs" (Hawes et al., 1995).
   c. Three types of licensed facilities (Clark, Turek-Brezina, Hawes, & Chu, 1994)
      (1) Homes serving patients with mental retardation or developmental disabilities
      (2) Homes serving patients with mental illness

(3) Homes serving a mixed population of physically frail older adults, cognitively impaired older adults, and persons with mental health problems. The majority of homes fall into this last category (Hawes et al., 1995).

d. Board and care facilities offer a good balance between independence and supervised nursing homes and may be the preferred residential setting for those stroke patients who cannot live alone and have the ability to pay for this alternative residential care setting.

e. Most board and care facilities are not covered by insurance, but in some cases a person may be able to use Social Security or veteran's benefits.

7. Day treatment care program (Jacelon, 2011)

   a. Day treatment care programs and adult day services provide supervised and therapeutic activities during daytime hours, rather than 24-hour supervision.

   b. This type of program is ideal for those patients who need a level of supervision a family member cannot provide during the day but that can be provided during evening and nighttime hours.

   c. This program usually is structured and can provide a variety of health, social, and related support services in a protective, safe setting.

   d. Elements of rehabilitative care are provided and the patient's impairments and limitations are taken into consideration when establishing individualized programs.

   e. The aim of the program often is to promote functional improvement and maintain the stroke patient's sense of control and self-determination while providing them a safe environment during the day when there is no one to supervise them (CARF International, n.d.).

   f. Most day treatment programs are federally or state funded, or are paid for with private funding. In some cases, private insurance may provide coverage.

8. Independent living center or senior living apartment (Jacelon, 2011)

   a. Independent living centers offer another postacute setting for those patients who have the ability to live alone but may need some additional resources or to share ADLs with other residents.

   b. Most are congregate facilities or senior living apartment settings including retirement and life-care communities. Independent living also can be set up in the stroke patient's home through an outside agency.

   c. There are usually shared activities that may include meals, community outings, transportation to medical appointments, housekeeping, religious services, and onsite healthcare clinics.

   d. "Health monitoring may or may not be included in this setting" (Jacelon, 2011, p. 510).

   e. Independent living centers are privately funded, although there may be state-funded senior assistance plans available to subsidize monthly rent and other services.

9. Outpatient rehabilitation services

   a. Outpatient therapy services are offered in a community setting such as a clinic, freestanding site, or hospital.

   b. Therapeutic modalities are prescribed by a physician. This prescription must include the type of therapy to be provided, the specific functional deficit to be addressed and treated, and the number of times the therapy is recommended on a daily and weekly basis.

   c. After a comprehensive evaluation is completed, therapies are then provided by a PT, OTR, or SLP. The outpatient care plan is developed with the patient and family with recommendations that are practical and within their ability to perform in the home and community (Jacelon, 2011).

d. For the patient who has had a stroke, outpatient therapy services may be targeted toward such functional deficits as self-care and mobility limitations, swallowing and communication disorders, or balance deficits.
e. Therapy treatment often occurs 3 to 5 times a week for no more than 1 hour and is less intense than what is offered in an IRF.
f. The stroke patient must not be homebound and must have transportation to and from the outpatient therapy center.
g. Services are covered by the patient's insurance provider, with a limitation on the number and duration of therapies to be provided. Services may be extended after the therapist submits a re-evaluation of functional deficits and further treatment needs to the insurance provider.
h. Outpatient services have been shown to prevent more costly hospitalizations and additional functional decline (Jacelon, 2011).

10. Home health care
    a. It is estimated that by 2025, more than 20% of the country's population will be older than 65 years. Couple this with the incidence of stroke and the need for home healthcare service will continue to grow.
    b. A *home healthcare agency* is a licensed community-based service that provides predominantly medically related services to patients in a home setting rather than in a medical facility.
    c. Services will vary according to the home healthcare agency.
    d. Services may include skilled nursing in addition to speech, occupational, and physical therapy.
    e. In many cases, services include assistance with cooking and other household chores.
    f. Nursing services often include monitoring of the patient's prescriptions and for possible medical complications. Other areas may include bladder and bowel management, disease management, skin care management, nutritional management, and pulmonary and cardiovascular management.
    g. Therapy in the home setting is provided at a less intense level than outpatient therapy services and is time limited. However, often it is meaningful for the stroke patient to undergo this treatment at home as he or she begins to navigate his or her home environment and the surrounding community.
    h. A physician's prescription is required to begin home healthcare services and to have specific therapeutic modalities evaluated and treated in the home setting. The conditions or issues for which the licensed nurse will need to monitor or provide care should be indicated by the physician.
    i. For some stroke patients, this is a temporary arrangement until their endurance improves or they are able to be transported to an outpatient facility. It is preferred that patients transition to outpatient therapies at the completion of home healthcare services to sustain functional gains.
    j. Medicare is the largest payer of home healthcare services, although many agencies accept private insurance funding. There are fewer agencies that will accept Medicaid, but this varies between states.

11. Private or personal care attendants
    a. In some cases, a stroke patient or their family may have the financial means to hire a private or personal care attendant (PCA).
    b. These attendants also are commonly known as caregivers, patient care assistants, personal support workers, and home care aides.
    c. This is a paid, employed person who helps persons who are disabled or chronically ill.
    d. A PCA may work for an agency or be hired on a private basis.
    e. Fees for service will vary depending on the individual's agency affiliation or private contract.
    f. Care plans may be established by a rehabilitation health practitioner, social worker, or other healthcare professional.
    g. Procurement of a PCA requires careful investigation on the part of the patient and family to ensure the aide is competent and trustworthy.
    h. A PCA can be valuable in assisting the stroke patient at home with ADLs, mobility, light housekeeping, and transportation.
    i. "The demand for PCA services is expected to rise sharply over the next 3 decades with population aging and rapid increases in the number of persons reaching the oldest age groups that need personal assistance and long-term care" (Organization for Economic Cooperation and Development, 2005).

Understanding Roles Within the Interdisciplinary Team

A. Rehabilitation in any setting includes an interdisciplinary approach, a focus on mutually accepted patient- and family-centered goals and outcomes, the attainment or maintenance of functional capacity, and nurses working on a team of professionals who understand the long-range needs of patients and who work together to ideally move the patient along the continuum of care.

B. A strong team of individuals is essential to the follow-up care of the stroke patient (**Figure 7-1**).

C. Stroke patients often have multiple complex problems along with varying degrees of physical and cognitive deficits. An interprofessional or interdisciplinary team is one of the most efficient ways of capitalizing on the collective knowledge and skills of multiple caregivers to address this complexity.

D. A strong interprofessional or interdisciplinary team pursues excellence in each specialty and recognizes the contribution of all disciplines as part of holistic care.

E. Team strategies may include daily or weekly team rounds or conferences (depending on the setting), a comprehensive patient and family orientation program, informal education at the bedside, peer support, patient and family meetings or conferences, and patient and family education or behavioral management sessions. The team also may meet periodically to discuss further program development and performance improvement measures.

F. The team includes two or more members from the medical team along with the patient and family or caregiver. It always includes a physician and a nurse. Other members vary depending on the complexity of the needed care and the setting.

G. Physical medicine and rehabilitation (PM&R) physicians or physiatrists (Jacelon, 2011; Physiatry and Rehabilitation Services, Inc., n.d.)
    1. The field of PM&R began in the 1930s to address musculoskeletal and neurological problems. Rehabilitation programs initially began in U.S. Veteran's Administration hospitals in the 1940s.

Figure 7-1. Typical Rehabilitation Team Composition

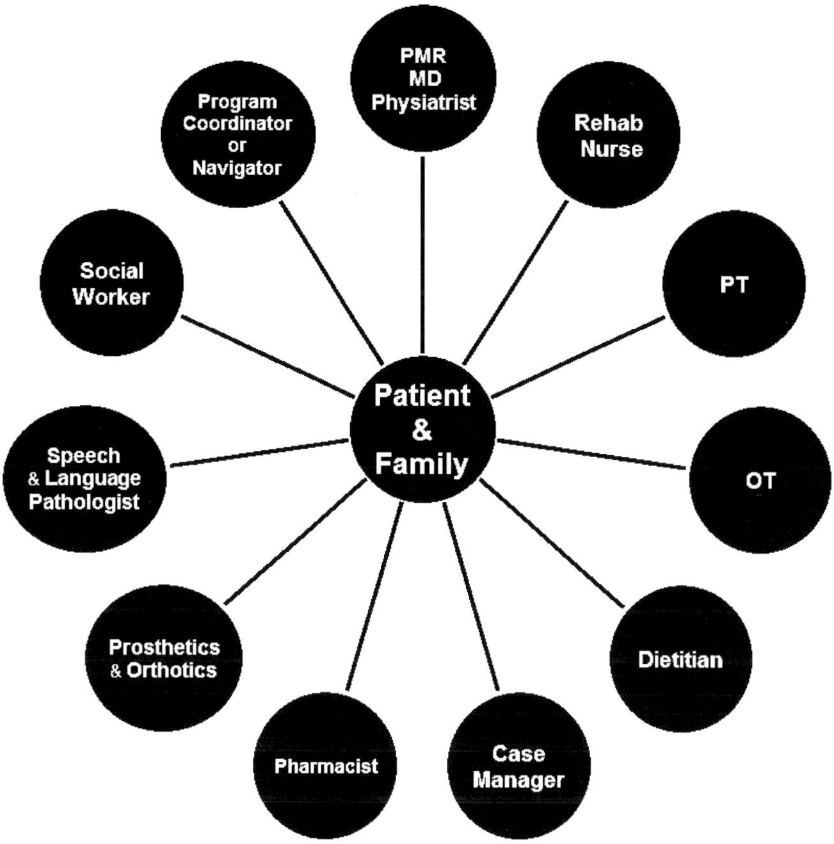

OT indicates occupational therapist; PMR, physical medicine and rehabilitation; PT, physical therapist.

2. "The term physiatrist was coined to describe a physician with specialized training in rehabilitation medicine" (Jacelon, 2011, p. 18). Most comprehensive rehabilitation centers employ at least one physiatrist. Many settings also assign an internal medicine physician to assist in the monitoring of medical comorbidities, unless the patient already has an assigned primary physician. Care of the stroke patient also may include other medical consultants, as needed.
3. PM&R physicians or physiatrists are board certified in PM&R, and many physiatrists have additional certifications in related specialties such as pain management or sports medicine.
4. The specialty of physiatry serves all age groups and treats problems that touch upon all of the major systems in the body. "As the population of America ages, as people survive conditions that once would have been fatal, and as quality of life is an increasing concern, the field of physiatry is moving to the forefront of medicine" (Physiatry and Rehabilitation Services, Inc., n.d.).
5. Settings that have a more acute or long-term care philosophy may not have a physiatrist on staff. In these cases, a primary physician may directly follow the patient, or there may be one physician assigned to oversee the medical management of all residents.
6. The physician is the medical leader of the interprofessional or interdisciplinary team.

H. Rehabilitation nurse (Jacelon, 2011)

1. The concept of rehabilitation nursing has been around since Florence Nightingale, who felt that nurses have a powerful influence on the lives of others. Her important work led to the philosophy of rehabilitation nursing care and how we as nurses "help individuals affected by chronic and disabling conditions, such as a stroke, adapt to disabilities, achieve their potential, and work toward productive and independent lives" (Jacelon, 2011, p.15).
2. The first formal nursing programs for rehabilitation nursing began in the 1950s; the first rehabilitation textbook, *Rehabilitation Nursing* by Alice Morrissey, also came out at this time (Jacelon, 2011). This comprehensive text emphasized that rehabilitation nursing include basic bedside nursing with "an emphasis on the importance of nutrition and activities of daily living" (Jacelon, 2011, p.18). The patient's future was emphasized and care plans addressing this were developed.
3. Over the years, rehabilitation nursing has developed into a specialty. In 1974, the Association of Rehabilitation Nurses (ARN) was formed and developed *The Standards and Scope of Rehabilitation Nursing Practice*. By 1984, ARN "developed a formal definition, philosophy, and conceptual framework of rehabilitation nursing and the association" (Jacelon, 2011, p.20). A certification exam for rehabilitation nurses was developed that same year, and now there are more than 12,000 rehabilitation nurses who hold the Certified Rehabilitation Registered Nurse (CRRN) certification (ARN, 2013a). ARN also publishes a specialty practice core curriculum, *The Specialty Practice of Rehabilitation Nursing*, which is currently in its sixth edition (Jacelon, 2011). This comprehensive text addresses all components of the practice of rehabilitation nursing across the continuum of care.
4. The value of rehabilitation nursing practice and related care concepts continues to be at the forefront of nursing practice as patient acuity increases, changing the basic scope of practice (Jacelon, 2011).
5. The rehabilitation nurse plays a key role on the interprofessional or interdisciplinary rehabilitation team and is in a position to provide nursing leadership and management to the team.
6. "The rehabilitation nurse, easily accessible to individuals, families, team members, and other concerned parties, and by virtue of specialized education, expertise, and interest in caring for individuals with chronic illness and disabilities, is considered the most qualified team leader and a key partner in a successful rehabilitation program" (ARN, 2013b).
7. Major roles of the rehabilitation nurse include, first and foremost, those of caregiver and expert practitioner. Other roles include teacher, coordinator of care, collaborator or liaison, counselor, case manager, and researcher.
8. The rehabilitation nurse will work with the stroke patient and his or her family to establish mutually accepted long- and short-term goals in the development of a comprehensive plan of care and provide a patient education program to assist the patient in transitioning to the next level of care or in sustaining function. This plan of care will be dependent on the setting and type of nursing service that is available to the patient.
9. Major roles of the rehabilitation nurse are illustrated in **Table 7-1** (Mauk, 2007).
10. The rehabilitation nursing team is always under the direction of the registered nurse and may include licensed vocational or practical nurses, certified nursing assistants, and patient care assistants.

Table 7-1. Nurse's Role on the Rehabilitation Team

- Provide holistic, well-rounded care to the client and caregiver.
- Establish collaborative goals with the rehabilitation team and implement interventions that result in the best possible outcome to meet the needs of the client and caregiver.
- Maintain a strong commitment to the rehabilitation team.
- Participate in the rehabilitation team process at team conferences and other team meetings, and offer input into team decision making.
- Communicate effectively and interact in a manner that facilitates the group process and team building.
- Reinforce the care provided by other team members.
- Coordinate team activities.
- Evaluate the effectiveness of the treatment plan on an ongoing basis.
- Advocate for the client and caregiver.
- Act as a resource to the rehabilitation team by possessing the specialized knowledge and clinical skills necessary to provide care for people with physical disabilities and chronic illness.
- Teach rehabilitation team members and reinforce the teaching done by specialists in rehabilitation and other healthcare disciplines.

Adapted from The Specialty Practice of Rehabilitation Nursing: A Core Curriculum *(5th ed.), by K. Mauk, 2007, Glenview, IL: Association of Rehabilitation Nurses. © 2007 by the Association of Rehabilitation Nurses. Adapted with permission.*

I. PT or physiotherapist
  1. "Physical therapists help people who have injuries or illnesses improve their movement and manage their pain. They are often an important part of rehabilitation and treatment of patients with chronic conditions or injuries" (U.S. Bureau of Labor Statistics, 2014a).
  2. The PT helps the patient who has had a stroke with his or her mobility and ability to navigate the surrounding environment. The PT works in collaboration with the rest of the interdisciplinary team.
  3. The PT is a licensed healthcare practitioner who often holds a doctorate degree and who can be employed in a variety of settings, including private offices and clinics, hospitals, and nursing homes (U.S. Bureau of Labor Statistics, 2014a).
     a. Although many work in hospitals, approximately 80% of PTs work in other settings, such as outpatient clinics or offices, IRFs, home healthcare agencies, SNFs, LTACHs, subacute facilities, private homes, education or research centers, schools, hospices, industrial/workplace/other occupational environments, and fitness centers or sports training facilities (American Physical Therapy Association [APTA], 2013).
  4. "Physical therapists have the opportunity to become certified as clinical specialists through the American Board of Physical Therapy" (APTA, 2013).
  5. The PT is an integral member of the interprofessional or interdisciplinary team and an expert in movement and movement disorders. The PT assists patients who have suffered a stroke recover, maintain, or improve their physical function.
  6. A PT seeks to identify and maximize quality of life and movement potential through prevention, intervention (treatment), promotion, habilitation, and rehabilitation (Nordqvist, 2009).
  7. A qualified PT is an expert in the examination and treatment of people with cardiothoracic, musculoskeletal, and neuromuscular diseases who focuses on conditions and problems that undermine the patient's ability to move and function effectively (Nordqvist, 2009).
  8. PTs teach patients how to prevent or manage their conditions so they will achieve long-term health benefits (APTA, 2013).

J. Physical therapy assistant (PTA)
   1. PTAs provide physical therapy services under the direction and supervision of a licensed PT (APTA, 2013).
   2. The PTA can assist the patient who has had a stroke by providing teaching exercises to improve mobility, strength, and coordination; training for activities such as walking with crutches, canes, or walkers; massages; and physical agents and electrotherapy such as ultrasound and electrical stimulation (APTA, 2013).
   3. Most states require a PTA to be licensed, registered, or certified. To work as a PTA, an individual must graduate with an associate degree from an accredited PTA program and then pass a nationally administered examination (APTA, 2013).

K. Occupational therapist (OTR)
   1. OTRs are registered and licensed healthcare practitioners who are integral members of the rehabilitation and postacute care teams. They work in collaboration with the rest of the interdisciplinary team.
   2. OTRs typically have a master's degree in occupational therapy. All states require OTRs to be licensed (U.S. Bureau of Labor Statistics, 2014b).
   3. The OTR can provide "comprehensive evaluations of the client's home and other environments (e.g., workplace, school), recommendations for adaptive equipment and training in its use, and guidance and education for family members and caregivers." See more at http://www.aota.org/about-occupational-therapy.aspx. (American Occupational Therapy Association, Inc. [AOTA], 2013).
   4. "Occupational therapy practitioners address the physical, cognitive, and emotional challenges brought on by a stroke, and they can help stroke survivors engage in the things they want and need to do" (AOTA, 2013).
   5. "Occupational therapists instruct patients on techniques and equipment that can make daily living and working easier" (U.S. Bureau of Labor Statistics, 2014b).
   6. Occupational therapists work on self-care with the stroke patient (**Table 7-2**).

L. Occupational therapy assistant or aide (OTA), certified occupational therapy assistant (COTA; U.S. Bureau of Labor Statistics, 2014b)
   1. The OTA or COTA works under the direction of the registered OTR.
   2. This valuable member of the team assists the OTR in treating patients with injuries, illnesses, or disabilities through the therapeutic use of everyday activities.
   3. The OTA or COTA helps stroke patients develop, recover, and improve the skills needed for daily living and working.
   4. This position requires an associate degree from an accredited occupational therapy assistant program. In most states, OTAs must be licensed (U.S. Bureau of Labor Statistics, 2014b).

M. SLP (U.S. Bureau of Labor Statistics, 2014c; American Speech-Language-Hearing Association [ASHA], 2014)
   1. An SLP (commonly referred to as a speech therapist) evaluates, diagnoses, and treats communicative, hearing, cognitive, and swallowing disorders in patients.
   2. An SLP often works in a hospital but also may work in a school or in the patient's home.
   3. The SLP is an integral member of the interprofessional or interdisciplinary team in the care of stroke patients. He or she works in collaboration with the rest of the interdisciplinary team, which may include teachers, physicians, audiologists, psychologists, social workers, rehabilitation counselors, and others.

Table 7-2. Occupational Therapist's Role

- Observe the stroke patient doing tasks, ask the patient questions, and review the patient's medical history.
- Use observations, answers, and medical history to evaluate the patient's condition and needs.
- Establish a treatment plan for the patient that details the types of activities to be done and specific goals to be accomplished.
- Help people with various disabilities with different tasks, such as helping an older person with poor memory use a computer.
- Demonstrate exercises that can help relieve pain, such as joint stretches, for people with chronic conditions.
- Evaluate a patient's home or workplace and identify how it can be better suited to the patient's health needs.
- Educate a patient's family and employer about how to accommodate and care for the patient.
- Recommend special equipment, such as wheelchairs and eating aids, and instruct patients how to use that equipment.
- Assess and record patients' activities and progress for evaluating clients, billing, and reporting to physicians and other healthcare providers.

Adapted from "Tips for Patients and Caregivers," by the American Occupational Therapy Association, Inc., 2014, www.aota.org/-/media/Corporate/Files/AboutOT/consumers/Adults/Stroke/Stroke%20Tip%20Sheet.pdf. © 2014 by the American Occupational Therapy Association. Adapted with permission.

4. Specific areas that the SLP may work on with stroke patients include articulation (pronunciation of words), fluency (stuttering), voice, receptive language (comprehension), expressive language, pragmatic language (social skills), oral motor skills, and swallowing.
5. SLPs typically must have a master's degree. They must be licensed in most states, although requirements vary by state (U.S. Bureau of Labor Statistics, 2014c).

N. Medical social worker or licensed clinical social worker (U.S. Bureau of Labor Statistics, 2014d; National Association of Social Workers, n.d.)

1. A social worker can be a direct-service social worker, who helps people solve and cope with problems in their everyday lives, or a clinical social worker, who diagnoses and treats mental, behavioral, and emotional issues.
2. The medical social worker (MSW) or licensed clinical social worker (LCSW) is an integral part of the interprofessional or interdisciplinary team in the care of stroke patients.
3. The MSW or LCSW uses social theories to understand human problems, help improve people's lives, and improve society as a whole.
4. The MSW or LCSW acts as an advocate for patients and their family. This includes providing education to teach them new skills and linking them to essential community resources.
5. The MSW or LCSW provides counseling to the patient who has suffered a stroke and provides support and assistance. The social worker helps the patient and family remedy any social issues and develop solutions to problems.
6. The MSW or LCSW can work in a variety of settings, including mental health clinics, schools, hospitals, and private practices.
7. "A bachelor's degree is required for most direct-service social work positions, but some positions and settings require a master's degree. Clinical social workers must have a master's degree. Licensure for social workers varies by state. Clinical social workers must be licensed" (U.S. Bureau of Labor Statistics, 2014d).

O. Rehabilitation nurse case manager (ARN, 2013b)
   1. The rehabilitation case manager is an integral part of the interprofessional or interdisciplinary team for the care of stroke patients.
   2. Case management is defined as "the process of assessing, planning, organizing, coordinating, implementing, monitoring, and evaluating the services and resources needed to respond to an individual's healthcare needs" (ARN, 2013b).
   3. The rehabilitation case manager practices in a variety of settings including hospitals; governmental or private agencies; and insurance-based agencies, whereby the individual is employed by a third-party payer (e.g., an insurance company), and in a variety of roles, including as an employer-based case manager, an independent case manager, a private case manager, or as a life care planner (ARN, 2013b).
   4. "The goal of case management is the provision of quality and cost-effective health and social care services. The rehabilitation nurse case manager realizes this goal by organizing rehabilitation and other necessary healthcare services to promote outcomes for the individual that will encourage the highest possible level of independence and quality of life" (ARN, 2013b).
   5. Effective rehabilitation case management is dependent on several key components of nursing practice. All team members contribute to this practice, however, the rehabilitation nurse serves in a specialized, unique role to provide this essential service (**Table 7-3**).
   6. Qualifications for a registered nurse who performs the rehabilitation case manager role include licensure as a registered nurse, preferably with a bachelor's degree in nursing (BSN) from an accredited school, or equivalent work experience, which ideally includes a minimum of 2 years of related clinical experience and experience in the rehabilitation of chronically or catastrophically ill or injured individuals. Certification as a CRRN is preferable.

P. Rehabilitation psychologist or neuropsychologist (Psychology Education Association, 2013; U.S. Bureau of Labor Statistics, 2014e)
   1. The psychologist is an integral part of the interprofessional or interdisciplinary team for the care of stroke patients.
   2. Rehabilitation psychologists evaluate and assist patients who have had a stroke and may be struggling with cognitive issues, chronic health conditions, emotional problems, or psychosocial problems.
   3. A rehabilitation psychologist holds a doctorate degree in psychology with additional clinical training in the care of patients with disabilities. A neuropsychologist has the same credentials but with additional clinical training in the care of patients with a neurological disorder. The latter is preferred in the comprehensive care of the stroke patient.
   4. After counseling interventions or assessments, rehabilitation psychologists also may assist patients with adapting to new situations, locating a support network, locating assistance and support services, and learning how to use technology to promote independent living.

Table 7-3. Essential Role Components of Rehabilitation Case Management for the Stroke Patient

Data Collection and Assessment	• Obtainment of necessary authorizations • Review and analysis of referral information • Review and assessment of patient's personal and medical history • Review of current status and development of treatment plan • Assessment of patient's learning needs related to diagnosis and prognosis • Contact treatment providers and review treatment plan • Assessment of family's knowledge base, health status, and expectations, and identification of a primary caregiver, if necessary
Data Analysis and Formulation of Nursing Diagnosis	• Identification of any temporary or permanent altercations in function • Identification of potential challenges or complications of physiological or psychosocial function • Identification of potential difficulties in community reintegration, where appropriate • Identification of learning needs of the patient and significant others • Consideration of vocational history prognosis for entering or re-entering the workforce
Establishment of Goals and Plan of Care	• Establishment of realistic goals to achieve optimal outcomes for the individual, done in collaboration with team members and available resources • Assistance to the individual, family, and team in identifying the variables that may influence the accomplishment of goals • Development of a comprehensive plan that includes short- and long-term goals and preventive treatment measures • Identification of alternatives for the individual's treatment when appropriate • Establishment of target dates for achievement of goals
Implementation of Plan of Care	• Use of rehabilitation principles to promote optimal outcomes for the individual • Ongoing assessment of the individual, family, and caregiver • Coordination of access to accelerated or alternative care options, when appropriate • Coordination of access to appropriate government and community programs and resources • Coordination and evaluation in a quality conscious, cost-effective manner of the individual's and family's use of medical equipment, supplies, medications, and the full spectrum of services; provision of instruction to the individual and family based on identified learning needs • Coordination of referrals for instruction or counseling as is agreeable to the individual and family, based on identified learning needs • Provision of education, guidance, and recommendations to the referral source regarding alternatives for care and services when appropriate • Prompt intervention to promote optimal functioning and prevent complications, when necessary • Facilitation and collaboration with the healthcare team for timely discharge planning to an alternative level of care or return to the individual's community when appropriate; and, coordination of the discharge plan with the healthcare team and providers
Collaboration	• Work with the healthcare team, payers, community agencies, providers, and legal representatives to ensure continuity of the individual's care through all healthcare settings • Promotion of effective communication among healthcare team members, including the individual, family, and payers and employer when appropriate • Participation in team meetings when indicated, incorporation of the recommendations and suggested services of the interprofessional team members into the plan of care, and communication with other case managers along the continuum of care for the coordination of the needs of the individual if case management involvement is limited by setting

continued

Table 7-3. Essential Role Components of Rehabilitation Case Management for the Stroke Patient continued

Documentation	• Provision of routine verbal and written documentation of the initial assessment and progress of the individual to the referral source or appropriate others on a timely, regular basis • Projection of costs and needs for the future and provision of cost analyses to the referral source as appropriate • Provision of a written summary of educational information for the individual, family, or referral source as appropriate.
Community Reintegration	• Assistance to the individual and family in anticipating needs and making plans for reentry to the home or an alternative living site • Recommendations for and coordination of home assessment services before discharge and reassessment after discharge, if necessary • Assistance with the selection of and arrangement for quality-conscious, cost-effective home care, equipment, and services • Monitoring of services for appropriate length and quality of service whether the patient will return home or transition to a different level of care • Arrangement for assessment of the setting as well as for reasonable adaptation of the site to meet the individual's needs • Assistance to the patient and family in anticipating needs and making plans for reentry into the community environment • Arrangement for special assessment by educational or vocational counselors when indicated • Assistance to the patient and family in planning for reentry to the school or work environment through collaboration with a vocational counselor (as appropriate) and through contact with the school system or employer representatives • Assistance to the patient and family with the identification of community activities and resources or volunteer placement when appropriate • Ensure funding is available for services through the referral source or other resources.
Evaluation	• Performance of periodic reassessments of the individual's and significant others' responses and progress toward treatment goals • Facilitation of and participation in conferences that provide ongoing evaluation of interprofessional dynamics, goal attainment, and treatment plan revisions • Facilitation of case closure based on the individual's response, progress toward treatment goals, and established criteria of the employing facility or agency, or at the request of the third-party payer, if appropriate • Determination of a final cost/benefit analysis for the agency or referral source at the close of the case.
Quality Assurance	• Provision for an evaluation of case management services • Incorporation of evaluative data in the provision of ongoing case management services • Adherence to established standards of practice as identified by ARN, American Nurses Association (ANA), and Case Management Society of American • Provision of case management services in accordance with ANA's Code of Ethics for Nurses.

Adapted from "Role Descriptions: The Rehabilitation Case Manager," by the Association of Rehabilitation Nurses, 2013, www.rehabnurse.org/pubs/role/Role-Rehab-Nurse-Case-Manager.html. © 2013 by the Association of Rehabilitation Nurses. Adapted with permission.

Rehabilitative Plan of Care

A. A comprehensive functional assessment is completed by every team member, including the nurse, and these assessments are incorporated into the stroke patient's plan of care.

B. Basic guidelines include the treatment of the underlying disease or disorder, prevention of secondary disability or illness, and treatment of the primary disability.

C. The rehabilitation system approach aims to restore function through reduction, substitution, and adaptation, and this is incorporated into the stroke patient's plan of care.

D. The rehabilitative plan of care must

  a. Include realistic goals that are mutually established between the patient and family and treating team member

  b. Emphasize functional independence for the stroke patient to enhance any residual function

  c. Take into consideration the attitudes of the patient and family, financial resources, environmental barriers, vocational barriers, and community resources

  d. Provide for adaptive tools to help the stroke patient alter their environment to promote the attainment of functional goals and recovery

  e. Recognize the various motivational and psychological factors of both the patient and family.

I. The specific areas of importance for the rehabilitation nurse in patient assessment, data collection, and care plan development are many and varied (**Table 7-4**).

Table 7-4. Areas of Importance for Rehabilitation Patient Assessment and Data Collection for Development of the Rehabilitation Patient Care Plan

• Physiological • Psychological • Cognitive • Behavioral • Social/Cultural • Family structure and dynamics	• Communicative ability • Educational background • Vocational status • Ability to perform activities of daily living • Functional ability

J. Specific areas of functional assessment and treatment in a post-acute setting involve evaluations by assigned team members and may include assessments of

1. Mobility
2. Self-care
3. Communication
4. Bladder and bowel management
5. Skin care management
6. Nutritional management
7. Pain management
8. Medication management
9. Management of medical issues
10. Safety awareness
11. Sexuality

K. Measuring function includes the assessment of all activities from basic care performance to community reintegration. Interventions then can be targeted to treatments and outcome measures at the level of impairment, limitations, and disability (Nagi, 1965).

L. Disablement models

1. The World Health Organization (WHO) first recognized Saad Nagi's work in the development of a disablement model in 1980. It described the care plan process for the person with a disability by first looking at the pathology and disease level (e.g., cerebral hemorrhage). Next, this model looked at how the person was affected at the organ level (e.g., right-sided hemiplegia). The model then went on to describe the resulting disability to identify how it may affect the patient at the personal level (e.g., difficulty with ADLs, mobility, communication). Finally, the model looked at how disablement might handicap the person in the community or society (e.g. affects return to work or school).
2. The WHO adopted the more widely used International Classification of Functioning, Disability, and Health (ICF) Scale in 2001 to further describe how a comprehensive functional rehabilitation care plan for the person with a disability (e.g., hemiplegia, aphasia, dysphagia) after suffering a severe stroke) is developed and designed.
3. The ICF Scale is divided into four distinct levels:
   a. Impairment—includes information about the functioning of basic body parts or organs
   b. Activity—includes information about the capacity of the person to do basic and complex actions
   c. Participation—includes information about the extent of the person's participation in society
   d. Environment—includes information about the impact of a person's environment
4. The ICF Scale is the preferred disablement model to guide members of the interprofessional or interdisciplinary team when developing a comprehensive rehabilitation plan of care because it incorporates concepts from the patient- and family-centered care approach and provides a biopsychosocial view of the health of the person with disabilities.
5. The ICF Scale has two parts, each with two components (**Table 7-5**). Part 1 assesses functioning and disability (body functions and structure, activities and participation), and part 2 assesses contextual factors (environmental and personal factors.

Table 7-5. Patient- and Family-Centered Care of the Stroke Patient Using the International Classification of Functioning, Disability, and Health Scale

Long-term goals as stated in own words by patient/family: "To get back to the way I was, to use my hands again and ride a bike."	**Patient perspective:** • Activity/participation— "I cannot button my shirt." • Body function/structure—"My left hand is very weak."
Environmental assessment: Patient resides in a second floor apartment with no elevator and a tub/shower; his mother lives in a single-story house.	**Clinical perspective:** • Activity/participation/resources—motivated; positive attitude; transfers • Activity/participation limitations—activities of daily living performance • Body function/structure/resources—coordination; balance; RUE and RLE motor control • Body function/structure/limitations—LUE and LLE motor control with loss of sensation

LLE indicates lower extremity; LUE, left upper extremity; RLE, right lower extremity; RUE, right upper extremity.

M. Functional assessment tools

1. The functional assessment tool that is chosen must be descriptive, evaluative, and predictive.
2. The functional assessment tool that is chosen must be practical, simple to administer, and yield meaningful results.
3. The functional assessment tool should measure disability, monitor progress, enhance communications, measure the effectiveness of treatment, and document the benefits of rehabilitation interventions.
4. Functional Independence Measure™ (FIM) measurement tool (Centers for Medicare & Medicaid Services [CMS], 2012a)
   a. The most widely used functional assessment tool in an IRF is the FIM. This functional independence measurement tool consists of 18 items that aim to measure self-care, bowel and bladder control, mobility, cognition, and communication. It is designed to be non-discipline specific so that any trained or certified team member can complete any line item. The FIM measures the burden of care and is very useful in the development of a comprehensive plan of care for the stroke patient who requires an inpatient rehabilitation program.
   b. FIM scoring must be accurate and must be reflected in the rehabilitation nurse's documentation of the patient's activities 24 hours a day, 7 days a week as part of justification for an inpatient rehabilitation stay. However, all team members contribute to the FIM scoring assessment and it is used as a guide for planning care and projecting an estimated length of stay in the IRF.
5. Inpatient Rehabilitation Facility Patient Assessment Instrument (IRF-PAI) (Jacelon, 2011)
   a. This is the data collection tool used in an IRF that is required by CMS for all Medicare Part A patients.
   b. The IRF-PAI has an FIM instrument as a component for further data collection and submission. It is completed upon admission and discharge. The admission rating determines a case mix group (CMG) level for projected payment and estimated length of stay targets. The CMG takes into consideration the patient's age, diagnosis, functional impairment, FIM levels, and comorbidities for the final CMG determination.
   c. In an IRF, there is usually a staff member responsible for the prospective payment system data collection and submission, along with careful oversight for compliance with all CMS guidelines.
6. CMS Minimum Data Set (MDS) (RTI International, 2013)
   a. "The MDS is a tool for implementing standardized assessment and for facilitating care management in nursing homes and non-critical access hospital swing beds" (The National Long Term Care Ombudsman Resource Center, 2013).
   b. The MDS "focuses on clinical assessment of nursing home residents to screen for common, often unrecognized or unevaluated, conditions and syndromes" (RTI International, 2013).
   c. The nursing home quality measures come from resident assessment data that nursing homes routinely collect on the residents at specified intervals during their stay. The assessment data is converted to develop quality measures that give consumers another source of information to show how well nursing homes are caring for their residents' physical and clinical needs. In turn, these quality measures are posted publicly for all consumers to evaluate (CMS, 2013).

7. Outcome and Assessment Information Set (OASIS; CMS, 2012b)
   a. This is a data set assessment used by home healthcare agencies.
   b. "The OASIS is a group of data elements that represents core items of a comprehensive assessment for an adult home care patient; and forms the basis for measuring patient outcomes for purposes of outcome-based quality improvement" (CMS, 2012b).
   c. The OASIS must be completed for all Medicare recipients of home healthcare services.
   d. "The OASIS is a key component of Medicare's partnership with the home care industry to foster and monitor improved home healthcare outcomes" (CMS, 2012b).
   e. The OASIS is a system of outcome measures for home health care and most OASIS items describe patient health and functional status.
8. Other functional measurement tools used in the postacute phase of stroke rehabilitation care (Jacelon, 2011)
   a. Other examples of ADL measurement scales
      (1) The Barthel Index uses a 0–100 scoring schema (from total independence to dependence) that assesses 10 self-care domains. The higher the score, the more dependent the patient.
         (a) The Barthel Index is more popular in European rehabilitation centers and is one of the oldest measures of ADL function.
      (2) The Kenny Self-Care Evaluation examines six domains: transfers, bed activity, personal hygiene, dressing, and locomotion. It uses a five-level scale from 0–4; the lower the score, the more dependent the patient.
      (3) The Katz Index of Independence in Activities of Daily Living (Katz, Ford, Moskowitz, Jackson, & Jaffe, 1963) uses letters from A (independent) to G (dependent) to score various functional abilities.
   b. Example of mental or cognitive functioning measurement tools
      (1) The Folstein Mini-Mental State Exam (MMSE; Folstein & Folstein, n.d.) often is used by the team psychologist or social worker.
      (2) It is a brief, 30-item survey that is used to screen for cognitive impairment following a stroke.
      (3) It takes approximately 10 minutes to administer and measures patient performance in such areas as arithmetic, memory, and orientation.
      (4) It is most useful for identifying early signs of dementia.
9. Rehabilitation nurses have an obligation to document the stroke patient's progress in a rehabilitation program, wherever it occurs. The nurse needs to document the patient's response to treatment and activities and the level of assistance they require.
10. Along with other interprofessional or interdisciplinary team members, the nurse participates in functional goal writing to guide the patient care plan.
11. The functional goal must first be mutually accepted by the stroke patient and family. It must be simple to understand for all team members; be practical and achievable; and must include the who, what, under what conditions or circumstances, and target or end date for goal achievement.
12. In addition, the registered nurse uses the nursing process to form nursing diagnoses that guide the plan of care for the stroke patient.
13. Early discharge planning and coordination of care with the entire team is paramount to successful patient outcomes of care.

Health and Wellness as a Way of Life

A. The postacute care plan should demonstrate the assistance of patients in maintaining and sustaining a healthy, productive lifestyle following a stroke.
   1. The definition of health is a state of complete physical, mental, and social well-being and is not merely the absence of disease.
   2. The definition of wellness is a dynamic process necessitating continuous balancing.
   3. The rehabilitation nurse helps the patient who has had a stroke to attain maximum functional abilities, adapt to an altered lifestyle, and learn ways to maintain optimal health and wellness.
   4. A continuum of care philosophy is practiced in rehabilitation and often is a lifelong plan for patients as they move through each transition or level of care following a stroke. It is dynamic and constantly changing to meet the needs of the person who has had a stroke, with the ultimate goal of living independently in the community whenever possible.

Specialized Innovative Rehabilitation Treatments After Stroke

A. Neuro-IFRAH® approach
   1. It is "a whole person approach to rehabilitation and habilitation. It is restoring function and making it functional to return to independent living and the resumption/assumption of life roles" (Neuro-IFRAH® Organization, n.d.).
   2. Neuro-IFRAH® stands for Neuro-Integrative Functional Rehabilitation and Habilitation. This innovative and integrative approach, originated by Waleed Al-Oboudi, MOT OTR/L, helps stroke patients relearn past skills as well as learn new ones (Neuro-IFRAH Organization, n.d.).
   3. This approach often is used by specially trained or certified occupational therapists and other trained staff (including nurses) when treating patients who have had a stroke or brain injury.

B. Constraint-induced movement therapy (CI or CIMT; Rickards et al., 2014)
   1. CIMT is a form of rehabilitation therapy developed by Dr. Edward Taub, a professor of psychology at the University of Alabama, that aims to improve the upper extremity function of patients who have had a stroke.
   2. The nonaffected side is constrained so that the patient is forced to use the affected side in an effort to promote functional and motor recovery.
   3. The theory behind this type of therapy is that nonuse sets in after a stroke because the patient does not want to use their weaker side because of clumsiness or poor control. In turn, recovery is delayed or dampened. However, repetitive use is thought to enhance motor recovery. If one is forced to use the affected side, a change occurs in the brain, forcing new neural pathways. This change is known as critical reorganization or neuroplasticity.
   4. The determination of the type of restraint used for this therapy depends on the required level of safety versus the intensity of the therapy as well as the tolerance of the patient. A sling or soft restraint often is used with the permission of the patient or family.
   5. There are seven components to the effective use of the CIMT method. If not all components are used, the method may be ineffective or underutilized (Pedlow, Lennon, & Wilson, 2014).
   6. Taub's therapy is "at the forefront of a revolution" in what is regarded possible in terms of recovery for stroke survivors (American Stroke Association, 2013).

C. Robotics (Brewer, McDowell, & Worthen-Chaudhari, 2007)
   1. "Rehabilitation robotics is a field of research dedicated to understanding and augmenting rehabilitation through the application of robotic devices" (Brewer et al., 2007).
   2. This field of biomedical engineering includes the development of devices tailored for assisting different sensorimotor functions (e.g., arm, hand, leg), development of different schemes of assisting therapeutic training, and assessment of sensorimotor performance (ability of the patient to move). In essence, a human-robot approach is used to promote motor recovery of a limb.
   3. For patients who have had a stroke, the use of robotics has been found to be an effective adjunct to other therapy modalities.
   4. Recent work in this field has shown great improvements in upper extremity function in self-care tasks as well as the improvement of upright stance for balance and gait (Carrera et al., 2011).

D. Neuro-optometrics (Politzer, n.d.)
   1. Vision-related side effects are common following a stroke and may include field cut loss, hemianopsia (loss of one half of the field of view to the right or left), quadranopsias (loss of about one quarter of the visual field), central or peripheral loss, photophobia, reading disorders, diplopia, or cranial nerve paralysis or weakness.
   2. The three side effects that cause the most impairment are visual field loss, intractable double vision, and visual/balance disorders.
   3. Neuro-optometrics, or visual rehabilitation, uses various therapeutic activities designed to minimize visual impairments.
   4. Teaching the stroke patient to scan the environment or possibly use prism glasses may minimize visual field loss.
   5. Prisms, special lenses, or intensive vision therapy may minimize double vision. Temporary spot patching with a blurring film also has been found to be helpful.
   6. "Visual balance disorders can be caused by a Visual Midline Shift Syndrome, oculomotor dysfunction in fixations, nystagmus, and disruptions of central and peripheral visual processing" (Politzer, n.d.). Lenses, prisms, and visual rehabilitation activities are used, depending on the visual diagnosis and cause. The therapist may be able to do vestibular rehabilitation retraining and therapy if there is a component of dizziness associated with this type of visual disorder following a stroke (Vestibular Disorders Association, n.d.).

E. Computer-assisted therapy for patients with aphasia or cognitive impairments
   1. The use of a computer to assist the stroke patient with aphasia can be an effective adjunct tool in assisting with word retrieval (ASHA, 2014).
   2. The use of virtual reality training combined with computer-based cognitive rehabilitation may be of additional benefit for treating cognitive impairment in stroke patients (Kim, Chun, Kim, & Park, 2011).
   3. The use of computers, software, and technology will continue to be useful adjuncts in therapeutic modalities to promote recovery following a devastating stroke. This will only continue to lend itself to improving the overall quality of life for these patients and their families.

F. Neurodevelopmental techniques (Miller et al., 2010)
   1. The Bobath concept focuses on postural control and recruiting typically uninvolved muscles to achieve movement using tactile and verbal cues to encourage or discourage movement.

G. Strength training and exercise including resistance training and exercise with elevated heart rate should be incorporated into poststroke rehabilitation when appropriate (Miller et al., 2010).

H. Adjuvant techniques (Miller et al., 2010)
  1. Functional electric stimulation is the use of neuromuscular electrical stimulation to stimulate sensory input and promote neural reorganization. Although thought to be effective over the short term, its efficacy in long-term rehabilitation is unclear.
  2. Virtual reality includes the use of computer simulation to provide a practice environment to confer multimodal sensory information.
  3. Biofeedback is provided through verbal, visual, or electromyography (EMG) biofeedback loops.

Managing Common Stroke Rehabilitation Obstacles

A. Cognitive and communication impairment (Miller et al., 2010)
  1. The etiology is multifactorial in stroke survivors.
  2. Diagnosis and management should be highly individualized.
  3. SLP are skilled at targeting aphasia and rehabilitative interventions for aphasia.
  4. Communication should be supplemented when possible with alphabet cuing, gestures, and other communication devices or boards.
  5. Attention retraining programs may be useful for managing anxiety.
  6. Neglect interventions include retraining to scan the environment, limb activation and trunk rotation, and passive sensory stimulation.

B. Shoulder pain and subluxation (Miller et al., 2010)
  1. Generally related to poor joint alignment, decreased active and passive shoulder range of motion, and reduced ligament and tendon function supporting the joint.
  2. Small trials suggest shoulder slings are effective at minimizing subluxation when appropriately fitted. Passive range of motion also may benefit.

C. Poststroke depression (Miller et al., 2010)
  1. Associated with higher mortality and poor functional recovery in stroke survivors
  2. Associated with social isolation in stroke survivors
  3. Patients should be assessed using an evidence-based scale.
  4. Treatment strategies aimed at stroke survivors are evolving and may include pharmacologic interventions, referral for psychotherapy, or a combination of interventions.

D. Chronic dysphagia interventions (Miller et al., 2010)
  1. Implement low-risk feeding strategies including self-feeding, modified diet consistency, reduced distractions during feeding, being fully awake during feeding, sitting upright while feeding, and encouraging small bites.
  2. The chin tuck or head rotation during feeding is a common intervention for dysphagia. The technique may not be appropriate or useful in patients with physical or cognitive issues. EMG biofeedback may improve the outcomes for chin tuck or head rotation strategies.
  3. Referrals should be made to the SLP for chronic dysphagia and aphasia management

E. Bowel and bladder dysfunction (Miller et al., 2010)
  1. Chronic urinary and fecal incontinence affects up to one half of stroke survivors.
  2. Bladder dysfunction etiology may be multifactorial, with factors including neurogenic bladder, urinary retention, and hyperreflexia with urge incontinence.
     a. Management includes a stepwise approach, beginning with training programs aimed at bedpan or commode offered every 2 hours while awake and every 4 hours

at night. Medication and surgical management may be indicated, depending on etiology.

3. Fecal incontinence and constipation also are common after stroke and often are related to decreased mobilization and access to the toilet.
   a. Management strategies should be aimed at the treatment of the underlying cause and include medications to increase motility and stool bulk.

F. Spasticity (Miller et al., 2010)
   1. Occurs in 35% of patients and may result in contracture and limited movement of limb.
   2. Management strategies include range of motion, heat therapy, electric stimulation, splinting, oral antispasmodics, intrathecal baclofen, botulism injections, and surgical release of the contracted muscle.

References

American Occupational Therapy Association, Inc. (2013). Tips for patients and caregivers. Retrieved from www.aota.org/-/media/Corporate/Files/AboutOT/consumers/Adults/Stroke/Stroke%20Tip%20Sheet.pdf

American Occupational Therapy Association, Inc. (2014). About occupational therapy. Retrieved from www.aota.org/about-occupational-therapy.aspx

American Physical Therapy Association. (2013, May 23). Who are physical therapists? Retrieved from www.apta.org/AboutPTs

American Speech-Language-Hearing Association. (2014). Careers in speech-language pathology. Retrieved from http://www.asha.org/careers/professions/slp

American Stroke Association. (2013). Constraint-induced movement therapy. Retrieved from http://www.strokeassociation.org/STROKEORG/LifeAfterStroke/RegainingIndependence/PhysicalChallenges/Constraint-Induced-Movement-Therapy_UCM_309798_Article.jsp

Assisted Living Federation of America. (2013). What is assisted living? Retrieved September 7, 2013, from http://www.assistedlivinginfo.com/Assisted-Living-Care/What-is-Assisted-Living

Association of Rehabilitation Nurses. (2008). *Standards and scope of rehabilitation nursing practice.* Glenview, IL: Author.

Association of Rehabilitation Nurses. (2013a). *The essential role of the rehabilitation nurse in facilitating care transitions.* Chicago, IL: Author.

Association of Rehabilitation Nurses. (2013b). Role descriptions: The rehabilitation nurse case manager. Association of Rehabilitation Nurses website. Retrieved from www.rehabnurse.org/pubs/role/Role-Rehab-Nurse-Case-Manager.html

Association of Rehabilitation Nurses. (n.d.). Role descriptions: The rehabilitation staff nurse. Retrieved from www.rehabnurse.org/pubs/role/Role-Rehab-Staff-Nurse.html

Brewer, B. R., McDowell, S. K., & Worthen-Chaudhari, L. C. (2007). Poststroke upper extremity rehabilitation: A review of robotic systems and clinical results. *Topics in Stroke Rehabilitation, 14*(6), 22–44. doi: 10.1310/tsr1406-22

CARF International. (n.d.). Quality standards. Retrieved September 15, 2013 from http://www.carf.org/Accreditation/QualityStandards/

Carrera, I., Moreno, H. A., Saltarén, R., Pérez, C., Puglisi, L., & Garcia, C. (2011). ROAD: Domestic assistant and rehabilitation robot. *Medical & Biological Engineering & Computing, 49*(10), 1201–1211. doi:10.1007/s11517-011-0805-4

Centers for Medicare & Medicaid Services. (2012a). The inpatient rehabilitation facility—patient assessment instrument (IRF-PAI) training manual. Retrieved from www.cms.gov/Medicare/Medicare-Fee-for-Service-Payment/InpatientRehabFacPPS/Downloads/IRFPAI-manual-2012.pdf

Centers for Medicare & Medicaid Services. (2012b). Outcome and assessment information set (OASIS). Retrieved from www.cms.gov/Medicare/quality-initiatives-patient-assessment-instruments/OASIS/background.htm

Centers for Medicare & Medicaid Services. (2013, September 20). Nursing home quality initiative. Retrieved from www.cms.gov/Medicare/Quality-Initiatives-Patient-Assessment-Instruments/NursingHomeQualityInits/index.html

Clark, R., Turek-Brezina, J., Hawes, C., & Chu, C. (1994). The supply of board and care homes: Results from the 1990 National Health Provider Inventory. Presented at the annual meeting of the Gerontological Society of America, Atlanta, GA.

Department of Health Care Services. (n.d.). Subacute care. Retrieved from www.dhcs.ca.gov/provgovpart/Pages/SubacuteCare.aspx

Folstein, M. F., & Folstein, S. E. (n.d.). *Mini Mental State Examination*, 2nd Ed. Retrieved from www.minimental.com

Hawes, C., Wildfire, J., Mor, V., Wilcox, V., Spore, D., Iannacchione, V., . . . U.S. Department of Health and Human Services Assistant Secretary for Planning and Evaluation. (1995, December). A description of board and care facilities, operators, and residents. Retrieved from http://aspe.hhs.gov/daltcp/reports/bcdesces.htm

Institute for Patient- and Family-Centered Care. (n.d.). Frequently asked questions. Retrieved from www.ipfcc.org/faq.html

Jacelon, C. (Ed.). (2011). *The specialty practice of rehabilitation nursing: A core curriculum* (6th ed.). Glenview, IL: Association of Rehabilitation Nurses.

Katz, S., Ford, A. B., Moskowitz, R. W., Jackson, B. A., Jaffe, M. W. (1963). Studies of illness in the aged. The index of ADL: A standardized measure of biological and psychosocial function. *Journal of the American Medical Association, 185*, 914–919.

Kim, B., Chun, M., Kim, L., & Park, J. Effect of virtual reality on cognition in stroke patients. *Annals of Rehabilitation Medicine, 35*(4), 450–459. doi: 10.5535/arm.2011.35.4.450

Matthews, J. L. (2013, March 3). Does Medicaid pay for assisted living? Retrieved from www.caring.com/questions/medicaid-pay-for-assisted-living

Mauk, K., Ed. (2007). *The specialty practice of rehabilitation nursing: A core curriculum* (5th ed.). Glenview, IL: Association of Rehabilitation Nurses.

McDaniel, G. (n.d.). Long term acute care hospital (LTACH). Retrieved from www.glgresearch.com/Dictionary/HC-Long-Term-Acute-Care-Hospital-(LTACH).html

Miller, E. L., Murray, L., Richards, L., Zorowitz, R. D., Bakas, T., Clark, P., . . . American Heart Association Council on Cardiovascular Nursing and the Stroke Council. (2010). Comprehensive overview of nursing and interdisciplinary rehabilitation care of the stroke patient: A scientific statement from the American Heart Association. *Stroke, 41*(10), 2402–2448. doi:10.1161/STR.0b013e7512b

Nagi, S. (1965). Some conceptual issues in disability and rehabilitation. In: Sussman M., editor. *Sociology and Rehabilitation*. Washington, DC: American Sociological Association; 100–113.

National Association of Social Workers. (n.d.). Social work organizations. Retrieved from www.socialworkers.org/swportal/swo1/

National Long-Term Care Ombudsman Resource Center. (2013). MDS 3.0. Retrieved from www.ltcombudsman.org/issues/MDS-3.0

National Institute of Neurological Disorders and Stroke. (n.d.). Post-stroke rehabilitation. Retrieved from http://stroke.nih.gov/materials/rehabilitation.htm

National Stroke Association. (n.d.). Stroke 101 fact sheet. Retrieved from www.stroke.org/site/DocServer/STROKE_101_Fact_Sheet.pdf?docID=4541

National Stroke Association. (2014). Recovery and rehabilitation. Retrieved from http://www.stroke.org/site/PageServer?pagename=rehabt

Neuro-IFRAH Organization. (n.d.). What is Neuro-IFRAH? Retrieved from www.neuro-ifrah.org/faq.aspx

Nordqvist, C. (2009, August 14). What is physical therapy (physiotherapy)? What does a physical therapist (physiotherapist) do? Retrieved from www.medicalnewstoday.com/articles/160645.php

Organization for Economic Cooperation and Development. (2005). Health policies and data: Long-term care for older people. Retrieved from www.oecd.org/document/50/0,3343,en_2649_33929_35195570_1_1_1_37407,00.html

Pedlow, K., Lennon, S., Wilson, C. (2014). The application of constraint induced movement therapy in clinical practice: An online survey. *Archives of Physical Medicine and Rehabilitation, 95*(2), 276–282. doi: 10.1016/j.apmr.2013.08.240

Physiatry and Rehabilitation Services, Inc. (n.d.). FAQs. Retrieved from www.rehabmedicine.org/FAQs/faqs.html

Politzer, T. (n.d.). Introduction to vision & brain injury. Retrieved from http://nora.cc/for-patients-main-menu-34/vision-a-brain-injury-mainmenu-64.html

Psychology Education Association. (2013). Rehabilitation psychologist. Retrieved from http://psychologycareercenter.org/rehabilitation-psychologist.html

Rickards, T., Sterling, C., Taub, E., Perkins-Hu, C., Gauthier, L., Graham, M., . . . Uswatte, G. (2014). Diffusion tensor imaging study of the response to constraint-induced movement therapy of children with hemiparetic cerebral palsy and adults with chronic stroke. *Archives of Physical Medicine and Rehabilitation, 95*(3), 506–514e.1. doi: 10.1016/j.apmr.2013.08.245

Roger, V. L., Go, A. S., Lloyd-Jones, D. M., Benjamin, E. J., Berry, J. D., Bravata, D. M., . . . American Heart Association Statistics Committee and Stroke Statistic Subcommittee. (2012, January). Heart disease and stroke statistics—2012 update. *Circulation, 127*(1), e6–e24. doi: 10.1161/CIR.0b013e31828124ad

RTI International. (2013). MDS 3.0 quality measures user manual (v8.0 04-15-2013) [data set user manual]. Retrieved from www.cms.gov/Medicare/Quality-Initiatives-Patient-Assessment-Instruments/NursingHomeQualityInits/Downloads/MDS-30-QM-User%E2%80%99s-Manual-V80.pdf

Treiger, T., & Fink-Samnick, E. (2013). COLLABORATE(c): A universal competency-based paradigm for the professional case management, part II: Competency clarification. *Professional Case Management, 18*(5), 219–243. doi: 10.1097/NCM.0b013e31829c8a3a

U.S. Bureau of Labor Statistics. (2014a). Occupational outlook handbook, 2012-13 edition, physical therapists. Retrieved from www.bls.gov/ooh/healthcare/physical-therapists.htm

U.S. Bureau of Labor Statistics. (2014b). Occupational outlook handbook, 2012-13 edition, occupational therapy assistants and aides. Retrieved from www.bls.gov/ooh/Healthcare/Occupational-therapy-assistants-and-aides.htm

U.S. Bureau of Labor Statistics. (2014c). Occupational outlook handbook, 2012-13 edition, speech-language pathologists. Retrieved from www.bls.gov/ooh/Healthcare/Speech-language-pathologists.htm

U.S. Bureau of Labor Statistics. (2014d). Occupational outlook handbook, 2012-13 edition, social workers. etrieved from www.bls.gov/ooh/community-and-social-service/social-workers.htm

U.S. Bureau of Labor Statistics. (2014e). Occupational outlook handbook, 2012-13 edition, psychologists. Retrieved from www.bls.gov/ooh/life-physical-and-social-science/psychologists.htm

Vestibular Disorders Association. (n.d.). What is vestibular rehabilitation therapy? Retrieved from http://vestibular.org/understanding-vestibular-disorder/treatment/treatment-detail-page

Chapter

8

Systems and Quality

Mary Straw, DHA RN ANP CNS; Mary Kelly, MBA RN CNRN

Individual stroke care should be delivered within a larger system of care. Stroke systems of care are based on established evidence, guidelines, and quality indicators developed by the Brain Attack Coalition (BAC), the American Stroke Association (ASA), the National Quality Forum (NQF), and the Centers for Medicare & Medicaid Services (CMS). Systems of care and quality improvement focus on customers, both internal and external, with the goal of improving the outcomes of patients suffering from stroke. Stroke systems of care extend across the continuum of stroke care. Quality should be measured in each area of the continuum, including community education, emergency medical intervention from the acute care setting, rehabilitation, and discharge. Evidence-based standards aim to improve the stroke quality of care.

Objectives

1. Summarize the rationale for standardization of care for the stroke population.
2. Identify protocols or pathways to care for the acute stroke population.
3. Outline quality improvement techniques to improve stroke outcomes.
4. Discuss the application of quality improvement techniques.
5. Identify criteria for stroke center certification.

The Stroke System of Care

A. Defining a stroke system of care
   1. In 2005, the ASA convened a task force to develop recommendations for the continued development of a stroke system of care. The task force concluded that a stroke system of care should include a coordinated range of stroke prevention, treatment, and rehabilitation services, including the following key components (Schwamm et al., 2005):
      a. Primordial and primary prevention
      b. Community education
      c. Notification and response of emergency medical services (EMS)
      d. Acute stroke treatment, including hyperacute and emergency department (ED) phases
      e. Subacute stroke treatment and secondary prevention
      f. Rehabilitation
      g. Continuous quality improvement activities
   2. Although elements of the stroke system of care listed previously exist in various levels of sophistication across the United States, the components often work in silos rather than forming a coordinated effort across the continuum of care (Schwamm et al., 2005).

B. Facilitating care within a stroke system of care
  1. Care within the stroke system of care should be organized, efficient, and evidence based.
  2. Efforts to organize care within stroke programs include
    a. Stroke program certification by external agencies and designation by some states
    b. Development and utilization of clinical practice guidelines (CPGs)
      (1) CPGs are a comprehensive review and summary of the literature with recommendations. CPGs generally are developed by national associations, societies, or groups of experts, and recommendations reflect a review of evidence and summary of current best practices by experts.
      (2) CPGs are often used to guide stroke program development and individual stroke care.
    c. Development of program tools to facilitate care according to the best understanding of evidence, including program protocols, policies, algorithms, guidelines, and work-flow maps. Multiple tools may be necessary to coordinate and standardize care within a program.
    d. Development and facilitation of a quality improvement program
      (1) Quality improvement and data monitoring may occur at the level of the stroke program, the hospital or healthcare system, regional or state systems, and national systems through national databases and metric reporting systems including the ASA's Get With the Guidelines program, the Paul Coverdale program, and CMS's Inpatient Quality Reporting Program, commonly known as core measures.
        (a) Data reporting may be tied to financial incentives and penalties.

C. Using protocols or pathways
  1. Serve as internal program guides and structure for the care of the stroke patient
  2. Developed by research-driven investigation, including a rigorous review of the literature coupled with evaluation of current practice when literature is scarce to guide practice
    a. Published in journals and by neurological organizations, including and not limited to
      (1) American Association Neuroscience Nursing (www.aann.org)
      (2) American Academy of Neurology (www.aan.com)
      (3) American Association of Neurological Surgeons (www.aans.org)
      (4) American College of Emergency Physicians (www.acep.org)
      (5) American Society of Neuroradiology (www.asnr.org)
      (6) Congress of Neurological Surgeons (www.neurosurgeon.org)
      (7) Society of Neurointerventional Surgery (www.asitn.org)
      (8) American Stroke Association (www.strokeassociation.org)
      (9) National Stroke Association (www.stroke.org)
      (10) National Institutes of Health (www.nih.gov)
      (11) National Institute of Neurological Disorders and Stroke (www.ninds.nih.gov)
      (12) Canadian Stroke Network (www.canadianstrokenetwork.ca)
      (13) Brain Attack Coalition (www.stroke-site.org)
      (14) Peer-reviewed journals
    b. May also be created by health systems
  3. A standardized and organized approach to the care of the stroke patient is associated with improved outcomes. To obtain external certification, stroke programs select stroke CPGs and design the stroke program to meet the needs of stroke patients according to published evidence by developing stroke treatment plans, initiating standardized stroke

order sets, and reviewing stroke patient outcomes. Many organizations use the following CPGs as the basis for their standardized stroke treatment plan of care. For each diagnosis, the organization should develop an organized approach to the following disease elements.

4. Key disease elements for program organization and outcome analysis
   a. Transient ischemic attack (TIA; Easton et al., 2009; Goldstein et al., 2011; Sacco et al., 2006)
      (1) Recommended guideline: *Guidelines for the Prevention of Stroke in Patients with Stroke or Transient Ischemic Attack* (Furie et al., 2011)
         (a) Hypertension management
         (b) Glycemic control
         (c) Statin therapy with intensive lipid-lowering effects is recommended to reduce risk of stroke and cardiovascular events among patients with ischemic stroke or TIA who have symptoms of atherosclerosis.
         (d) Support tobacco cessation efforts if the patient is smoking or has smoked in the past year
      (2) Patients with ischemic stroke or TIA who are heavy drinkers should eliminate or reduce their consumption of alcohol.
      (3) Increase physical activity.
      (4) Initiation of antiplatelet agents or oral anticoagulation
      (5) Evaluate for and treat the following:
         (a) Extracranial carotid disease
         (b) Extracranial vertebrobasilar disease
         (c) Atrial fibrillation
         (d) Acute myocardial infarction and left ventricular thrombus
         (e) Cardiomyopathy
         (f) Prosthetic heart valve
         (g) Native valvular heart disease
         (h) Arterial dissections
         (i) Patient foramen ovale
         (j) Hyperhomocysteinemia
         (k) Inherited thrombophilias
         (l) Antiphospholipid antibodies
         (m) Sickle cell disease
         (n) Cerebral venous sinus thrombosis
         (o) Fabry disease
         (p) Pregnancy
         (q) Postmenopausal hormone therapy
   b. Acute ischemic stroke (Acker et al., 2007; Adams et al., 2007; Pugh et al., 2012; Summers et al., 2009)
      (1) Recommended guideline: *Guidelines for the Early Management of Patients with Acute Ischemic Stroke* (Jauch et al., 2013)
         (a) EMS evaluation and transport to primary stroke center or comprehensive stroke center
         (b) Education of all stroke system of care providers on recognition of stroke signs and symptoms
         (c) Possible use of telemedicine for emergent stroke care
         (d) Rapid triage in ED

1) Patient history
2) Neurological assessment
3) Use of National Institutes of Health Stroke Scale (NIHSS)
4) Diagnostic testing and imaging
5) Goals for treatment implementation
   a) ED-based care (Bock, 1996; Jauch, 2013)
      i. Action time
         i. Door to physician ≤10 minutes
         ii. Door to stroke team ≤15 minutes
         iii. Door to computed tomography (CT) initiation ≤25 minutes
         iv. Door to CT interpretation ≤45 minutes
         v. Door to alteplase (intravenous [IV] tissue plasminogen activator [TPA]) ≤60 minutes
         vi. Door to stroke unit admission ≤3 hours

(e) Access to neurological expertise (i.e., neurologist)
(f) Evaluation for alteplase (IV TPA) and appropriate monitoring
   1) Less than or equal to 3 hours of symptom onset
   2) 3–4.5 hours of symptom onset (del Zoppo et al., 2009)
(g) Evaluation for advanced stroke rescue (i.e., neurointervention [clot removal, coiling])
(h) General supportive care
   1) Temperature
   2) Blood pressure
   3) Glucose
   4) Fluids
   5) Oxygen
   6) Positioning
(i) Cardiac monitoring
(j) Care on a stroke unit
   1) Venous thrombosis prophylaxis
   2) Antiplatelet
   3) Anticoagulation
   4) Statin
(k) Risk factor evaluation and management
(l) Stroke education
(m) Consideration for rehabilitation

c. Hemorrhagic stroke with differentiation between subarachnoid hemorrhage (SAH) and intracranial hemorrhage (ICH)
   (1) SAH (Connolly et al., 2012; Pugh et al., 2012; Summers et al., 2009)
      (a) EMS rapid transport to an ED equipped to care for SAH
         1) Urgent evaluation and treatment of acute onset of severe headache
         2) Consider high-volume hospital with more than 35 cases of SAH/year
      (b) Non-contrast head CT followed by lumbar puncture if CT is not diagnostic
      (c) Determination if aneurysm is amenable to clipping or coiling with digital subtraction angiography and three-dimensional rotational angiography
      (d) After repair of the rupture, diagnostic imaging
      (e) Determination of clinical severity using a valid scale such as the Hunt and Hess scale

(f) Control of hypertension
(g) Nimodipine to increase neurologic outcomes
(h) Assess and treat
1) Vasospasm
2) Symptomatic hydrocephalus (acute and chronic)
3) Glucose
4) Fever
5) Fluid volume
6) Electrolyte imbalance
(i) After hospital stay, an evaluation should be conducted for cognitive behavioral and psychosocial issues.
(j) Aggressive management of risk factors
(k) Screen first-degree relatives

(2) ICH (Morgenstern, 2010; Pugh et al., 2012; Summers et al., 2009)
(a) EMS rapid transport to an ED equipped to care for ICH
(b) Rapid diagnosis with neuroimaging (CT or magnetic resonance imaging [MRI])
(c) Medical treatment of homeostasis/antiplatelets/deep venous thrombosis prophylaxis
1) If severe coagulation factor deficiency or severe thrombocytopenia, consider factor replacement therapy or platelets, respectively
2) Withhold warfarin; when indicated give vitamin K
3) Lower extremity intermittent pulsation devices
a) In patient management and prevention of secondary brain injury
i. Monitor ICH in intensive care unit (ICU)
ii. Glucose control
iii. Manage and treat hydrocephelus
iv. Treat seizures with antiepileptic
v. Clot retrieval
vi. Manage blood pressure
vii. Prevent recurrent ICH, risk factor management
viii. Consider end-of-life issues

5. Integration of CPGs
a. Organizational leadership must review CPGs yearly and upon changes in CPG
(1) Choose appropriate CPG based on the stroke patient population served at the organization.
(2) Develop a process to integrate CPG into stroke program and care of the patient, which may include organizational protocols, decision algorithms, order sets, or standing orders.
(3) Ensure CPGs are available to all members of the stroke patient care team.
(4) Review care compliance with CPG.
(5) Review stroke patient outcomes when CPGs are used.

Acute Stroke Setting, Team, and Survival

A. Quality improvement initiatives according to inpatient levels of care
1. ED
a. First point of contact with stroke team for most patients
b. ED should have well-established communication with EMS and a process to alert the stroke team once prehospital notification is received.

c. Personnel educated and trained in the diagnosis and treatment of all stroke types
d. Protocols for the rapid triage and treatment of all stroke types including the use of alteplase and management of elevated intracranial pressure (ICP)
e. ED personnel may be part of acute stroke team

2. ICU
   a. Care for unstable stroke population or patients needing intensive neurological nursing management
   b. Continuous cardiac monitoring
   c. Management of multiple IV medications
   d. Management of airway
   e. Management of elevated ICP
   f. Management of temperature
   g. Management of craniectomy patients
   h. Nurses need to recognize neurological complications and deterioration.
   i. Train staff in the use of appropriate neurological assessment tools.
   j. Nurse-to-patient ratio should be 1:2 for the first 24 hours or while the patient is neurologically unstable.
   k. Use of evidence-based protocols for all stroke types
3. Stroke units/step-down units
   a. Stable stroke population, but needs advanced neurologically trained nursing management
   b. Continuous cardiac monitoring
   c. Staff trained in use of neurological assessment tools
   d. Nurse-to-patient ratio, 1:4
   e. Use of evidence-based protocols for all stroke types
   f. Active rehabilitation services on unit (possible satellite gym on unit)
   g. Active discharge planning
4. Medical unit
   a. Stable stroke population near discharge
   b. Noncardiac involvement for stroke patient population
   c. Staff trained in the use of neurological assessment tools
   d. Active rehabilitation services on unit
   e. Active discharge planning
5. Rehabilitation
   a. Outpatient
      (1) Outpatient clinic–based care
      (2) Appointment based
      (3) Intensive rehabilitation
      (4) Depending on the facility, team members may include physicians, physical and occupational therapists, speech-language pathologists, psychologists, therapeutic recreation specialists, and vocational rehabilitation counselors.
      (5) Patients need transportation to facility.
   b. Acute
      (1) Inpatient care
      (2) Team members may include physicians, physical and occupational therapists, rehabilitation nurses, speech-language pathologists, psychologists, therapeutic recreation specialists, care managers, and vocational rehabilitation counselors.

(3) Coordinated care between team members, patient, and family
(4) Ability for active involvement in rehabilitative services for a specified time each day (designate by current standards)

c. Subacute
(1) Inpatient care
(2) Often in free-standing nursing homes
(3) Team members may include nurses, physical and occupational therapists, speech-language pathologists, and care managers.
(4) In some facilities additional team members may include psychologists, therapeutic recreation specialists, and vocational rehabilitation counselors.

d. Long-term care
(1) Nursing home care
(2) Team members include nurses and care managers
(3) In some facilities additional team members include physical and occupational therapists and speech-language pathologists.

6. Acute rehabilitation team (**Table 8-1**)

Table 8-1. Healthcare Providers Commonly Part of the Stroke Rehabilitation Team

Discipline	Website	Description
Certified rehabilitation counselors	www.crccertification.com	Assist individuals with disabilities to maximize their vocational and avocational living goals in the most integrated setting possible through the application of the counseling process, including vocational and counseling, case management, referral, and service coordination; identifying and addressing employment and attitudinal barriers; and job analysis, development, and placement services.
Neuropsychologists	www.apa.org	Specialize in brain-behavior relationships and have extensive training in anatomy, physiology, and neuropathology. They identify and treat cognitive and neurobehavioral dysfunction, and through assessment also monitor recovery and thereby enhance community reintegration.
Occupational therapists (OT)	www.aota.org	Focus on the "skills of living" necessary for independent and satisfying living. OT services include customized treatment programs to perform daily activities, comprehensive home and jobsite evaluations and adaptation recommendations, performance skills assessment and interventions, adaptive equipment recommendations and training, and family and caregiver education.

continued

Table 8-1. Healthcare Providers Commonly Part of the Stroke Rehabilitation Team continued

Discipline	Website	Description
Rehabilitation nurses (RN)	www.rehabnurse.org	Manage complex medical issues, provide ongoing patient and caregiver education, and establish care plans to maintain optimal wellness. RNs use a holistic approach to fulfill patients' medical, environmental, spiritual, vocational, and educational needs via principles from other disciplines and their own unique medical expertise (bowel, bladder, and skin management). In all care settings, RNs function as coordinators/case managers, collaborators, and counselors. A registered nurse with at least 2 years of practice in rehabilitation who passes the Association of Rehabilitation Nurses examination can earn the Certified Rehabilitation Registered Nurse distinction.
Physical therapists (PT)	www.apta.org	PTs are experts in examining and treating neuromuscular problems that affect the abilities of individuals to move. PTs practice in many settings and with all age groups.
Physicians	www.aapmr.org	Usually coordinate the rehabilitation team and manage medical conditions pertaining to stroke and comorbidities. A physician may be a physiatrist (i.e., specializing in physical medicine and rehabilitation and thus restoration of function in individuals with problems that range from simple physical mobility to more complex cognitive issues).
Recreational therapists	www.atra-online.com	Provide treatment services and recreation activities to individuals with disabilities to facilitate independent physical, cognitive, emotional, and social functioning by enhancing individuals' current skills and assisting new skill development for daily living and community function. Besides discharge planning for community reintegration, they help individuals develop or redevelop social, discretionary time, decision-making, coping, self-advocacy, and basic skills to enhance overall quality of life.
Social workers	www.naswdc.org	Assist individuals, groups, or communities restore or enhance their capacity for social functioning, while creating societal conditions favorable to their goals. Requires knowledge of human development and behavior; social, economic, and cultural institutions; and interactions among these factors. Social workers help prevent crises; counsel individuals, families, and communities to facilitate coping with everyday stresses; and identify resources to allow individuals with disabilities to remain in the community.
Speech and language pathologists (SLP)	www.asha.org	Assess speech, language and other cognitive functions, as well as swallowing, and provide interventions and counseling/education to address language and speech disorders (e.g., aphasia, apraxia of speech, dysarthria, and cognitive-communication impairment). SLPs also intervene when swallowing and cognitive disorders exist. They provide services to all age groups and in all care settings.

Reprinted from "Comprehensive Overview of Nursing and Interdisciplinary Rehabilitation Care of the Stroke Patient," by E. L. Miller, L. Murray, L. Richards, R. D. Zorowitz, T. Bakas, P. Clark, and S. A. Billinger, 2010, Stroke, 41, *pp. 2402–2448. © 2010 by American Heart Association/American Stroke Association. Reprinted with permission.*

B. Acute stroke team (AST)
   1. Formation of AST for ED and inpatient care areas
      a. AST staffed by a variety of healthcare personnel, including
         (1) Personnel with experience and expertise dealing with cerebral vascular disease
         (2) One physician and one other healthcare provider
      b. AST must be available 24 hours/day, 7 days/week.
         (1) At bedside within 15 minutes
         (2) AST should respond to the ED and other hospital patient care units.
   2. Role of AST
      a. Responsible for responding to patients with acute stroke in ED and other hospital wards
      b. AST should follow an organized process for rapid assessment.
      c. AST initiates diagnostic testing and immediate care.
      d. The AST is the key element in screening and delivery of acute therapies.
      e. Team members must be familiar with and have expertise in the recognition, diagnosis, stabilization, and acute care of all stroke types.
      f. AST should use evidence-based protocols for all types of stroke.
      g. AST should keep a log of all triage data elements and review for quality improvement activities.

C. Stroke leadership
   1. Administration
      a. Institutional commitment and support
         (1) Organization
         (2) Infrastructure
         (3) Funding
      b. Stroke registry with outcomes
      c. Quality improvement activities
      d. Educational programs
         (1) Public
         (2) Professional
      e. Commitment to certification process
   2. Medical director
      a. Designated medical director who has training and expertise in cerebrovascular disease
      b. Examples include neurologists, vascular neurologists, and neurosurgeons
      c. Provide administrative leadership
      d. Provide clinical guidance
   3. Stroke coordinator
      a. Expertise in neurological, neurological, and cerebrovascular disease
      b. Participate in development of stroke program
      c. Manage daily program activities
      d. Participate in quality improvement activities

D. Point of care for survival: ASA Chain of Survival (**Table 8-2**)
   1. Call 911
      a. Recognition of stroke signs and symptoms
      b. Early activation of EMS
      c. Use of prehospital stroke identification scale
      d. Dispatch of EMS should happen in the shortest time possible based on local resources.

2. EMS prehospital evaluation
   a. EMS response should be rapid and within the same goals established for other acute events (i.e., acute myocardial infarction or trauma)
   b. Use of tool for recognition of stroke signs and symptoms
   c. Use of algorithms and protocols that reflect the most current stroke treatment
   d. Establish "Last Known Well"
   e. Rapid transport to stroke center
3. Prehospital notification
   a. Prehospital notification results in preparation for the arrival of the stroke patient at the receiving hospital
   b. Activates in-hospital notification of stroke team members
   c. Allows for hospital allocation of resources
   d. Results in faster treatment upon arrival to the hospital
4. Hospital door to needle in less than 60 minutes
   a. Early administration of alteplase is associated with better outcomes.
   b. Treatment of stroke less than 60 minutes from arrival
   c. Development of protocols for rapid triage
      (1) Arrival to AST ≤15 minutes
      (2) Arrival to CT scan ≤25 minutes
      (3) Arrival to CT scan results available ≤45 minutes
      (4) Arrival to administration of alteplase ≤60 minutes

Table 8-2. Stroke Chain of Survival

Detection	Recognition of stroke signs and symptoms
Dispatch	Call 911 and priority emergency medical services dispatch
Delivery	Prompt transport and prehospital notification to hospital
Door	Immediate emergency department (ED) triage
Data	ED evaluation, prompt laboratory studies, and computed tomography imaging
Decision	Diagnosis and decision about appropriate therapy
Drug	Administration of appropriate drugs or other interventions

Reprinted from "The Links in the Chain of Survival," by the American Heart Association, 2008, www.americanheart.org/presenter.jhtml?identifier=3012016. © 2008 by the American Heart Association/American Stroke Association. Reprinted with permission.

Quality Improvement Techniques to Improve Stroke Outcomes

A. Quality improvement
   1. Definition: According to the Agency for Healthcare Quality and Research (AHRQ), quality in health care is doing the right thing at the right time, in the right way, to achieve optimal results (2003). In addition, quality is having the correct balance in services provided. Quality improvement is the systematic process of improving healthcare quality (Rivard, Parker, & Rosen, 2013).
   2. History
      a. Healthcare quality is often traced to Florence Nightingale and Ernest Amory Codman, early leaders in quality and process improvement.
      b. 1927–1940: Dr. E. Deming developed quality improvement methodology.
      c. 1980: Avedis Donabedian published a detailed description of The Donabedian Model.
         (1) Process, structure, outcomes

(2) Specific to health care

d. National Committee Quality Assurance (NCQA): Founded in 1990, NCQA is a private nonprofit dedicated to improving healthcare quality.

e. CMS developed standards charging hospitals to develop and implement performance improvement programs as conditions of participation (CoP; Rogers, 2007).

3. Framework

a. The most common framework for healthcare quality improvement is the Donabedian model (Donabedian, 1987).

(1) Structure is viewed as the context in which care is being provided as it relates to process and outcomes.

(2) Process is identifying whether evidence-based care is being followed.

(3) Outcomes are the effects or impact on care.

4. The Institute of Medicine's (IOM) six domains should be taken into consideration when developing a quality plan (IOM, 1999).

a. Safe—avoid injury to the patient

b. Effective—evidence-based medicine

c. Patient centered—care that takes into consideration the patients wants and needs

d. Timely—reducing waits and delays in care

e. Avoid waste—this includes supplies, energy, equipment, ideas

f. Equitable—care that does not deviate in its quality due to gender, ethnicity, or socioeconomic status

B. Examples of techniques and tools used in rapid cycle performance improvement

1. PDSA—plan, do, study, act

a. Plan—develop a plan to test a change

b. Do—carry out the plan or test

c. Study—observe and learn from the consequences of the plan or change

d. Act—decide if modifications should be made to the plan

2. Six-Sigma/LEAN (Institute for Healthcare Improvement, 2005)

a. Six Sigma (DMAIC [define, measure, analyze, improve, control])—an improvement system for existing processes falling below specification and looking for incremental improvement

b. LEAN—elimination of non–value-adding processes or techniques

3. Root cause analysis—retrospective analysis of an adverse event or error, including data collection and data analysis

C. Why use these quality improvement techniques

a. Quality improvement must follow a set process to determine if interventions and care improve the healthcare status of patients. Integrating evidence-based medicine in care processes improves the health care of the stroke population.

D. Across the continuum of care

1. Prehospital

a. Communication with ED by EMS

b. Documentation of time of symptom onset, also known as last known well

c. Laboratory results such as glucose

d. Cincinnati Stroke Scale or equivalent performed

2. ED

a. Door to physician

b. Door to CT scan

c. Door to laboratory

3. Critical care
   a. Complications: infection, conversion, deterioration, NIHSS, processes
4. Stroke unit
   a. NIHSS, assessment intervals, complications, length of stay, processes
5. Rehabilitation
   a. Team assessments and interventions
   b. Use of Modified Rankin Score (mRS)
6. Ancillary departments
   a. Assessments, interventions, processes

E. Team responsibilities for quality improvement
1. Executive level
   a. Supports the certification process
   b. Responsible for recourses
   c. Responsible for quality of care
2. Quality level
   a. Develop performance improvement plan.
   b. Ensure the provision of a comparable level of quality of care to all patients.
   c. Perform an ongoing systematic review of the services provided by the stroke center to maintain stable processes and identify opportunities for improvement.
   d. Develop and implement effective solutions to identified problems and opportunities for improvement.
   e. Ensure that important functions are coordinated with all relevant departments through collaborative efforts.
   f. Develop or participate in a stroke registry that will track the number and type of stroke patients seen, their treatments, timelines for receiving treatments, and the impact indicators selected to measure outcomes.
   g. Comply with state and federal requirements.
3. Departmental level
   a. Successful implementation of performance improvement plan
   b. Critical in data analysis, review, and comparison to best practices
   c. Distribution of data to point-of-care practitioners
4. Ancillary department members
   a. Physicians, physician assistants, nurses, rehabilitation therapists, pharmacists, respiratory therapists, dietitians, case managers, radiology staff, and endovascular staff

Criteria for Stroke Center Certification

A. Early research
1. Early pioneers
   a. BAC—a group of professional, voluntary, and governmental entities dedicated to reducing the occurrence, disabilities, and death associated with stroke. The goal of the coalition is to strengthen and promote relationships among its member organizations to help people who have had a stroke or are at risk for a stroke (Alberts et al., 2005).
   b. National Institute of Neurologic Disorders and Stroke (2013)—its mission is to reduce the burden of neurological disease, a burden borne by every age group, every segment of society, and people all over the world.
   c. National Stroke Association—national nonprofit healthcare organization focusing 100% of its resources and attention on stroke

d. ASA—its mission is to build healthier lives, free of cardiovascular diseases and stroke.

B. Paul Coverdale Study—The mission of the Paul Coverdale National Acute Stroke Registry is to

1. Measure, track, and improve the quality of and access to care for stroke patients from onset of stroke symptoms through rehabilitation and recovery
2. Decrease the rate of premature death and disability from acute stroke
3. Eliminate disparities in care
4. Support development of stroke systems of care that emphasize quality of care
5. Improve access to rehabilitation and opportunities for recovery after stroke
6. Increase the workforce capacity and scientific knowledge for stroke surveillance within stroke systems of care (CDC, 2013)

C. Levels of certification

1. Stroke-ready facility
   a. Requirements vary according to state and region
      (1) Ability to triage, treat, and transfer acute stoke patients
      (2) Written care protocols
      (3) EMS
      (4) ED care
      (5) Cerebral and cerebral vascular imaging
      (6) Cardiac imaging
      (7) Administrative and organizational support
      (8) Outcomes and quality improvement
      (9) Educational programs
   b. Reporting data
      (1) January 2013—CMS required eight stroke core measures
2. Primary stroke center
   a. Requirements
      (1) Acute stroke team
      (2) Written care protocols
      (3) EMS
      (4) ED care
      (5) Stroke unit care
      (6) Cerebral and cerebral vascular imaging
      (7) Cardiac imaging
      (8) Rehabilitative services
      (9) Administrative and organizational support
      (10) Outcomes and quality improvement
      (11) Educational programs
      (12) Certification
   b. Reporting data
      (1) January 2013—CMS required eight stroke core measures
3. Comprehensive Stroke Center
   a. Requirements
      (1) Acute stroke team
      (2) Written care protocols
      (3) EMS
      (4) ED care

(5) Advanced neurointerventional capacities
(6) Advanced neurosurgical services
(7) Neurocritical care
(8) Neurointensivist
(9) Stroke unit care
(10) Cerebral and cerebral vascular imaging
(11) Cardiac imaging
(12) Rehabilitative services
(13) Depression screening
(14) Administrative and organizational support
(15) Outcomes and quality improvement
(16) Educational programs
(17) Patient and family assessment
(18) Patient and family education
(19) Discharge planning
(20) Certification

b. Reporting data
   (1) January 2013—CMS required eight stroke core measures
   (2) Proposed The Joint Commission comprehensive measures
   (3) Healthcare Facilities Accreditation Program (HFAP)

D. Development of certification standards
1. The Joint Commission (2013)—Certified programs must demonstrate a systematic approach to care delivery and a commitment to performance improvement through ongoing data collection and analysis. Requirements address three areas:
   a. Consensus-based national standards, which cover
      (1) Program management
      (2) Clinical information management
      (3) Delivering or facilitating care
      (4) Supporting self-management
      (5) Measuring and improving performance
   b. Effective use of evidence-based clinical practice guidelines to manage and optimize care
   c. An organized approach to performance measurement and improvement activities
2. Det Norske Veritas (DNV)
   a. Stroke certification programs incorporate elements from DNV's NIAHO® hospital accreditation standards, as well as requirements from the guidelines of the Brain Attack Coalition and recommendations of the ASA. The emphasis these programs place on deploying a disciplined management system, combined with the relevant clinical best practices, sets DNV stroke certifications apart from other programs .
   b. Hospitals seeking and maintaining a Stroke Center Certification must participate in the Medicare program and be in compliance with the CoPs, which may be demonstrated by maintaining accreditation with DNV or another CMS-approved accreditation organization.
3. HFAP
   a. A hospital seeking Primary Stroke Center certification through HFAP shall comply with the following requirements before its application will be considered:
      (1) "The hospital shall have current hospital accreditation through an entity with CMS deeming authority.

(2) Healthcare facilities seeking HFAP Primary Stroke Center certification must comply with all HFAP primary stroke center standards. Patients eligible for the stroke center protocol include those who, following a CT scan, have a diagnosis of ischemic stroke, hemorrhagic stroke, or TIA.

(3) The hospital shall have a minimum of 12 consecutive months' of stroke data" (HFAP, 2013, 2014).

E. State certification—as of 2010 (CDC, 2011)

1. Enacted legislation—14 states: Delaware, Florida, Georgia, Illinois, Kentucky, Missouri, New Jersey, New Mexico, North Dakota, Oklahoma, Rhode Island, Texas, Virginia, and Washington
2. Pending legislation—two states: Massachusetts (a study was ordered) and West Virginia
3. Non-legislative (administrative) policy—five states: Connecticut, Maryland, Massachusetts, New York, and Oklahoma. States with primary stroke center administrative rules clarifying legislation include Florida, New Jersey, Oklahoma, and Texas.
4. Both enacted legislation and non-legislative policy—one state: Oklahoma
5. No primary stroke center policy—31 states and the District of Columbia. Of those, some had passed supporting legislation.
6. Supporting legislation—16 states (as of July 2010): Arkansas, Alabama, California, Colorado, Illinois, Indiana, Louisiana, Maryland, Mississippi, Nevada, North Carolina, Ohio, Rhode Island, South Carolina, Tennessee, and Texas

F. Benefits of certification

1. According to The Joint Commission website, certification by The Joint Commission (2013)
   a. Improves the quality of patient care by reducing variation in clinical processes. The Joint Commission's standards and emphasis on clinical practice guidelines help organizations establish a consistent approach to care, reducing the risk of error.
   b. Provides a framework for program structure and management. Certification standards help organize the disease management program. This helps to maintain a consistently high level of quality, using effective data-driven performance improvement.
   c. Provides an objective assessment of clinical excellence
   d. Creates a loyal, cohesive clinical team. Certification provides an opportunity for staff to develop their skills and knowledge. Achieving certification provides the clinical team with concrete validation of their combined efforts.
   e. Promotes a culture of excellence across the organization
   f. Facilitates marketing, contracting, and reimbursement. Certification may provide an advantage in a competitive healthcare marketplace and improve the ability to secure new business.
   g. Strengthens community confidence in the quality and safety of care, treatment, and services
   h. Makes a strong statement to the community about an organization's efforts to provide the highest quality services.
   i. Is recognized by select insurers and other third parties. In some markets, certification is becoming a prerequisite to eligibility for insurance reimbursement, or participation for managed care plans and contract bidding.
   j. Can fulfill regulatory requirements in select states. Certification may meet certain regulatory requirements in some states, which can reduce duplication on the part of certified organizations.

2. NCQA
   a. Receive market advantage
   b. High standards of quality
   c. Recognition from key contractors

G. Core Measures
   1. 2013—CMS mandatory stroke core measures (American Recovery Act: stage 1 meaningful use; **Table 8-3**)
   2. Proposed comprehensive metrics by ASA task force (**Table 8-4**; Liefer et al., 2011)
   3. Meaningful Use—American Recovery and Reinvestment Act of 1009
      a. Goals

Table 8-3. Clinical Quality Measures for Eligible Hospitals and Clinical Access Hospitals Beginning with FY 2014

NQF Number	Stroke Measure	Numerator Statement
NQF 0435	Stroke-2 ischemic stroke—discharged on antithrombotic therapy	Ischemic stroke patients prescribed antithrombotic therapy at hospital discharge
NQF 0436	Stroke-3 ischemic stroke—anticoagulation therapy for atrial fibrillation/flutter	Ischemic stroke patients with atrial fibrillation/flutter who are prescribed anticoagulation therapy at hospital discharge
NQF 0437	Stroke-4 ischemic stroke—thrombolytic therapy	Acute ischemic stroke patients who arrive at this hospital within 2 hours (120 minutes) of time last known well and for whom IV t-PA was initiated at this hospital within 3 hours (180 minutes) of time last known well
NQF 0438	Stroke-5 ischemic stroke—antithrombotic therapy by end of hospital day two	Ischemic stroke patients administered antithrombotic therapy by the end of hospital day two
NQF 0439	Stroke-6 ischemic stroke—discharged on Statin Medication	Ischemic stroke patients with LDL greater than or equal to 100 mg/dL, or LDL not measured, or, who were on a lipid-lowering medication prior to hospital arrival are prescribed statin medication at hospital discharge
NQF 0440	Stroke-8 ischemic or hemorrhagic stroke—stroke education	Ischemic or hemorrhagic stroke patients or their caregivers who were given educational materials during the hospital stay addressing all of the following: activation of emergency medical system, need for follow-up after discharge, medications prescribed at discharge, risk factors for stroke, and warning signs and symptoms of stroke
NQF 0441	Stroke-10 ischemic or hemorrhagic stroke—assessed for rehabilitation	Ischemic or hemorrhagic stroke patients who were assessed for rehabilitation services

IV indicates intravenous; LDL, low-density lipoprotein; t-PA, tissue plasminogen.

Reprinted from "EHR Incentive Programs," by the Centers for Medicare & Medicaid Services, 2014, www.cms.gov/Regulations-and-Guidance/Legislation/EHRIncentivePrograms/Downloads/2014_CQM_EH_FinalRule.pdf.

Table 8-4. Summary of Metrics for Comprehensive Stroke Centers

Metric	Core Metric	Ischemic Stroke, TIA, or Asymptomatic Cerebrovascular Stenosis	SAH and Nonruptured Aneurysm	ICH and AVM (With or Without Hemorrhage)
Metric 1: Percentage of patients who have an ischemic stroke or who have a TIA with a deficit at the time of the initial admitting note or neurology consultation note for whom an NIHSS score is documented.	Yes	Ischemic stroke, TIA		
Metric 2: Percentage of ischemic stroke patients eligible for intravenous thrombolysis who receive it within the appropriate time window.	Yes	Ischemic stroke seen within 4.5 h of patient last being seen at baseline		
Metric 3: Percentage of patients who are treated for acute ischemic stroke with intravenous thrombolysis whose treatment is started ≤60 minutes after arrival.	Yes	Ischemic stroke treated with intravenous thrombolysis		
Metric 4: Median time from arrival to start of multimodal CT or MR brain and vascular imaging (MRI/MRA or CT/CTA) for ischemic stroke patients arriving within 6 hours of the time that they were last known to be at baseline, if 1 of these studies is ordered.	Yes	Ischemic stroke seen within 6 h of patient last being known to be at baseline		
Metric 5: Percentage of ischemic stroke patients seen within 6 hours of the time they were last known to be at baseline who have documentation that an endovascular recanalization procedure either was performed or was considered and deemed not to be appropriate or possible. A reason should be documented if an endovascular procedure was not performed.	No	Ischemic stroke seen within 6 h of patient last being known to be at baseline		

continued

Table 8-4. Summary of Metrics for Comprehensive Stroke Centers continued

Metric	Core Metric	Ischemic Stroke, TIA, or Asymptomatic Cerebrovascular Stenosis	SAH and Nonruptured Aneurysm	ICH and AVM (With or Without Hemorrhage)
Metric 6: Median time from arrival to start of treatment for acute ischemic stroke patients undergoing an endovascular intervention.	No	Ischemic stroke treated with endovascular intervention		
Metric 7: Percentage of patients treated with intravenous thrombolysis who have a symptomatic intracranial hemorrhage within 36 hours of treatment.	Yes	Ischemic stroke treated with intravenous thrombolysis		
Metric 8: Percentage of acute ischemic stroke patients treated with endovascular interventions who develop significant intracranial hemorrhage within 36 hours of treatment.	Yes	Ischemic stroke treated with endovascular intervention		
Metric 9: Percentage of acute ischemic stroke patients who are treated with intravenous thrombolysis or who undergo endovascular interventions for whom there is documentation of a 90-day mRS score.	Yes	Ischemic stroke treated with intravenous thrombolysis or endovascular procedure		
Metric 10: Percentage of patients undergoing CEA, or carotid angioplasty or stenting, with stroke or death within 30 days of the procedure.	No	CEA or stenting		
Metric 11: Percentage of patients undergoing intracranial angioplasty and/or stenting for atherosclerotic disease with stroke or death within 30 days of the procedure.	No	Intracranial angioplasty and/or stenting		
Metric 12: Percentage of SAH, ICH, and AVM patients for whom initial severity measures are documented.	Yes		Hunt and Hess scale if SAH	ICH score if ICH (whether or not AVM); Spetzler-Martin for all AVM

continued

Table 8-4. Summary of Metrics for Comprehensive Stroke Centers continued

Metric	Core Metric	Ischemic Stroke, TIA, or Asymptomatic Cerebrovascular Stenosis	SAH and Nonruptured Aneurysm	ICH and AVM (With or Without Hemorrhage)
Metric 13: Median time from admission to start of procedure intended to obliterate a ruptured aneurysm by surgical clipping or endovascular coiling for patients who arrive within 48 hours of the hemorrhage that led directly to admission.	Yes		SAH	
Metric 14: Percentage of patients with aneurysmal SAH arriving within 48 hours of hemorrhage for whom a coiling or clipping procedure was not started within 36 hours of arrival who have a documented reason for not having undergone coiling or clipping within 36 hours of arrival.	No		SAH	
Metric 15: Percentage of patients with documented aneurysmal SAH for whom nimodipine treatment (60 mg every 4 hours or 30 mg every 2 hours) is started within 24 hours of diagnosis and for whom such treatment is continued until 21 days after the hemorrhage or until discharge if they are discharged <21 days after the SAH.	Yes		SAH	
Metric 16: Percentage of SAH patients with diminished level of consciousness and ventriculomegaly who are treated with EVD.	No		SAH	

continued

Table 8-4. Summary of Metrics for Comprehensive Stroke Centers continued				
Metric	**Core Metric**	**Ischemic Stroke, TIA, or Asymptomatic Cerebrovascular Stenosis**	**SAH and Nonruptured Aneurysm**	**ICH and AVM (With or Without Hemorrhage)**
Metric 17: Median frequency of noninvasive monitoring performed for surveillance for vasospasm in patients with aneurysmal SAH during the period between 3 and 14 days after SAH.	No			
Metric 18: Complication rates for aneurysm coiling and clipping.	No		All	
Metric 19: Median time from arrival to start of treatment to reverse the INR with a procoagulant preparation (eg, fresh frozen plasma, recombinant factor VIIa, prothrombin complex concentrates) for patients with warfarin-associated ICH and an elevated INR (INR >1.4).	Yes			ICH (if warfarin-associated)
Metric 20: Percentage of patients undergoing surgical or endovascular treatment of an AVM with stroke or death within 30 days of the procedure.	No			AVM
Metric 21: Percentage of patients with ischemic or hemorrhagic stroke or TIA transferred from another hospital to the CSC with documentation of the time from the first call from the transferring hospital to the CSC (to a member of a stroke program or to a centralized transfer center) to arrival time at the CSC.	No	All patients transferred from another hospital	All patients transferred from another hospital	All patients transferred from another hospital

continued

Table 8-4. Summary of Metrics for Comprehensive Stroke Centers continued

Metric	Core Metric	Ischemic Stroke, TIA, or Asymptomatic Cerebrovascular Stenosis	SAH and Nonruptured Aneurysm	ICH and AVM (With or Without Hemorrhage)
Metric 22: Percentage of patients admitted to each type of unit to which patients with ischemic or hemorrhagic stroke or TIA are initially admitted (eg, neurological/neurosurgical ICU, medical ICU, surgical ICU, general ICU, coronary care unit, burn ICU, stroke unit, other intermediate-level-of-care unit, neurology floor, or other floor). A separate percentage should be calculated for each type of unit.	No	All	All	All
Metric 23: Percentage of patients with stroke or death within 24 hours of diagnostic neuroangiography.	Yes	If diagnostic angiogram is performed	If diagnostic angiogram is performed	If diagnostic angiogram is performed
Metric 24: Percentage of patients who have a diagnosis of ischemic or hemorrhagic stroke who undergo EVD and then develop ventriculitis.	No	If patient has EVD	If patient has EVD	If patient has EVD
Metric 25: Median number of days from admission to completion of evaluations for physical therapy, occupational therapy, speech-language pathology, and rehabilitation medicine, unless there is documentation on admission that some or all of these evaluations are not needed or that the patient cannot tolerate them because of medical instability.	No	All	All	All

continued

Table 8-4. Summary of Metrics for Comprehensive Stroke Centers continued

Metric	Core Metric	Ischemic Stroke, TIA, or Asymptomatic Cerebrovascular Stenosis	SAH and Nonruptured Aneurysm	ICH and AVM (With or Without Hemorrhage)
Metric 26: Percentage of patients admitted with diagnoses of ischemic stroke, SAH, AVM, intracranial hemorrhage, extracranial cervical stenosis, intracranial stenosis, or TIA who are enrolled in a clinical research study.	No	All	All	All

AVM indicates arteriovenous malformation; CEA, carotid endarterectomy; CSC, comprehensive stroke center; CT, computed tomography; CT/CTA, computed tomography/computed tomography angiography; EVD, external ventricular drainage; ICH, intracerebral hemorrhage; ICU, intensive care unit; INR, international normalized ratio; NIHSS, National Institutes of Health Stroke Scale; MR, magnetic resonance; MRI/MRA, magnetic resonance imaging/angiography; mRS, modified Rankin Scale; SAH, subarachnoid hemorrhage; and TIA indicates transient ischemic attack.

Reprinted from "Metrics for Measuring Quality of Care in Comprehensive Stroke Centers: Detailed Follow-Up to Brain Attack Coalition Comprehensive Stroke Center Recommendations: A Statement for Healthcare Professionals from the American Heart Association/American Stroke Association," by D. Leifer, D. M. Bravata, J. J. Connors III, J. A. Hinchey, E. C. Jauch, S. Claiborne Johnston … R. Zorowitz, 2011, Stroke, 42, *pp. 849–877.*

(1) The use of a certified electronic health record (EHR) in a meaningful manner, such as e-prescribing
(2) The use of certified EHR technology for electronic exchange of health information to improve quality of health care
(3) The use of certified EHR technology to submit clinical quality and other measures

b. Implementation for stroke patients
(1) Stage 2 reporting began January 1, 2014. Reporting clinical quality measures include
(a) NQF 0435: Stroke 2 ischemic stroke patients prescribed antithrombotic therapy at hospital discharge
(b) NQF 0436: Stroke 3 ischemic stroke patients with atrial fibrillation/flutter who are prescribed anticoagulation therapy at hospital discharge
(c) NQF 0437: Stroke 4 acute ischemic stroke patients who arrive at this hospital within 2 hours (120 minutes) of time last known well and for whom IV t-PA was initiated at this hospital within 3 hours (180 minutes) of time last known well
(d) NQF 0438: Stroke 5 ischemic stroke patients administered antithrombotic therapy by the end of hospital day 2
(e) NQF 0439: Stroke 6 ischemic stroke patients with LDL greater than or equal to 100 mg/dL, or LDL not measured, or, who were on a lipid-lowering medication prior to hospital arrival are prescribed statin medication at hospital discharge.

(f) NQF 0440: Stroke 8 ischemic or hemorrhagic stroke patients or their caregivers who were given educational materials during the hospital stay that addressed all of the following: activation of EMS, need for follow-up after discharge, medications prescribed at discharge, risk factors for stroke, and warning signs and symptoms of stroke.

(g) NQF 0441: Stroke 10 ischemic or hemorrhagic stroke patients who were assessed for rehabilitation services

References

Acker, J. E., Pancioli, A. M., Crocco, T. J., Eckstein, M. K., Jauch, E. C., Larrabee, H., ...Stranne, S. K. (2007). Implementation strategies for emergency medical services within stroke systems of care: a policy statement from the American Heart Association/American Stroke Association Expert Panel on Emergency Medical Systems and the Stroke Council. *Stroke, 38*, 3097–3115.

Adams, H. P., del Zoppo, G. J., Alberts, M., Bhatt, D., Brass, L., Furlan, A., ... Wijdicks, E. F. (2007). Guidelines for the early management of adults with ischemic stroke. *Stroke, 38*, 1655–1711.

Agency for Healthcare Research & Quality. (2003). Your guide to choosing quality healthcare. Retrieved from www.ahrq.gov/consumer/qnt

Alberts, M. J., Latchaw, R. E., Selman, W. R., Shephard, T., Hadley, M. R., Brass, L. M., ... Walker, M. D. (2005). Recommendations for comprehensive stroke centers: A consensus statement from the Brain Attack Coalition. *Stroke, 36*(7), 1597–1616.

Bock, B. F. (1999). Proceedings of a National Symposium on Rapid Identification and treatment of Acute Stroke: Response System for Patients Presenting with Acute Stroke. (NIH Publication No. 97–4239). Retrieved from www.ninds.nih.gov/news_and_events/proceedings/stroke_proceedings/bock.htm

Centers for Disease Control and Prevention. (2011). *A summary of primary stroke center policy in the United States*. Atlanta: U.S. Department of Health and Human Services.

Centers for Disease Control and Prevention. (2013). Paul Coverdale National Acute Stroke Registry. Retrieved from www.cdc.gov/dhdsp/programs/stroke_registry.htm

Centers for Disease Control and Prevention. (2014). Eligible Hospital & Critical Access Hospital Clinical Quality Measures (CQMs). Retrieved from www.cms.gov/Regulations-and-Guidance/Legislation/EHRIncentivePrograms/Downloads/2014_CQM_EH_FinalRule.pdf

Connolly, E. S. Jr, Rabinstein, A. A., Carhuapoma, J. R., Derdeyn, C. P., Dion, J, Higashida, R. T., ... Council on Clinical Cardiology. (2012). Guidelines for the management of aneurysmal subarachnoid hemorrhage: a guideline for healthcare professionals from the American Heart Association/American Stroke Association. Retrieved from http://stroke.ahajournals.org/content/early/2012/05/03/STR.0b013e3182587839.full.pdf+html. *Stroke, 43*(6), 1711–1737.

del Zoppo, G. J., Saver, J. L., Jauch, E. C., & Adamas, H. P. (2009). Expansion of the time window for treatment of acute ischemic stroke with intravenous tissue plasminogen activator: a scientific advisory from the American Heart Association/American Stroke Association. *Stroke, 40*(8), 2945–2948.

Donabedian, A. (1987). Commentary on some studies of the quality of care. Heath Care Financing Review, 75.

Easton, J. D., Saver, J. L., Albers, G. W., Alberts, M. J., Chaturvedi, S., Feldman, E., ... Sacco, R. L. (2009). Definition and evaluation of transient ischemic attack: A scientific statement for healthcare professionals from the American Heart Association/American Stroke Association Stroke Council; Council on Cardiovascular Surgery and Anesthesia; Council on Cardiovascular Radiology and Intervention; Council on Cardiovascular Nursing; and Interdisciplinary Council on Peripheral Vascular Disease. *Stroke, 40*(6), 2276–2293.

Furie, K. L., Kasner, S. E., Adams, R. J., Albers, G. W., Bush, R. L., Fagan, S. C., ...Wentworth, D. (2011). Guidelines for the prevention of stroke in patients with stroke or transient ischemic attack. *Stroke, 42*, 227–276. doi:10.1161/STR.0b013e3181f7d043

Goldstein, L. B., Bushnell, C. D., Adams, R. J., Appel, L. J., Braun, L. T. Chaturvedi, S., Creager, M. A., ...Pearson, T. A. (2011). Guideline for the primary prevention of stroke: A guideline for healthcare professionals. *Stroke, 42*, 51–584. doi:10.1161/STR.0b013e3181fcb238

Healthcare Facilities Accreditation Program. (2013). *Stroke certification guide*. Chicago: Author.

Healthcare Facilities Accreditation Program. (2014). Primary stroke center certification program. Retrieved from www.hfap.org/AccreditationPrograms/stroke.aspx.

Institute for Healthcare Improvement. (2005). *Going Lean in Health Care*. IHI Innovation Series white paper. Cambridge, MA: Author.

Institute of Medicine. (1999). *To Err Is Human*. Washington, DC: National Academy Press.

Jauch, E. C., Saver, J. L., Adams, H. P., Bruno, A., Connors, J. J., Memaerschalk, B. M., ... Council on Clinical Cardiology. (2013). Guidelines for the early management of adults with ischemic stroke. *Stroke, 44*, 870–947. doi:10.1161/STR.0b013e318284056a

The Joint Commission. (2013). *Certification review process guide: Disease specific care certification*. Washington, DC: Author.

The Joint Commission. (2014). Advanced certification for primary stroke centers. Retrieved from www.jointcommission.org/certification/primary_stroke_centers.aspx

Leifer, D., Bravata, D. M., Connors, J. J., Hinchey, J. A., Jauch, E. C., Johnston, S. C., … Zorowitz R. (2011). Metrics for measuring quality of care in comprehensive stroke centers: detailed follow-up to brain attack coalition comprehensive stroke center recommendations: a statement for healthcare professionals from the American Heart Association/American Stroke Association. *Stroke, 42*, 857.

Miller, E. L., Murray, L., Richards, L., Zorowitz, R. D., Bakas, T., Clark, P., Billinger, S. A., (2010). Comprehensive overview of nursing and interdisciplinary rehabilitation care of the stroke patient. *Stroke, 41*, 2402–2448. doi:10.1161/STR.0b013e3181e7512b

Morgenstern, L. B., Hemphill, J. C., Anderson, C., Becker, K., Broderick, J. P., Connolly, E. S., … Tamargo, R. J. (2010). Guidelines for the management of spontaneous intracerebral hemorrhage: A guideline for healthcare professionals from the American heart Association/American Stroke Association. *Stroke, 41*, 2108–2129. doi:10.1161/STR.0b013e3181ec611b

National Institute of Neurologic Disorders and Stroke. (2013). Home page. Retrieved from www.ninds.nih.gov

Pugh, S., Mathiesen, C., Meighan, M., Summers, D., & Zrelak, P. (2012). *Guide to the care of the hospitalized patient with ischemic stroke* (2nd ed). AANN Clinical Practice Guideline series. Glenview, IL: American Association of Neuroscience Nurses.

Rivard, P. E., Parker, V. A., & Rosen, A. K. (2013). Quality improvement for patient safety: Project level versus program level learning. *Health Care Management Review, 38*(1), 40–50. doi:10.1097/HMR.0b013e318245019f

Rogers, L. M. (2007). Meeting the Center for Medicare & Medicaid Services requirements for quality assessment and performance improvement: A model for hospitals. *Journal of Nursing Care Quality, 21*(4), 325–332.

Sacco, R., Adams, R., Albers, G. W., Alberts, M., Benavente, O., Furei, K. et al. (2006). Guidelines for the prevention of stroke in patients with ischemic stroke or transient ischemic attack: A statement for healthcare professionals from the American Heart Association/American Stroke Association Council on Stroke: Co-sponsored by the Council on Cardiovascular Radiology and Intervention: The American Academy of Neurology affirms the value of this guideline. *Stroke, 37*, 577–617.

Schwamm, L., Pancioli, A., Acker, J. E., Goldstein, L. B., Zorowitz, R. D., & Shephard, T. J. (2005). American Stroke Association taskforce on the development of stroke systems: Recommendations for the establishment of stroke systems of care. *Stroke, 36*, 690–763. doi:10.1161/STR.0000158165.42884.4F

Summers, D., Leonard, A., Wentworth, D., Saver, J. L., Simpson, J., Spilker, J. A., ... American Heart Association Council on Cardiovascular Nursing and the Stroke Council. (2009). Comprehensive overview of nursing and interdisciplinary care of the acute ischemic stroke patient: A scientific statement from the American Heart Association. *Stroke, 40*(8), 2911–2944.

Index

G

H

I

J

K

L

M

N

O

P

Q

R

S

T

U

V

W

X

Z